CANCER ETIOLOGY, DIAGNOSIS AND TREATMENTS

PALLIATIVE CARE TO THE CANCER PATIENT

THE MIDDLE EAST AS A MODEL FOR EMERGING COUNTRIES

Cancer Etiology, Diagnosis and Treatments

Additional books in this series can be found on Nova's website under the Series tab.

Additional e-books in this series can be found on Nova's website under the e-book tab.

CANCER ETIOLOGY, DIAGNOSIS AND TREATMENTS

PALLIATIVE CARE TO THE CANCER PATIENT

THE MIDDLE EAST AS A MODEL FOR EMERGING COUNTRIES

MICHAEL SILBERMANN
EDITOR

nova publishers
New York

For permission to use material from this book please contact us:
Telephone 631-231-7269; Fax 631-231-8175
Web Site: http://www.novapublishers.com

Library of Congress Cataloging-in-Publication Data

ISBN: 978-1-63117-709-5

Library of Congress Control Number: 2014936325

Published by Nova Science Publishers, Inc. † New York

CONTENTS

PREFACE

Michael Silbermann[*]*, D.M.D., Ph.D.*

Technion- Israel Institute of Technology and the Middle East Cancer Consortium,
Haifa, Israel

OVERVIEW

Most of the Middle Eastern countries are categorized as low- and middle-income countries, and, as other developing countries, they suffer from the increased burden of cancer. The most recent global cancer statistics (2012) indicate that 56.8% of the 14.1 million estimated new cases of cancer that year, and 64.9% of the estimated 8.2 million cancer deaths, occurred in less developed regions of the world [1].

Unfortunately, health systems in many countries in the Middle East are ill-prepared to deal with this new and rapidly growing challenge [2]. Some 70% of all cancer patients in the Middle East are diagnosed when the tumor has already reached stage III or IV and is no longer curable. For these patients the only treatment option left is palliative care. However, most of the currently used opioids – morphine, oxycodone and fentanyl – are unavailable to the majority of cancer patients in the region, the result of regulatory and pricing obstacles, lack of knowledge, or false beliefs. Moreover, government policies in the majority of countries in the region still do not recognize palliative care as an essential component of health care. An added element in this problematic situation is that along with the moderate-to-severe pain that most cancer patients (60%-90%) suffer at some point along the trajectory of the illness, about a third of the patients will also suffer from depression or anxiety. Therefore, benzodiazepine-type anxiolytics and sedative hypnotics are also indispensable medications for the treatment of cancer-related mental disturbances, yet these medications too, are largely unavailable in the region.

In Western societies curative procedures are often prioritized ahead of palliative care, reflecting a cultural non acceptance of death. By contrast, in Islamic societies, which comprise the majority of the Middle East population, patients are more accepting of death and

* Address for correspondence: Dr. Michael Silbermann, Professor, Executive Director, Middle East Cancer Consortium, 15 Kiryat Sefer Street, Haifa 3467630, Israel; Tel: 972-4-824-4794; Fax: 972-4-834-6338; E-mail: cancer@mecc-research.com

live in coexistence with the realization of the inevitability of death. This attitude has an important impact on how the patient and the family view death.

An additional cultural barrier to the delivery of palliative care in the region is the general association of such care with "giving up" on life rather than providing quality of life for the patient who is suffering from a terminal illness.

A recent report of the International Narcotics Control Board (2010) points to large disparities in opioid consumption among Middle Eastern countries, with Israel showing a level of 3,482 S-DDD per million inhabitants per day, while Turkey and Cyprus have a level of 600 S-DDD per million inhabitants per day, Saudi Arabia, Jordan and Lebanon under 200 S-DDD per million inhabitants per day, Egypt 49 S-DDD, and Iraq and Pakistan 10 S-DDD. Clearly, these medicines continue to be unavailable and inaccessible to meet the medical needs of the populations in most countries in the region. The result is massive inequities in access to pain relief, with over 99% untreated and painful deaths occurring in these developing countries.

Working Toward Solutions

One of the main obstacles to the provision of satisfactory palliative care and pain management is the paucity of training of health professionals, which explains the practitioners' reluctance to prescribe opioids. Hence, instruction in the basic principles of palliative care should be mandatory in all graduate and specialty training programs for physicians and nurses. Toward that goal, the Middle East Cancer Consortium (MECC) has given special emphasis to the importance of training programs throughout the Middle East with a strong community-based orientation. In a recent, as yet unpublished, Middle Eastern survey on palliative care we were surprised and pleased to learn that over 90% of the participants in the Middle East (most of them nurses and physicians) are familiar with the concept of palliative care, and that pain relief and symptom management are provided to over 70% of cancer patients in the region [3]. Therefore, it is very encouraging to know that the Middle East has taken a big step forward to overcome the problem of lack of awareness within the medical profession, in contrast to the public at large, so that there is less of justification for patients to be deprived of such care.

Teaching Palliative Care in the Middle East

The lack of availability of opioids is supported in part by patients' and families' traditional fear of addiction to pain medications, assessed at 80% of the Middle Eastern populations [3,4]. Moreover, as in many other countries worldwide, communication difficulties between health care professionals and patients and families are widespread in most Middle Eastern countries. Much of this can be traced to the way medicine is taught. The curricula in most medical schools attach relatively little importance to issues related to doctor-patient communication, as this aspect of health care is still considered an adjunct to medical training rather than a core concept, in view of the prevailing paradigm that death is equated to failure [5]. Hence, inexperienced doctors are left to fumble through critical conversations pertaining to end-of-life, with little guidance. Overall, palliative care services in the Middle East are rarely integrated into the care plan for seriously ill patients.

By the same token, the region lacks teaching programs for staff support in caring for terminally ill patients. Yet, professional education programs in palliative care are in great demand by doctors and health care providers. Palliative care has been designated as part of national cancer control programs in some countries. Therefore, these programs should include palliative care programs in their primary healthcare programs, with an emphasis on the community. Unfortunately, governments in the Middle East do not seem inclined to change legislation concerning palliative care policies [4]. Hence, progress in palliative care has largely been driven by NGOs, including the Anticancer Society and the Cypriot Association of Cancer Patients and Friends in Cyprus, the Israel Cancer Association, Al-Sadeel Society in Palestine, and the Oman Cancer Association, Princess Lalla Salma Foundation in Morocco. The Lebanese Cancer Society, which all promote public awareness and community care services, two areas that are sorely neglected.

Cultural norms in the region are such that palliative care consultations are still complex and for the most part patients and families are not part of the decision-making process. Moreover, cultural, religious and/or spiritual beliefs influence end-of-life care, and patients and families avoid discussions about dying and death.

Community health resources are still very limited in most countries in the Middle East, yet, the Republic of Cyprus has been a remarkable success story in setting up community palliative care services, offering a model for other Middle Eastern countries to follow. The Cypriot Anticancer Society and the Cypriot Association of Cancer Patients and Friends (PASYKAF) set up a system of home-based care services in Nicosia, with specialized palliative-care nurses operating an outstanding service. The Cypriot experience shows that efficient palliative care is possible in even the most constrained financial settings.

A core issue in implementing good palliative care services both in hospitals and in the community relates to improved communication between caregivers, patients and their families. At least half the regional caregivers admit to a lack of essential communication skills (breaking bad news, family meetings negotiating the goal of care, prognosis). Open discussions between caregivers and patients/families are viewed increasingly as essential for effective and genuine care. International organizations such as MECC, Oncology Nursing Society (ONS) and American Society of Clinical Oncology (ASCO) have adopted the mission of training professionals in the region through individualized courses in specific countries, regional workshops, and exchange programs with palliative care institutions in the United States.

How Many People Need Palliative Care?

Of the total number of new cancer cases in developed countries in the year 2012, an average of 47.3% died, while in the developing countries the rate was 66.4%.

Table 1. Global rates of cancer incidence and deaths in 2012[1]

	Global	Developed countries	Developing countries
Number of new cancer cases ASR (W)	182.3	268.3	147.7
Number of deaths ASR (W)	102.4	108.5	98.4
Mortality/Incidence rates	0.56	0.40	0.66

ASR- Age Standardized Incidence Rates (World) per 100,000 world population

In any given population, the starting point for estimating the need for palliative care is the number of deaths per year [6]. A minimum of 63% of all deaths may require palliative care [7]. Notably, there is a distinct difference between palliative care needs in the last few weeks of life, which may largely include primary care professionals and community-home based services, as compared to needs earlier in the illness trajectory, which may include palliative care specialists. By and large, a knowledge of the annual population numbers in need of such services is invaluable for service planning and development.

Treatment Priorities

Due to the growing prevalence of cancer [1], the overall cost of medical care has risen steeply. Recent criticism suggests that a shift is needed to limit intensive second- and third-line chemotherapies with little proven benefit regarding survival [8]. Approximately a quarter of all health care expenditure is incurred by people in the last year of life. In this context, a relevant question is what the patient's view and the public view is regarding palliative care. It is important to understand how patients' priorities are influenced by personal characteristics and by country in terms of culture, religious beliefs, the provision of palliative care services, and legal frameworks.

To answer some of these questions, a recent survey was conducted in seven European countries aiming to examine health care professionals' and patients' preferences and views when faced with questions concerning palliative care services, and to identify overall and country-specific views and recommendations [8]. The results showed that the most popular priority was quality of life (QoL), which, of course, has direct implications for cancer treatment and care. Accordingly, the treatment of cancer will have to shift focus to a greater emphasis on the improvement of quality of life. This, in turn, will necessitate the improvement of clinicians' skills in symptom management and communication. MECC, ONS and ASCO have been involved in promoting this kind of training to physicians and nurses throughout the Middle East.

A small minority of respondents in the European survey were more interested in life extension over improving QoL. These patients were also the ones who preferred death at home.

It would be of great interest to explore the general patterns on such issues in Middle Eastern populations, and associated influential factors such as religion, tradition and culture.

Considering the cultural diversity in the Middle East, one would assume that dissimilarities exist between countries and between populations. Such findings would have implications when caring for patients in different parts of the region, and would highlight the need for both country-specific and individualized approaches to care. Population-based studies would provide the essential evidence necessary to reorient cancer treatment in line with patient and family priorities regarding palliative care.

Home Care and Preference of Place of Death

Well-organized home care is still a distant reality for the majority of cancer patients in the Middle East, even though it is viewed as the preferred place for care, especially at the end of life. Accumulated evidence about the benefits of home care suggests that holistic wellbeing is greater at home, and that this is the patients' and families' first choice. Since families in the Middle East comprise an integral part of the palliative care team, there is increased recognition of the need to further empower the family by instruction in treatment approaches, care goals, and the decision-making process. Evidence from systemic reviews suggests that home palliative care results in higher caregiver and patient satisfaction [9], as patients and their families attach a high value to being at home. The home provides a familiar environment where they can sustain control and have greater freedom than in a hospital or other inpatient facilities. An active advocacy program in the community can augment home-based palliative care service, and with this increase the proportion of home deaths.

What Do People Actually Want?

There is consistent evidence across many studies that home is the main preference for place of death (25%-87%) favoring home deaths, depending on whether the question was asked of patients, caregivers or the general population) [9]. In a recent survey of 9,344 citizens across seven European countries, the home preference ranged from 51% (Portugal) to 84% (The Netherlands). Since different cultures and ethnicities affect people's preferences, a similar survey in the Middle East would be of great value in anticipating the interplay of different cultural factors on patients' and families' preferences. By way of example, research has shown that patients from lower socio-economic groups living in poorer areas in Europe are less likely to die at home. Similarly, Pakistani, Indian, Bangladeshi, Black African, Black Caribbean and Chinese patients living in the UK are significantly more likely than white patients to die in hospital [10].

With regard to the current situation in Middle Eastern countries, more data is needed in order to determinate prevailing preferences, along with a better understanding of the factors associated with death at home in the various local communities. We still do not know whether in the Middle East, dying at home is preferable to dying in hospital, taking into account the conditions available in the health care system vis-à-vis the community. It is believed, however, that the psychological, social and holistic measures of the patient's wellbeing are better met at home than in an institutional setting [11-13].

According to a recent report in the *Guardian* [14], almost three-quarters of the cancer patients in England who die in hospital would have preferred to die at home. Furthermore,

63% of those whose loved one died at home rated the overall quality of home care as excellent or outstanding, compared with only 37% of those whose loved one died in hospital. A Macmillan Cancer Support survey found that 41% of people with terminal cancer were not always treated with dignity and respect by hospital doctors [14].

Approximately 50% of the incidence of cancer in developing countries occurs in individuals below age 65. The impact of cancer on all populations is devastating, but is especially so for the poor, vulnerable and socially disadvantaged, who get sicker and die sooner as a result of cancer [15]. The Middle East needs more research monitoring the public's preferences as to place of care and death. Such research will provide needed scientific support for future national programs by revealing emergent population priorities, and developing responsive palliative care services and clinical practice accordingly. Furthermore, factors influencing cancer risks suggest that basic inequities and unmet needs still exist, such as distance to quality care facilities.

Yet, while public health programs in the region have focused largely on preventing and treating infectious diseases and malnutrition, more attention has been given recently to improving quality of life for patients and their families when dealing with cancer. Accordingly, MECC, ONS and ASCO began introducing palliative care to familiarizing professionals throughout the Middle East (with palliative care). Since then, hundreds of physicians, nurses, pharmacists, social workers, and psychologists have been trained in basic and advanced palliation protocols [16-20]. Moreover, since palliative care has become an immediate need, it has been seen as an entry point to initiating and setting up cancer control plans and programs in the individual countries. Having undertaken this mission, we feel that in some way we are an avantgarde in palliative care, promoting such care in the region, while facilitating additional regional academic activity [21-23].

The goal of the MECC palliative care initiative is first, to decrease the suffering of cancer patients and their families, while treating the disease itself. This goal can be achieved regardless of cultural differences. People will embrace palliative care if it is introduced with a cultural-sensitive approach, while recognizing that it is a fundamental human right [24].

In Summary

The benefits of palliative care include improved ability of function and enjoyment in life, and even prolonged survival for the terminally ill [25]. Palliative care, therefore, can and should be delivered while patients receive treatment for disease. However, to date there are two major stumbling blocks that hinder the practice of palliative care in the Middle East:

1. The widespread misunderstanding of palliative care by the public, which wrongly equates it with end-of-life, and
2. A severe shortage of doctors and nurses trained in palliative care.

Distressing symptoms such as pain, shortness of breath and fatigue, which often accompany cancer, can and should be prevented and managed by the trained family physician and/or the trained community nurse in a patient's own home. No less important, palliative care also includes help in accessing additional community services, while trying to find out what is most important to a patient's quality of life and how these goals might be achieved

[25]. Nurses play a pivotal role in extending such services in the community while helping patients and their families navigate complex needs.

REFERENCES

[1] International Agency for research on Cancer. World Cancer Report, 2012; Lyon: IARC 2013.

[2] Scaling up cancer diagnosis and treatment in developing countries: what can we learn from the HIV/AIDS epidemic? Editorial, Annal. Oncol. 21:680-682, 2010.

[3] Current state of palliative care in Middle Eastern countries. An ONS-MECC survey. Unpublished data.

[4] Cleary, J., Silbermann, M., Scholten, W., Cherny, N. Formulary, availability and regulatory barriers to accessibility of opioids for cancer pain in the Middle East: A report from the Global Opioid Policy Initiative (GOPI). Ann. Oncol. 24: (XI)51-59, 2013.

[5] Shetty, P. The parlous state of palliative care in the developing world. The Lancet 376: 1453-1454, 2010.

[6] Higginson, I.J. Health care needs assessment: Palliative and terminal care. In: Health Care Needs Assessment, Stevens, A. & Raftery J. eds. Oxford Radcliffe Medical Press, 1997, pp 1-28.

[7] Mutagh, F.E.M., Bausewein, C., Verne, J., Groenvald, E.I., Kaloki, Y.E., Higginson, I.J. How many people need palliative care? A study developing and comparing methods for population-based estimates. Palliative Medicine online 21, May 2013. Doi: 10.1177/0269216313489367 http://www.sagepublications.com.

[8] Higginson, I.J., Gomes, B., Calanzani, N., Gao, W. et al. Priorities for treatment, care and information if faced with serious illness: A comparative population-based survey in seven European countries. Palliative Medicine, Nov. 13, 2013. Doi: 10.1177/0269216313488989 http://pmj.sagepub.com

[9] Higginson, I.J., Sarmento, V.P., Calanzani, N., Benalia, H., Gomes, B. Dying at home - is it better: A narrative appraisal of the state of the science. Palliative Medicine, online 22 May, 2013. http://pmj.sagepub.com/content/early/2013/05/22/0269216313487940.

[10] Coupland, V.H., Madden, P., Jack, R.H., et al. Does place of death from cancer vary between ethnic groups in South East England? Palliat. Med. 25:314-322, 2011.

[11] Wright, A. A., Keating, N.L., Balboni, T.A. et al. Place of death with cancer and predictors of bereaved caregivers' mental health. J clin Oncol 28:4457-4464, 2010.

[12] Neergaard, M.A., Vedsted, P., Olesen, F. et al. Associations between successful palliative trajectories, place of death and GP involvement. Scand J Health Care 28: 138-145, 2010.

[13] Yao, C.A., Hu, W.Y., Lai, Y.F. et al. Does dying at home influence the good death of terminal cancer patients? J Pain Symptom Manag 34: 497-504. 2007.

[14] Most cancer patients want to die at home, report says. The Guardian, 28 October 2013. http://www.theguardian.com/society/2013/oct/28/most-cancer-patients-want…

[15] World Cancer Day 2014: Myth 2-cancer is a disease of the wealthy, elderly and developed countries- http://www.worldcancerday.org/myth-2-cancer-disease-wealthy-elderly-and…

[16] Silbermann, M. MECC workshop on psycho-oncology: Alleviation of fear, frustration and sense of loss through non-pharmacological treatment modalities. J. Pediatr. Hematol. Oncol. 32:22-82 (Guest Editor, 2010).

[17] Silbermann, M. MECC workshop on palliative care services in the Middle East. J. Pediatr. Hematol. Oncol. 33:S1-80 (Guest Editor, 2011).

[18] Silbermann, M. MECC workshop on cancer pain, suffering and the complexities of evidence-based intervention in cancer care. J. Pediatr. Hematol. Oncol. 33:S81-161 (Guest Editor, 2011).

[19] Silbermann, M., Arnaout, M., Abdel Rahman, H., Ashraf, S., Ben Arush, M., El-Shami, M., Al-Hadad, S., Huijer, H., Pitsillides, B., Taeyildiz, N., Shad, A. Pediatric palliative care in the Middle East. In: Pediatric palliative care: Global Perspectives. Knapp, C., Madden, V., Flower-Kerry. S., eds. Springer Science, pp.127-159, 2012.

[20] International Symposium on Palliative Care and the Geriatric Patient. Silbermann, M., Balducci, L., Schrijuers, D. eds. Ann. Oncol. 24 VII 1-55, 2013.

[21] Advanced ASCO-MECC International Development and Education Course in Palliative Care: Approaches for oncology integrated palliative care in Middle Eastern countries. Silbermann, M., Balducci, L., Schrijvers, D. eds. Ann. Oncol. 23:S1-79, 2013.

[22] Ben Arie, E., Ali-Shtayeh, M.S., Nejmi, M., Schiff, E., Hassan, E., Mutafoglu, K., Afifi, F., Jamoas, R.M., Lev, E., Silbermann, M. Integrative oncology in the Middle East: Wearing traditional and complementary medicine in supportive cancer care. Supportive Care in Cancer 19: 2011. Doi: 10.1007/200520-1121.

[23] Silbermann, M., Arnaout, M., Daher, M., Nestoros, S., Pitsillides, B., Charalmbous, H., Gultekin, M., Abdulla, R.M.F., Mostafa, K.A.H., Khleif, A.D. Manasrah, N., Oberman, A. Palliative care in Middle Eastern countries: Accomplishments and challenges. Ann. Oncol. 23: S14-27, 2012.

[24] Crane, K. Palliative care gains ground in developing countries. JNCI 102: 1613-1615, 2010.

[25] Brody, J.E. The treatment that respects pain. The New York Times. Dec. 3, 2013, p. D7.

In: Palliative Care to the Cancer Patient
Editor: Michael Silbermann

ISBN: 978-1-63117-709-5

Chapter 1

PALLIATIVE CARE IN CYPRUS: CURRENT STATUS

Haris Charalambous**, B.M., M.R.C.P., F.R.C.R.,
Barbara Pitsillides, R.G.N., M.Sc.Pall.
and Sophia Nestoros, M.D., M.Sc.Pall.
[1]Bank of Cyprus Oncology Center, Nicosia; Cyprus
[2]Cyprus Association of Cancer Patients and Friends (PASYKAF), Nicosia, Cyprus
[3]Cyprus Anti-Cancer Society, Nicosia, Cyprus

INTRODUCTION

Cyprus is the third largest island in the Mediterranean after Sicily and Sardinia. Cyprus has been an independent state since 1960. In 1974 the island partitioned into two parts; the area under the effective control of the Republic of Cyprus, comprising about two thirds of the island's area, and the Turkish-controlled area in the north. In 2004 the Republic of Cyprus joined the European Union and in 2008 it joined the Euro. According to the 2011 latest census, the population is 838.897 inhabitants [1] with 659.350 Cypriot citizens and 176.547 foreign citizens (112.424 from the European Union).

Cyprus has developed as a centre in the Eastern Mediterranean for offshore businesses, financial services, shipping and tourism, and is considered to be among the world developed countries with very high Human Development Index [2]. Currently however Cyprus is in the middle of a major financial crisis, necessitating financial bailout from the European Union, the European Central Bank and the International Monetary Fund. The latest estimate per capita GDP (adjusted for purchasing power) before the financial crisis at 28,961 USD (2010 estimate), is around the average of the European Union (EU27) [3].

There is currently no National Health Care system to provide universal health care cover for all citizens in Cyprus, although there are currently plans to implement such system in 2015. Health care is delivered within a large Public Health Care sector (free for almost 80% of the population) and a smaller Private Health Care sector. Private Health Care is partly covered by private medical insurance, although a significant part is covered by "out of pocket

* Address for correspondence: haris.charalambous@bococ.org.cy

contributions". Another limitation of the Cyprus Health Care system, is the absence of an organized Primary Care level, with only a few General Practioners operating in Cyprus, essentially resulting in patients' care provided by the secondary and tertiary level providers. Finally in terms of health care spending, in 2011 Cyprus spent 7.3% of its GDP towards health care, which is lower than the 8.9% average of the European Union [4].

In 2008 (last year with records from the Cyprus Cancer Registry), there were 2844 new patients diagnosed with cancer in Cyprus, whilst about 1050 cancer patients die each year due to their disease [5]. Treatment of all patients with cancer is free of charge in the two public / government oncology units, located in the Nicosia and Limassol General hospitals and also in the Bank of Cyprus Oncology Centre (BOCOC). The BOCOC is a not for profit organization, co-founded and co-funded by the Bank of Cyprus and the Cyprus Government, and is the only tertiary Oncology referral centre in Cyprus (providing comprehensive specialized non surgical oncology services, including Radiotherapy). Even when patients opt to have treatment privately, they receive all chemotherapy drugs free [6,7].

The Cancer services as a result are based in Nicosia (radiotherapy and chemotherapy) and Limassol (chemotherapy). In terms of geographical citing, Nicosia is in the middle of the island. North of Nicosia is the occupied part of Cyprus controlled by Turkey (See Figure 1. Map of Cyprus underneath: blue line: border since 1974). In terms of distances that patients have to travel to Nicosia, the furthest east town of Paralimni is 75-85 km away, in the south the town of Larnaca and Limassol are less than 70 Km away, whilst the furthest away district by far is in the west of the island, Paphos, is around 120 Km away. Between all main towns in Cyprus (Nicosia, Larnaca, Limassol, Paphos and Paralimni) there are new, modern, dual carriage motorways, allowing for both safe and fast travel between the main towns.

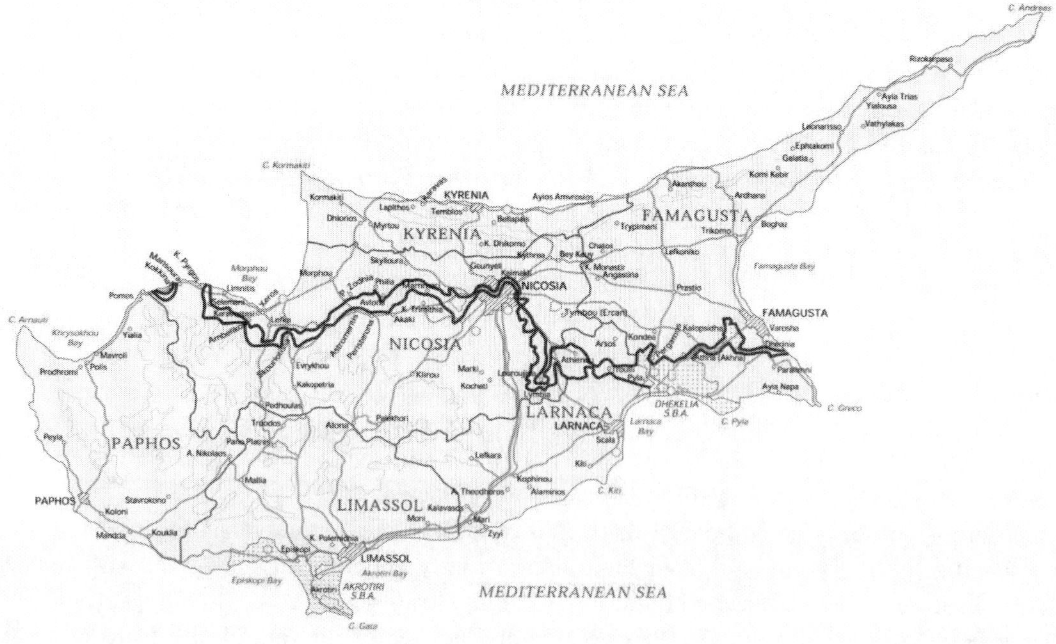

Figure 1. Map of Cyprus.

Palliative Care (PC) in Cyprus has its origins in the establishment of the two main not-for profit NGOs (Non Government Organizations), the Cyprus Anti-Cancer Society (CACS) in 1971 and the Cyprus Association of Cancer Patients and Friends (PASYKAF) in 1986 [6,7,8]. Unfortunately the Public Health Care system, which caters for most patients, has no organized public PC services, hence PC is provided predominantly by the NGOs [6,7,8].

THE CURRENT SERVICES

The current services provide almost exclusively to adult cancer patients, there are no organized paediatric PC services [6,7,8]. Patients with other life-threatening but non- cancer related conditions, are rarely referred to these PC services.

PC services in the Government of Cyprus controlled area, are provided predominantly by the Cyprus Anti Cancer Society (CACS) [9] and the Cyprus Association of Cancer Patients and Friends (PASYKAF) [10]. There are also the "Friends of Life" Limassol [11], and "Friends of the Hospice" Paphos [12] NGOs (run by expatriates from the U.K.) fundraising and helping with PC especially in the districts of Limassol and Paphos. Supportive and PC, sometimes extending to end of life care, is also provided by the two Public Hospital Oncology Units in Nicosia and Limassol and by the BOCOC. In table 1, there is a list of all the services provided across the Government of Cyprus controlled part of island.

Table 1. Palliative Care Provision in Cyprus, 2013

Organization delivering service	Hospice / PC Unit	Hospital Support Team	Psycho/ Social Service	Home Care Team	Day Care	Supportive-PC Unit / Drop in Centre	Grand Total
PASYKAF			1	1	1		3
C ACS	1		1	1	1	2	6
Government oncology units:							
Nicosia General Hospital Oncology Unit						1	1
Limassol General Hospital Oncology Unit						1	1
Non for profit NGO:							
Bank of Cyprus Oncology Centre (co-funded by the BOC)		1	1			1	3
Total	1	1	3	2	2	5	14

In the Turkish controlled area of Cyprus, there are two NGOs, the "Kemal Saracoglu Foundation for Children with Leukemia and Fight Against Cancer" and the 'Help Those With Cancer Association". Since 2003, Turkish Cypriots could access for free all PC and hospital services in the Government of Cyprus controlled areas, although new legislation enforced since August 2013 as a result of the financial crisis, is likely to impact negatively on new Turkish-Cypriot patients receiving treatment for free in the Government of Cyprus hospitals.

The Cyprus Anti-Cancer Society (CACS) [9]

The CACS was established in 1971. Their emphasis has been on inpatient hospice care, centered around the Arodafnousa hospice. CACS runs the following services:

- the hospice of Arodaphnousa in Nicosia (main hospice in Cyprus),
- a newly founded Supportive and PC Unit / Drop in Centre, Evagoreio in Limassol,
- a Home Care Service (community PC) in all districts, with experienced PC nurses, all of them with certificates in PC from the Princess Alice Hospice (Wales) visiting patients at home
- a day care service in all districts (once a week),predominantly for patients to socialize and receive emotional / psychosocial support
- a psychosocial service offering support to patients and families either at home or at any hospital, and
- a transportation service (providing free transport of patients from their districts to the Oncology centres, especially to the BOC Oncology Centre in Nicosia, for treatment).

Since 2012, due to the increasing workload of the BOCOC, patients can receive supportive day care treatment, e.g., blood transfusions, intravenous (iv) rehydration, iv bisphosphonates, iv antibiotics, and general symptom control measures, following referral from the BOCOC, in the Arodafnousa hospice in Nicosia and in the Evagoreio centre in Limassol. In Arodafnousa this service is offered three times a week, with 369 patients treated in 2012, whilst 455 patients were treated at Evagoreio in Limassol during the same period.

In table 2, there are estimates of the number of patients that have used these services in 2012, compared to 2010 and 2000, showing a marked increase over time.

Table 2. Number of patients accessing CACS's Services per year

	2000	2010	2012
Arodaphnousa Hospice (in-patient)	158	176	315
Supportive Care / Drop in Centre	N/A	N/A	824
Home Care (5 daytime teams)	304	1244	1760
Day Care (once a week)	60	75/centre / week	75/centre/ week
Outpatient Visits	12	Approx 100	Approx 150
Psychosocial service	578	821	975
Physiotherapy	N/A	394	524

The Cyprus Association of Cancer Patients and Friends (PASYKAF) [10]

PASYKAF was established in 1986 by a number of Cyprus Cancer patients, their families and their friends, hence their name. Its mission and philosophy was to provide supportive and palliative care services that improve the quality of life of cancer patients and their families at all stages of the disease, with emphasis on home based supportive and PC, with psychological support being equally as important as nursing care.

PASYKAF runs the following services:

- a comprehensive home care service in all districts in Cyprus, which is truly multidisciplinary, including specialist PC nurses, physiotherapists, social workers and psychologists in patients' homes / in the community.
- day centres in all districts in Cyprus
- psychosocial support service in all districts
- physiotherapy service in all districts and finally
- a transportation service from all districts to the Oncology Centre in Nicosia.

In table 3, there are estimates of the number of patients that have used these services in 2012, compared to 2010 and 2000, again showing a marked increase over time.

Table 3. Number of patients accessing PASYKAF's Services per year

	2000	2010	2012
Home Care Service (5 teams) - new patient referrals	700	791	974
Home Care workload (i.e., both new and old patients)	816	1226	1660
Day Care (5 units) (each opens weekly)	-	57 centre/ week	57 centre/week
Psychosocial support service	877	1534	1762
Physiotherapy	-	366	407

Both CACS and PASYKAF are also involved in organizing public awareness programs and campaigns to promote Cancer prevention and early Cancer detection in Cyprus, and they have both advocated/worked towards the improvement of both diagnostic and therapy Oncology services, as well as research in Cyprus.

Other NGO's include:

- The Friends of Life Limassol [11] is a registered charitable association founded in 2007. Until recently they provided the funds for the running of 3-4 inpatient hospice beds in Chrysovalantou private clinic in Limassol.
- The Friends of the Paphos Hospice [12] is a small voluntary organization, founded in 2006, member of the worldwide Hospice movement. Until recently they have supported the existence of a 3-5 inpatient hospice unit in the Evangelismos private hospital in Paphos.
- ELAZO is an organization supporting cancer patients from the Nicosia Hospital.

Non Cancer NGO's:

- K.Y.F.A (Kentron Ypostirixis Foreon AIDS)[13] the Support Centre For People with HIV or AIDS was founded in 2000 with the aim to support people living with HIV/AIDS. K.Y.F.A. maintains a day centre in Limassol, providing psychosocial support, information and legal advice if needed for people with HIV/AIDS. K.Y.F.A also runs a free telephone line, again providing information and support.

Finally there are no private (fee paying) PC services in Cyprus.

Inpatient Palliative Care Services/Hospices

The main hospice in Cyprus, the Arodaphnousa Hospice is located in Nicosia. It was set up in 1976 and was fully renovated with charity donations at a cost close to half a million euros in 2011. The Arodafnousa hospice accepts referrals from all organizations and physicians, and from all over Cyprus, including the Northern part, which is no longer under the effective control of the republic of Cyprus. It has 15 beds, 13 single rooms and one double room. As a result of the financial crisis, resulting in considerably decreased fundraising and a significant financial budget deficit, the CACS had to lay off staff, with the resultant closure of three (3) hospice beds in Arodafnousa, hence currently only twelve (12) inpatient beds are open.

Also as a result of the current financial crisis in Cyprus, the two small hospice units in Limassol, at Chrysovalantou Clinic paid by the Friends of Life (Limassol) NGO, and in Pafos at the Evangelismos Hospital, funded by the Friends' of the Paphos Hospice NGO, ceased to operate in 2013. Instead Friends for Life Limassol NGO is making a financial contribution to the CACS towards the running of the Arodafnousa Hospice, whilst Friends for Hospice in Paphos is trying to open a limited number (3-6) PC inpatient beds in Paphos at the St Georges private clinic, towards the end of the year.

Hence as a result of the financial crisis, there are currently only twelve (12) inpatient hospice beds available in Cyprus, as per the table 4 below. This needs to be contrasted to the 2011 figure of twenty-four (24) beds. The current capacity of only twelve (12) hospice beds is clearly inadequate to cover the needs of a population close to one (1) million, when compared with the European guidelines in the EAPC (European Association of Palliative Care) White Paper [14], where the original need for 50 PC care beds needed per million population has been upgraded to 80-100 beds per million population in view of the needs of non-cancer patients and the prevalence of chronic diseases due to the European population growing older.

The acute shortage of hospice beds in Cyprus has resulted in an intensified effort to implement a previous policy of the Arodafnousa Hospice to meet patients and families, before the admission and explain the reason for the admission at the hospice, the goals of care and discharge planning procedures (e.g., that once symptoms are controlled patients are going to return home). This has helped to reduce lengthy in-patient stays, and has resulted in an increased number of patient admissions per year (see table 2).

Table 4. Hospice/Palliative care Beds For Cyprus 2011 compared to 2013

Name	District	Beds [8] 2011	Beds 2013	Population [1] (approximately)
Arodaphnousa Palliative Care Centre	Nicosia / Larnaca/ Ammochostos	15	12	515.000
Chrysovalantou Clinic	Limassol	4	Closed	235.000
Pafos Hospice (Evaggelismos Hospital)	Paphos	5	Closed	90.000

As a result of the scarcity of inpatient hospice beds, oncology beds are often being used instead for cancer patients, unable to be looked after at home. Hence when no inpatient hospice beds are available, patients with palliative care needs, including end of life care, are accommodated at the Oncology centres (BOCOC and the Oncology Units in Nicosia and Limassol General Hospitals), where they originally received their oncology treatment. In the past, there was also the problem of patients or families refusing admission to the Arodafnousa hospice, which was associated with the stigma of death, however this is now less of a problem, possibly due to earlier contact of patients and families with PC doctors and nurses, and more open communication and less collusion in discussions of patients with their health care professionals [15].

Finally, there is currently a new initiative to open a new purpose built hospice, including facilities for children with cancer, Archangel Michael Hospice in Mesa Chorio village in Paphos [16]. Whilst this is in the final stages of completion, this facility however again due to the financial crisis will not be able to take patients until the time that sufficient funds are in place to ensure the smooth running of the facility in the future.

Outpatient Palliative Care in Cyprus

Predominantly this is provided by community based / home care teams (along the examples of the UK and Australia), with experienced PC nurses, some with post-graduate degrees in PC working alongside psychologists, social workers and physiotherapists. There is excellent multi-disciplinary team working for both NGOs, whilst the absence of PC physicians working with PASYKAF is covered by dedicated / trained (or in training) PC physicians from both the Limassol Oncology Unit and the BOCOC.

There are currently dual home care teams in each district by the two main NGOs (CACS and PASYKAF), and as a result both home care services offer a limited service over weekends and public holidays as well as no service for 14 hours from 6 p.m. to 8 a.m. every day [8]. During this period, emergency calls from patients and their families are directed to the Oncology Centre / General Hospital Oncology Units.

More recently, there have been a number of initiatives relating to outpatient PC in the BOC Oncology Centre (BOCOC) in Nicosia. Firstly since 2010, the two PC physicians from the CACS run a specialist PC clinic once a week at the BOCOC. This helps both to improve patients' difficult to control symptoms, but also encourages earlier introduction of PC in patients with advanced / metastatic cancer. Furthermore, since 2012 with two physicians in the BOCOC receiving specialist training in PC, there has been the ability to form a hospital

PC team and run daily a supportive/ PC unit /drop in centre, to address urgent symptom control problems for cancer patients attending the BOCOC.

Also in 2012, with the opening of a new purpose built facility in Limassol by the CACS, the Evagoreio supportive-PC Unit / Drop in Centre, and the employment of a third physician, there has been the ability to run daily a more comprehensive outpatient PC service in Limassol, in addition to the available service in Nicosia.

Current Human Resources / Staffing in PC

There are currently only two (2) physicians fully trained in PC in Cyprus; both work at the Arodafnousa hospice. Furthermore there is an oncologist with a diploma in Palliative Medicine, working in the Oncology Unit of the Limassol General hospital. Finally there are also currently three (3) physicians undergoing specialist PC training in a three (3) year training program with the Institute of Palliative Care (formerly based in the San Diego Hospice, now in Ohio) in the USA. Two of them work at the BOCOC in Nicosia, and the other one works with the CACS in the Evagoreio Centre in Limassol.

For all PC staff, including nurses, psychologists, social workers and physiotherapists, working in PC in Cyprus, see table 5.

Table 5. PC Staff in Cyprus

Organization	Physicians	Nurses	Psychologists	Social Workers	Physio-Therapists
CACS	3 (1 in training)	13 full time (All certificate PC)	3	2	2
PASYKAF	0	13 full /7 part time (2MSc/1 diploma PC)	3 full time / 3 part time	4	1 full time/ 5 part time
BOCOC	2 (in training)	No specialized PC nurses	1	0	0

Opioid Availabilility/Regulations/Consumption and Pain Management in Cyprus

Availability of Opioids and Regulatory Barriers in Cyprus

Regarding the availability of opioids in Cyprus in comparison to the essential drugs list of the WHO [17] and the International Association for Hospice and Palliative Care (IAHPC) list of essential medicines for palliative care [18], all four opioids on the WHO list are available, i.e., codeine, oral morphine immediate and controlled release forms and injectable morphine, whilst from the IAHPC list there is also availability of fentanyl transdermal patches, methadone, and oxycodone [19]. See table 6.

Until recently methadone was only available for prescription by psychiatrists, hence there is limited experience / expertise using this drug, whilst oxycodone immediate release is available, but patients in Cyprus have to pay for this* (despite the fact that the long release preparation is provided for free, as are all other opioids for cancer patients in Cyprus). There is however no availability of buprenorphine and hydromorphone in Cyprus.

Table 6. Availability of Opioids in Cyprus According to WHO and IAHPC Lists

	WHO	IAHPC	Cyprus
Codeine, oral	Yes	Yes	√
Morphine, oral immediate release	Yes	Yes	√
Morphine, oral controlled release	Yes	Yes	√
Injectable morphine	Yes	Yes	√
Oxycodone, oral immediate release	No	Yes	√*
	WHO	IAHPC	Cyprus
Fentanyl, transdermal patch	No	Yes	√
Methadone, oral immediate release	No	Yes	√

Regarding benzodiazepine availability, most benzodiazepines including diazepam, lorazepam and midazolam, are available, with no restrictions to prescribe in Cyprus. In fact Cyprus has the highest benzodiazepine consumption per capita in the Middle East [8].

Examining the current legal framework in Cyprus for prescription of opiates compared to the guidelines for assessment of national opioid regulations of the World Health Organization [20], there is no significant overregulation for opioids in Cyprus [23], however there is no legal framework to facilitate emergency prescribing and dispensing [19]. See table 7.

Table 7. Regulatory Restrictions to Accessibility of Opioids in Cyprus

Requirement for registration of patients to receive opioids prescriptions	Not required
Requirement for physicians to have a license to prescribe opioids.	Not required
Requirement for duplicate or triplicate prescriptions	Not required
Requirement for special prescription form	Yes. Separate pink prescription form used. (Does not have to be used exclusively by a specific physician / any physician can use)
Prescription duration	Up to 30 days
Dose limits	No limit to the maximum dose that can be prescribed.
Limitations on dispensing privileges	None exist. (All pharmacies can dispense opioids).
Provision for opioid prescribing in emergency situations	No regulation to allow physicians to prescribe by telephone or to fax a prescription to the pharmacist, or for nurses and pharmacists to issue a limited emergency prescription.
Pharmacist privilege to correct technical error on a prescription	A pharmacist is not allowed in Cyprus to correct a technical error even at the direction of the prescribing physician.
Use of stigmatizing terms for opioid analgesics in regulations	No use of stigmatizing terms (e.g., drugs of addiction, dangerous drugs or as poisons) for opioid analgesics

In summary there is easy and free availability for most opioids (and in all forms: i.e., oral, transdermal patches and subcutaneous use in syringe drivers) and benzodiazepines in both hospitals and in the community in Cyprus, with no significant regulatory restrictions.

Opioid Consumption in Cyprus

Data for annual opioid consumption from the Pain and Policy Studies Group from Wisconsin, for Cyprus between 2006 and 2010 expressed as total Morphine Equivalence (ME) in mg per person ranged between 10 to 17.9 mg/person per year [21]. This is considerably less than the ME of other Southern Europe countries, ranging from 91 to 298 mg/person, and although higher than that of other Middle East countries, it is still considerably lower than that of Israel at 144.0 mg/person [22]. See table 8.

Table 8. Morphine Equivalence (ME) Data for Mediterranean and Middle East Countries

Country	ME mg/person
Spain	298.1
Portugal	154.1
Italy	143.8
Greece	91.5
Turkey	11.5
Jordan	5.7
Lebanon	5.0
Egypt	1.2
Israel	144.0

Differences in opioid consumption are often due to excessive regulatory restrictions / differences in opioid availability [23], and doctor / patient factors to prescribe / accept opioids. Given that there are no significant regulatory restrictions and no problems with opioids availability to account for the underuse of opioids in Cyprus, doctors / patients factors, i.e., negative attitudes of patients and their families toward opioid medications, or inadequate knowledge and attitudes of the prescribing physicians regarding opioids are likely to blame [19].

Pain Management for Cancer Patients in Cyprus

In view of this low opioid consumption in Cyprus, three studies were enacted to examine physicians' prescribing habits for cancer pain both within and outside the BOCOC [19]. Data were collected regarding the presence and severity of pain and prescription of analgesia in a cross-sectional study of 141 patients receiving outpatient chemotherapy at the BOCOC, in a retrospective study of 90 new Lung Cancer patients referred to one Oncologist in the BOCOC, and in a prospective study of 100 new cancer patients referred to the BOCOC [19]. In the first study, the results reflected the prescribing habits of oncologists within the Oncology centre, whilst the second and third studies reflected the prescribing habits of physicians outside the oncology centre. The results showed that respectively 56.0%, 48.1% and 57.7% of patients with pain were prescribed analgesia, with the majority of patients being prescribed paracetamol and non steroidal anti-inflammatory drugs, and respectively only 8.6%, 11.5% and 0 % of patients were prescribed strong opioids [19]. In the last two studies, following their oncology appointment the prescription of analgesia to patients with pain, increased to 80.8% and 73.1% respectively, whilst the prescription of strong opioids, to 28.8% and 34.6%, reflecting oncologists' practice [19].

Table 9. Results from Analgesia Prescribing Habits Studies in Cyprus

Study	Patients with pain	Patients with pain prescribed analgesia		Patients with pain prescribed strong opioids	
		Onset	After Onc appointment	Onset	After Onc appointment
Cross sectional Chemotherapy	116/141(82.3%)	65/116 (56.0%)	-	10/116 (8.6%)	-
Lung cancer Retrospective	52/90 (57.8%)	25/52 (48.1%)	42/52 (80.8%)	6/52 (11.5%)	15/52 (28.8%)
Prospective all diagnoses	26/100 (26%)	15/26 (57.7%)	19/26 (73.1%)	0/26	9/26 (34.6%)

Reproduced with permission from Charalambous H, et al. Ann Oncol 2012 Suppl 3:79-83 [19].

The above studies confirm both the under-treatment of pain and the underuse of opioids for cancer patients in Cyprus. Possible reasons for this are physicians' inadequate training or experience and negative pre-conceptions in relation to opioids by both patients and physicians. Support for the presence of opioid phobia comes also from the high use of Fentanyl patch and Oxycodone (together for 2010 accounting close to 70% of opioid use in Cyprus[21]), and the low use of morphine in Cyprus (about 20% for 2010[21]), possibly due to the fact that patients do not realise and are not told that Fentanyl and Oxycodone are opioids.

Education/Training of Staff in PC

Both CACS and PASYKAF NGOs see education and training as an important part of their work. Both are members of the European Association for Palliative Care (EAPC) and encourage their staff to attend EAPC conferences and training programmes[7]. Furthermore CACS in the late 90's and early 2000's, funded two (2) physicians to complete Master's courses in PC in the UK, both of them work at the Arodafnousa hospice, whilst currently funding a third one. PASYKAF funded also another physician to obtain a diploma in PC. Both organizations have also funded distance learning post-graduate degrees and diplomas in PC for a number of nurses to become specialist nurses in PC.

Systematic high quality training courses in PC for Oncology and PC staff in Cyprus were initiated by the Middle East Cancer Consortium (MECC) [24]. MECC is an intergovernmental organisation, which was set up in 1996 by the governments of Cyprus, Egypt, Israel, Jordan, the Palestinian Authority and the U.S., through the National Cancer

Institute (NCI). The goal of MECC is to "raise cancer awareness in the Middle East and, ultimately, to reduce the burden of cancer in the region" [25]. MECC under the guidance of professor Silbermann organised a number of PC courses on an annual basis for health care professionals from its constituent members working predominantly in the Oncology or PC field with the first one taking place in 2004, in Larnaca, Cyprus [25]. The last course was on Paediatric Pain and PC Master Class again in Larnaca, taking place between the 28th of November and 1st of December, 2011.

Another important training initiative relates to physicians currently undergoing specialist training in PC. The MECC courses helped to bring attention towards the need to improve PC services in Cyprus and the need to have more PC physicians working in Cyprus. As a result both the Board of Trustees of the BOCOC and of the CACS agreed to the funding of three (3) scholarships for specialist training in PC. These scholarships were offered to two (2) internal medicine / general physicians already working in the BOCOC and a general physician working at the CACS. Their training started in 2012 at the Institute of Palliative Medicine in San Diego (now Ohio) in the US [26], with one (1) month of training in the US for every 6 months of training / practice in Cyprus, and a yearly visit from the US team in Cyprus (first one took place in February 2013). Currently all three (3) physicians continue to work in Cyprus, whilst progressing with their specialist PC training both in Cyprus and the US.

Finally an advanced Communication Skills Training course was undertaken in March 2011 by Professor Leslie Fallowfield's team in Cyprus [27] for twenty (20) Oncologists, PC physicians, psychologists and nurses. Following the success of this first course, the aim is to continue with similar courses, and the training to be provided by Cypriot facilitators.

Training in PC of Health Care Professionals Not Working in PC

Currently the Cyprus Institute of Technology, the European University, the University of Nicosia and Frederick University, offer nursing degrees to graduate level in Cyprus. Within their nursing undergraduate curricula, there is dedicated time for Oncology nursing, with clinical attachments in the Oncology wards (with exposure to patients with PC needs). All nursing universities also offer a PC module, which is optional in the fourth year, consisting of lectures, case studies and workshops, and also a pain management module, which is an integral part of the curriculum. In terms of post-graduate curricula, nurses on the one year post-graduate community nursing course, spend time with the NGOs home care teams to gain experience in home care nursing of cancer patients, whilst the University of Nicosia provides a full Pain module for their MSc Nursing course.

There are only three (3) Medical Schools in Cyprus. The first Medical School was set up by the St George's Medical School from London in conjunction with the University of Nicosia in 2011, whilst in the autumn of 2013 both the University of Cyprus and European University are planning to start Undergraduate Medical Courses. In terms of undergraduate medical training in PC, at this early stage, there have been no specific plans to include PC in their curricula, although this may change in the future. Equally these medical schools, given that they have so recently been set up, have so far not contributed to post-graduate PC training / Continued Medical Education (CME) activities of physicians in Cyprus.

The NGOs, CACS, PASYKAF, the BOCOC and the Marianna Lordos Memorial Foundation have been involved in organizing lectures, seminars or conferences relating to

Oncology and PC in Cyprus, open to all health care professionals in Cyprus. The biggest of those is the CACS bi-annual conference in Oncology and PC, with the last one in 2011 attended by more than 320 attendees, and with twenty (20) invited foreign speakers from Europe and the USA [28].

In December 2011, a targeted initiative to provide PC training to public hospitals staff, took place. The Ministry of Health, in conjunction with the two main NGOs (CACS and PASYKAF) and the BOCOC, organized a thirty (30) hour, five (5) day PC course in Nicosia with faculty from the Institute of Palliative Medicine, from San Diego, led by Dr Frank Ferris. This included training of fifty (50) members of staff predominantly from the public hospitals. The aim for this course was firstly to provide training in PC to public hospitals' staff, who had never in the past any PC training, secondly to improve collaboration between public hospital staff with the PC staff from the NGOs and finally to identify committed public hospitals staff to become the pioneers to set up PC teams within the public hospitals. Whilst the first two goals were met, unfortunately the financial difficulties in Cyprus, did not allow for the Ministry of Health to support the setting up of PC teams within public hospitals.

Multidisciplinary Cancer Care in Cyprus: Progress and Challenges

Cancer care has been traditionally about team work and multidisciplinary care, given the need for different medical specialties to help with the diagnosis, staging, disease directed therapy, supportive and palliative care of cancer patients. PC has also embraced this approach, especially in view of the fact that patients with advanced / metastatic cancer have complex physical, psychosocial and religious /spiritual needs, as a consequence of their disease and its treatment. These needs cannot be met by just one health care professional, hence there is a need of an extended team of health care professionals including doctors, palliative care nurses, psychologists, social workers, chaplains or spiritual guides, able to deal with different problems according to their different areas of expertise (see figure 2).

In Cyprus multidisciplinary care for cancer patients has been gradually adopted in the last 6-7 years, with patients increasingly being treated by specialist Multi-Disciplinary Teams (MDTs) and management decisions being taken within MDT meetings. The first MDT meeting in Thoracic Cancer was set up in 2006 at the BOCOC and subsequently MDT meetings in Breast, Gastro-intestinal and Gynecological Cancer were set up. These teams have however been restricted to core members of oncologists, surgeons and sometimes radiologists, whilst the attendance is not compulsory, and especially for lower volume surgeons from the private sector it is not practical or feasible to attend.

Furthermore, as a proof of the improvement in multidisciplinary and between organizations (NGOs and the BOCOC) collaboration involving PC, since February 2013, a weekly Multi-Disciplinary Team (MDT) meeting involving oncology and PC professionals (oncologist, PC nurses, physicians training in PC, BOCOC nurses, pharmacists, psychologist and a Christian Orthodox priest), has been set up at the BOCOC. This is a first step to offer a more comprehensive multidisciplinary care for patients with advanced cancer (by involving earlier the appropriate members of the multidisciplinary team to meet the complex needs of patients with advanced cancer) and to improve collaboration and communication between hospital and community teams.

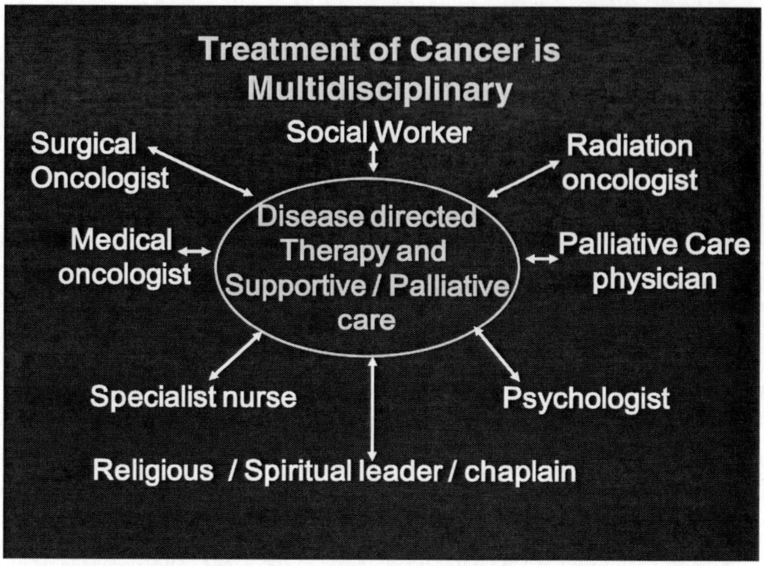

Figure 2. Multidisciplinary Cancer Care.

Despite the availability of PC services, not all oncologists refer to the multidisciplinary PC team [29]. Hence adopting a more comprehensive, multi-disciplinary model of care with an increased involvement of more health care professionals especially in relation to PC and Psychosocial support (i.e., including the PC physicians/nurses, psychologists and chaplains) has been more challenging. The problem of under-referral to PC or avoiding to use the PC MDT, may relate to the perceptions of some oncologists, that they can do all this by themselves or that there is nothing further that can be done for their patients [30]. This is often due to the lack of training of Oncologists in PC, or lack of contact with other specialties and members of the MDT, hence oncologists are not aware of the potential impact of PC as well as of other members of the MDT to meet the complex needs of patients with advanced cancer [31].

Overall in Cyprus the predominant oncology practice used to be of disease directed therapy very much until the end of life, and then referral to the hospice or in fact patients would often die in hospital (as there was a stigma attached to going to the hospice, as the place "where you go to die"). Whilst PC teams existed in the community organized by the two NGOs, there was little communication or collaboration between the PC and oncology teams. Equally the two PC physicians in the past were strictly present in the hospice with little contact with the oncologists in the main tertiary oncology centre in Cyprus, at the BOCOC. This however has changed with an increased presence of PC physicians in the BOCOC over the last three years, with the two physicians at the BOCOC now training in PC and with more combined training and lectures attended by both PC and Oncology staff, resulting in a gradual change in terms of attitudes of oncologists and their approach to PC, with both increased and earlier referrals from oncologists to PC. This is evidenced by the increased cancer patients receiving PC under the care of both NGOs in 2012 compared to 2010 (see tables 2 and 3).

CURRENT PC SERVICES IN CYPRUS: STRENGTHS AND LIMITATIONS

The biggest strength of PC services in Cyprus, is the training, experience and dedication of PC staff both at the CACS and PASYKAF organizations. Both organizations have shared a major commitment for continuous training and education, and have encouraged their staff beyond attending training courses, also to work and attain higher degrees in PC [7]. Through consistent training and education of PC staff, they have been able to provide high quality service to cancer patients in Cyprus, both in the Arodafnousa hospice and in the community. Equally training in PC is now taking place for staff within the BOCOC.

There are however significant problems with PC in Cyprus. A major issue is the lack of organized PC services for Paediatric Cancer patients. The biggest problem however is that currently there are no PC services within the main public hospitals, i.e., there are no specialized hospital PC teams, either with dedicated PC physicians or specialist PC nurses [8]. As a result patients in the public hospitals have no input from specialist PC teams, and this applies both for cancer patients and also patients with other life threatening illnesses. Finally the other main problem of PC services is that there is little co-operation between the two main NGOs in terms of provision of community PC services, resulting in a duplicated and fragmented service, where currently each home care service only covers the patients at home between 8 am to 6 pm [8].

BARRIERS FOR THE DEVELOPMENT OF PC IN CYPRUS

In a review of PC in the Six (6) MECC countries by Clark and Bingley [32] from the International Observatory on End of Life Care and in another review in the EAPC Atlas of Palliative Care in Europe [33,34], the main barriers for PC in Cyprus were considered to be the following:

1. Model of provision of PC services completely reliable on NGOs, whilst NGOs have no stable and predictable funding, apart from limited grants from the government.
2. No government provision to include PC in the general health care system, and no PC teams in public hospitals.
3. Lack of awareness and understanding of PC needs at public, government, and professional levels
4. Lack of specialists in PC
5. Lack of core education and training for health care professionals (non PC staff) in PC resulting among others in underuse of opioids for cancer pain
6. Lack of education of patients about PC and opioids

Since both these two publications, apart from an improvement in educational and training initiatives for health care professionals, not much has changed especially in relation to the public/government services and commitment to invest / develop PC. In order therefore to improve PC services it is necessary to tackle all these different issues / barriers. All organizations involved in PC would need to work hard to educate / raise awareness and lobby for continual support for PC services at the government level (to invest to develop PC services in the public hospitals, and provide more funding towards the NGOs), at the health professional level so that PC awareness and training improves and finally at the society and patients level, again to improve awareness and dispel myths and fears about cancer and PC. There is also an urgent need to maintain the momentum, which has just now been established after many years of relative inactivity in the PC field in Cyprus.

Stage of PC Development in Cyprus and the Vision/Plans for the Future

Four stages of development of PC are recognized, associated progressively with more comprehensive PC services. The 1st stage is when no Services are identified, the 2nd stage is that of Capacity Building, the 3rd stage of Localized provision and the final /4th stage is that of Approaching Integration [32]. Cyprus meets the main criteria for both capacity building (i.e., awareness of PC needs, being registered with key organizations e.g., EAPC/ WHO / MECC, having links with/visits to other PC/hospice organizations, conference participation, education and training initiatives, preparation of development strategy) and also localized provision [32] (i.e., local campaigning and publicity, initial capacity building, services set up and funding established, government legislation in progress, opioids available, external training courses, developing academic links and research activity). It is therefore accepted that Cyprus in terms of PC services is approaching integration [32].

There is still however a need to improve PC services on a number of fronts. A proposal for a new model of PC services for Cyprus, based on the UK / Australian practice, has been made [8] and was incorporated in the Cyprus National Cancer Plan [35]. This has however not been implemented as yet, possibly as a result of the financial crisis.

The vision for PC services development in Cyprus entails the following:

1. Set up public hospitals' PC teams: With the help of the NGOs, the government would need to invest in the training and then employment of a core team of professionals in each general hospital in the five districts (with a specialist PC care doctor, PC specialist nurse and psychologist or social worker). These teams would work within hospitals offering a consultant service to improve patients' symptoms, and facilitate their transfer to the community, whilst for more complicated cases facilitate referral to hospice care.
2. Set up Home Care PC teams with 24 hour cover: This should be achieved by uniting the home care teams of the two NGOs (+/- recruitment of a few more PC nurses), so that with increased capacity, a true 24 hour service can be provided to patients and their families, enabling them to stay at home for as long as possible.
3. Expand Inpatient (hospice) PC services: Ideally three (3) hospices are needed to cover geographically all districts in Cyprus. Arodafnousa hospice to continue covering the district of Nicosia, a second hospice to cover the districts of both Larnaca with Ammohostos, and finally a third hospice to cover both the districts of Limassol and Paphos. This should be associated with expansion of palliative care

beds in the first instance to about forty (40), and then work towards having 80-100 PC beds/ million population, as suggested by the EAPC guidelines [14].

4. Aim to train and then appoint specialist PC physicians in each district: having dual appointments in hospices and local hospital / oncology centres-units, who are going to be central in coordinating care and improve integration of PC within standard oncology care. Whilst being involved in the direct management of hospice inpatients and lead home care teams in the community, they are also going to provide advice and leadership for public hospitals' / oncology units-centres' PC teams (see figure 3). Furthermore they would have a valuable role in providing education and training to a variety of professional groups to improve the standard of general PC provided by non PC physicians and nurses, and finally become involved in PC research in Cyprus.

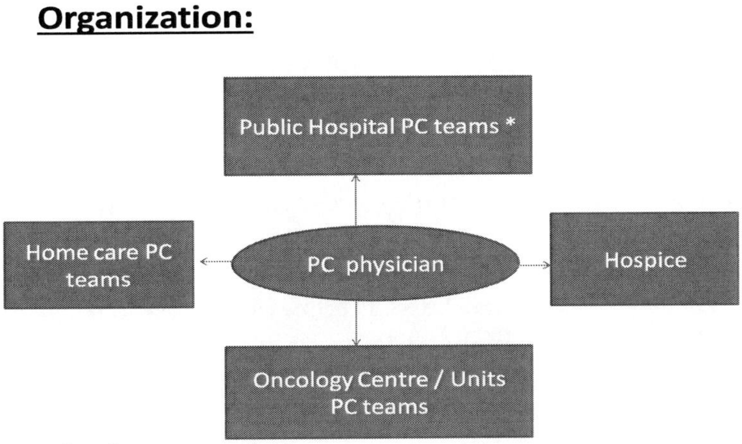

*Should cater not just for cancer patients.

Figure 3. Organization of PC services around the PC physician.

Conclusions

Until today NGOs have been the main providers of PC in Cyprus, providing both inpatient (hospice) and outpatient (home care) community PC services. In the recent past, significant improvements have been made to the access rate of cancer patients to high quality PC, through better collaboration between Oncology services, especially at the BOCOC and PC NGOs and their staff, by working together in the Oncology centre, and by joint training and educational events. Overall quality of PC has also improved as a result of the dedication and training/expertise of PC staff, gained especially via MECC training initiatives, culminating in a new initiative to train three (3) new physicians as specialists in PC in the US. Furthermore with the set up of three (3) new Medical Schools in Cyprus in the last couple of years, there is hope that both academic and also educational/continuing professional development activities in the field of PC are going to expand.

Limitations and challenges of PC services in Cyprus however include the lack of both Paediatric PC services and PC services within public hospitals, as well as the lack of collaboration between the two main NGOs providing PC services. Furthermore due to the financial crisis in Cyprus, the NGOs face significant financial problems due to decreased fundraising resulting in budget deficits, with the viability of their services being threatened in the immediate/short term. This financial crisis however represents an opportunity for the Government of Cyprus and the Ministry of Health to invest in PC in Cyprus. Beyond improving patients' care/experience and families support, this can also potentially result in decreased health care costs through savings relating to decreased aggressive End of Life care and by facilitating care for patients in the community as opposed to care provided in the hospitals and the oncology units/centre.

REFERENCES

[1] http://www.cystat.gov.cy/mof/cystat/statistics.nsf/All/32DCF1B1D5F73997C22579730 03704DF?OpenDocument&sub=2&sel=1&e=&print accessed 8th of October 2013.

[2] http://hdr.undp.org/en/statistics/ (Human Development Index) accessed 8th of October 2013.

[3] http://www.gfmag.com/gdp-data-country-reports/287-cyprus-gdp-country-report.html#axzz1sYmGJiRR accessed 8th of October 2013

[4] MERCER report: http://www.hio.org.cy/docs/mercer_report_october2013.pdf accessed 1st November 2013

[5] http://www.moh.gov.cy/MOH/MOH.nsf/0/A0B4FEC0AC7BB073C22579C7002A9683/$file/%CE%88%CE%BA%CE%B8%CE%B5%CF%83%CE%B7%20%CE%A0%CF%81%CE%BF%CF%8C%CE%B4%CE%BF%CF%85%20%CE%B3%CE%B9%CE%B1%20%CF%84%CE%BF%20%CE%AD%CF%84%CE%BF%CF%82%202011%20(%CE%A3%CF%84%CE%BF%CE%B9%CF%87%CE%B5%CE%AF%CE%B1%202006-2008).pdf accessed 12th October 2013. Cyprus Cancer Registry: Progress Report for 2011.

[6] Malas S. The current Status of Palliative Care in Cyprus: Has it improved in the last years? J Pediatr Hematol Oncol 2011; 33: S47-51.

[7] Cyprus Country report from the International Observatory for End of Life Care, University of Lancaster, UK. http://www.lancaster.ac.uk/shm/research/ioelc/international/pdf/cyprus_country_report.pdf accessed 9th October 2013

[8] Silbermann M, Arnaout M, Daher M et al. Palliative cancer care in Middle Eastern countries: accomplishments and challenges. *Ann. Oncol.* 2012; Suppl 3:15-28.

[9] http://www.anticancersociety.org.cy/anticancer1/page.php?pageID=1&langID=0 accessed 9th of October 2013

[10] http://www.pasykaf.org/en accessed 9th of October 2013.

[11] http://www.friendsforlife.org.cy accessed 9th of October 2013.

[12] http://www.paphoshospice.org accessed 9th of October 2013.

[13] http://www.kyfahivcenter.com/en/ accessed 30th October 2013.

[14] Standards and Norms for Hospice and Palliative Care in Europe-The EAPC White Paper. Lukas Radbruch, Sheila Payne and the Board of Directors of the European Association for Palliative Care (EAPC) http://ukz.katolik.cz/texty%20sokrates/eapc.pdf accessed 9th of October 2013.

[15] Charalambous H, Koukides A, Avgousti V, Gavrielidou V. Cancer patients preferences for information in Cyprus. Support Care Cancer 2012; 20 (Suppl 1): S 241.

[16] http://archangel-michael-hospice.com accessed 9th of October 2013.

[17] World Health Organization. Geneva. Switzerland: World Health Organization; 2007. The selection and use of essential medicines.

[18] De Lima L. International Association for Hospice and Palliative Care list of essential medicines for palliative care. *Ann. Oncol* 2007;18(2):395-399.

[19] Charalambous H, Protopapa E, Gavrielidou D, Avgousti V. Physicians' prescribing habits for cancer pain in Cyprus. *Ann. Oncol.* 2012 Apr;23 Suppl 3:79-83.

[20] World Health Organization. Achieving Balance in National Opioids Control Policy: Guidelines for Assessment. Geneva, Switzerland: World Health Organization; 2000.

[21] http://www.painpolicy.wisc.edu/sites/www.painpolicy.wisc.edu/files/country_files/morphine_equivalence/cyprusME.pdf accessed 8th of October 2013

[22] http://www.painpolicy.wisc.edu/countryprofiles accessed 8th of October 2013

[23] Cherny NI, Baselga J, De Conno F et al. Formulary availability and regulatory barriers for accessibility of opioids for cancer pain in Europe: a report from the ESMO/EAPC Opioid Policy Initiative. *Ann. Oncol* 2010; 21: 615-626.

[24] http://www.mecc.cancer.gov/ accessed on the 20th of October 2013.

[25] http://www.mecc.cancer.gov/pc.html accessed on the 20th of October 2013.

[26] http://www.palliativemed.org/International-Palliative-Medicine-Fellowship accessed on the 20th of October 2013.

[27] http://www.bococ.org.cy/index.php?s_id=38&a_id=1469 accessed on the 20th of October 2013.

[28] http://www.anticancersociety.org.cy/anticancer1/page.php?pageID=89&mpath=/114 accessed on the 20th of October 2013.

[29] Silbermann M, Pitsillides B, Al-Alfi N et al. Multidisciplinary care team for cancer patients and its implementation in several Middle Eastern countries. *Ann. Oncol.* 2013; 24 Suppl 7:vii41-47.

[30] Abrahm JL. Integrating palliative care into comprehensive cancer care. *J. Natl. Compr. Canc. Netw.* 2012; 10(10):1192-8.

[31] Charalambous H, Silbermann M. Clinically based palliative care training is needed urgently for all oncologists. *J. Clin. Oncol.* 2012; 30 (32):4042-3.

[32] Bingley A, Clark D. A comparative review of palliative care development in six countries represented by the Middle East Cancer Consortium (MECC). *J. Pain Symptom. Management.* 2009 Mar;37(3):287-96

[33] Centeno C, Clark D, Lynch T et al. EAPC atlas of Palliative Care in Europe, 2007 ISBN 0-9758525-5-8.

[34] http://www.eapc-taskforce-development.eu/documents/national/cyprus.pdf accessed 9th of October 2013

[35] Cyprus National Cancer Plan – from the Cyprus National Cancer Committee in Greek (Εθνική Επιτροπή για τον Καρκίνο). 2012.(Document can be requested through the Ministry of Health in Cyprus)

In: Palliative Care to the Cancer Patient
Editor: Michael Silbermann

ISBN: 978-1-63117-709-5

Chapter 2

PALLIATIVE CARE IN EGYPT: AWARENESS IS THE PROBLEM

Khaled Abdelhmeed Mostafa, M.D., Dipl. Card., Dipl. Q.M.H.C.*
National Cancer Institute, Cairo University, Cairo, Egypt

INTRODUCTION

Egypt, at the northeast corner of Africa on the Mediterranean Sea, is bordered on the west by Libya, on the south by the Sudan, and on the east by the Red Sea and Israel. It is nearly one and one-half times the size of Texas. Egypt is divided into two unequal, extremely arid regions by the landscape's dominant feature, the northward-flowing Nile River. The Nile starts 100 mi (161 km) south of the Mediterranean and fans out to a sea front of 155 mi between the cities of Alexandria and Port Said. Land area: 384,344 sq mi (995,451 sq km. Population (2012 est.): 83,688,164 (growth rate: 1.92% Cairo, 10,902,000, Alexandria, 4,387,000; Giza, 2,597,600 and the country is divided into 26 governorates (1).

Regarding care of cancer patients, there are cancer care centers affiliated to the ministry of health in 12 governorates. Also, all faculties of medicine (10 in number) and military hospitals have sectors for cancer care. In fact, the biggest and more specialized center is the National Cancer Institute (NCI), which is affiliated with Cairo University. NCI carries on research, education and clinical responsibilities and is considered to be the main reference in Egypt regarding cancer.

Palliative care in Egypt is in an early stage of development with very few palliative care activities available even in all of the above specialized centers. At this stage, research is crucial to develop suitable palliative care models with respect to the needs, culture, and resources in Egypt.

Opioid consumption figures in Egypt are among the lowest worldwide indicating largely inadequate cancer pain control. Based on the data published in the most recent annual report of the International Narcotics Control Board, the average opioid consumption in Egypt during

* Address for correspondence: k24mostafa@hotmail.com

2008-2010 was 62 defined daily doses for statistical purposes (S-DDD) per million inhabitants per 5 days. With this Figure Egypt was ranked 115th among 184 countries (2).

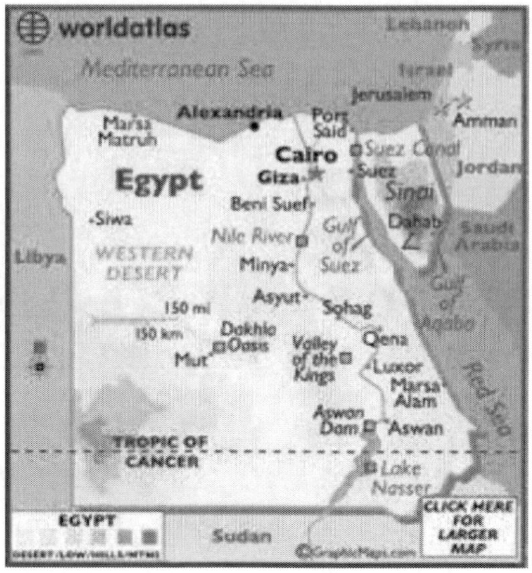

Figure 1. Map of Egypt.

In 2011, I did a fishbone analysis to discover the root cause(s) of this very low morphine consumption, as shown in the following figure.

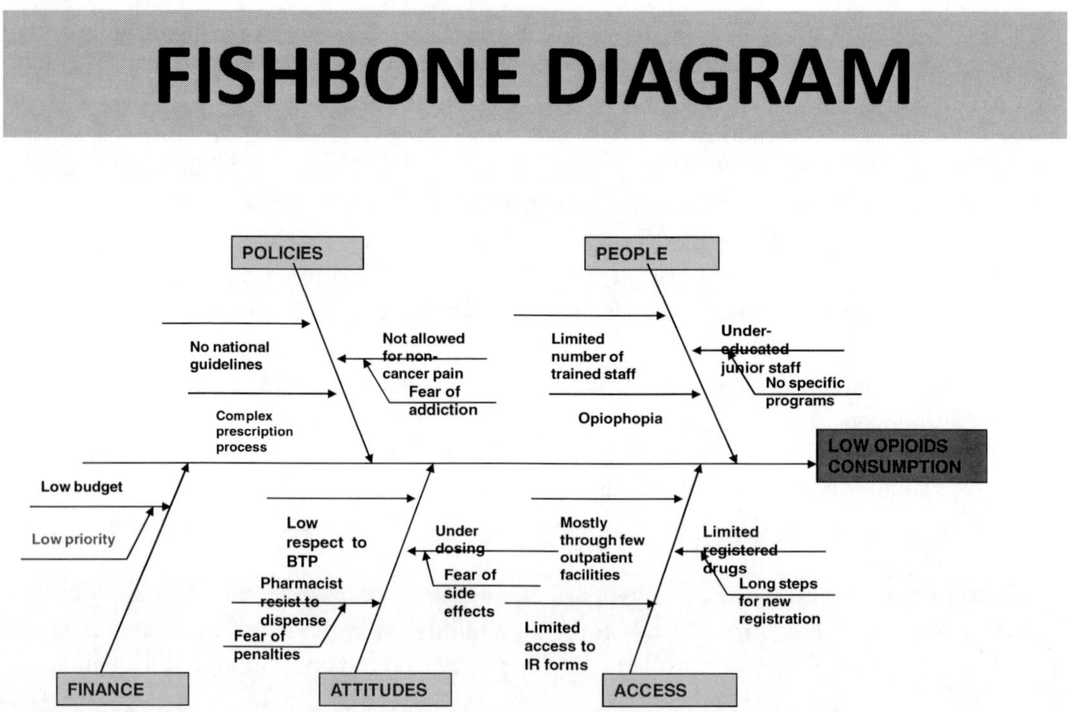

Figure 2. Fishbone Diagram Analysis for Low Opioids Consumption.

Low awareness among government, physicians, pharmacists and the community was found to be the root cause of underuse of opioids.

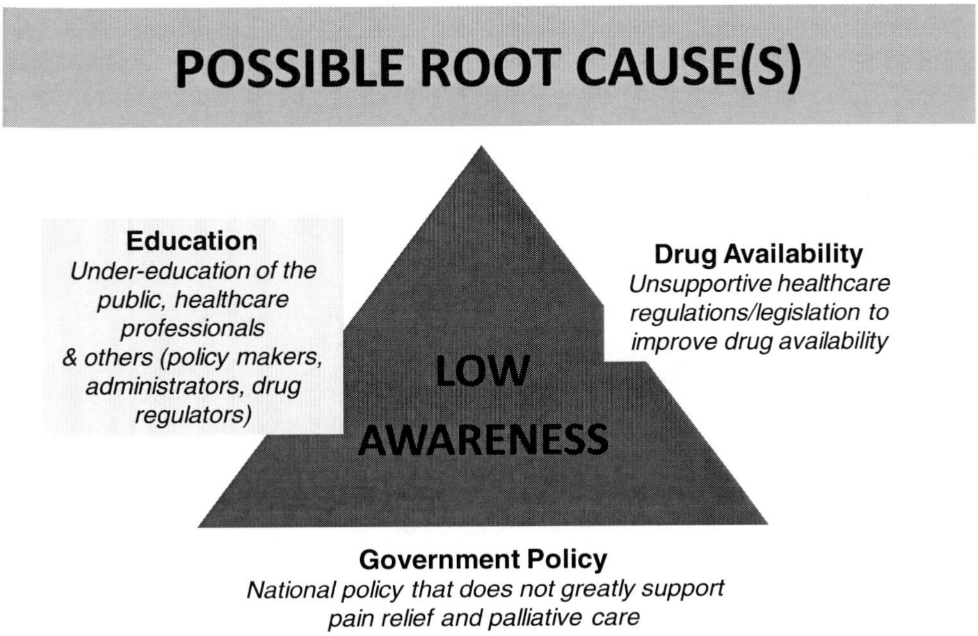

Figure 3. Low awareness is the root cause.

National Cancer Institute of Egypt

- NCI has started providing its service since 1969
- NCI provides free service for more than 80% of cancer patients in Egypt.
- Outpatient clinics receive about 700 patients per day for treatment or follow up
- Number of new patients in 2010 was about 18,156, 70% of them with advanced disease
- Starting from October 2008, they have been providing a one-day-per-week palliative care service (out-patient clinic) for adult patients.

Faced Problems in NCI program

- There is no applied national program.
- Insufficient communication with concerned departments
- Poor understanding and awareness of the role of palliative care in the community
- A well-trained nursing staff and volunteers are not available for palliative care service
- Insufficient supplies and equipment
- Difficulties in access and continual care (weekends)
- No available inpatient service

As a result of the increasing lists of patients waiting to attend palliative clinics in NCI of Cairo, they are faced with the problem of providing high quality pain-care service through its outpatient pain clinic. The program was intended to provide a 24/7 outpatient cancer pain management service as rapidly accessible, high-quality care to patients with complex pain and palliative care symptom burdens. In addition, this model avoids inpatient hospital admissions.

Features of High Quality Service in NCI Palliative Outpatient Facilities

1 Accurate identification of the patient and his/her illness in all care settings.
2 Easy and accurate scheduling and follow-up systems.
3 Easy access to ancillary departments.
4 Adequate number of staff with a comfortable working environment.
5 Organize policy & procedures and guidelines of standards.
6 Safety and effective opioid therapy.
7 Highly educated and trained providers available during work hours and on-call.
8 Easy communication and collaboration between staff member with other specialities.
9 Active involvement in palliative care literature reviews and scientific activities towards the goal of maintaining best practice protocols for clinical use.
10 Continuous and careful monitoring for periodic re-evaluation of the service.

Our experience in NCI, Cairo University, demonstrated that urgent, high-intensity cancer pain management and palliative care services may be delivered with great efficiency in an outpatient setting that avoids the use of emergency rooms and inpatient wards. We have not attempted to assess explicit patient and family satisfaction about this particular issue in a scientifically validated manner. However, we received a great deal of anecdotal feedback from patients and families; these comments often compare our model favorably with clinical settings that lack a 24/7 infusion area. In particular, feedback centers on our easy access of services and our responsive and expert staff. In addition, patients and their families stress that avoiding unnecessary hospital admissions minimizes the impact of urgent pain/symptom management on the activities of daily life (3).

What Do We Need?

1 A national governmental home-based palliative care program to cover awareness, education with evident guidelines and a reasonable policy for availability of opioids and their disposal.
2 Encourage the community's share in the program by money donations, hospice places, volunteers and training .
3 Organize a national master or diploma degree in palliative care with reasonable training hours.

References

[1] *EGYPT CIA—The World Factbook*. April 6, 2011. Accessed: April 18, 2011.

[2] International for Narcotics Control Board. *Narcotic drugs: Estimated world requirements for 2011; statistics 2009*. 2011. United Nations, New York

[3] Hameed KA. Optimizing pain care delivery in outpatient facilities: experience in NCI, Cairo, Egypt. *J Pediatr Hematol Oncol Apr 2011*;33 Suppl 1:S19-22.

In: Palliative Care to the Cancer Patient
Editor: Michael Silbermann
ISBN: 978-1-63117-709-5

Chapter 3

PALLIATIVE CARE IN IRAQ

Salma Abbas Al-Hadad, M.D.[1*], Mazin Faisal Al-Jadiry, M.D.[1] and Claudia Leftko[2]

[1]Children's Welfare Teaching Hospital, Baghdad College of Medicine, Baghdad, Iraq

[2]MAEd, the Iraqi Children's Art Exchange Foundation, US

INTRODUCTION

There is a growing awareness and recognition by the international medical, humanitarian aid and development community that cancer and other non-communicable diseases deserve more attention. The high-level meeting of the General Assembly of the United Nations on the Prevention and Control of Non-Communicable Diseases (September, 2011), and publications including *Closing the Cancer Divide:* call for the more developed countries to share information, strategies, and human and financial resources with those on the other side of the development gap. [1] Iraq is classified as a low/medium income country (LMIC); some two-thirds of worldwide cancer deaths occur in countries in this category. We recognize the importance of international collaboration; we need help. We also recognize the challenge of cross-cultural and language issues to deliver and accept such help. Palliative care is particularly delicate in that it concerns quality of life issues which, while broadly understood to respond to our common humanity, are subject to different interpretations in different cultures and communities.

As pediatric oncologists at Children's Welfare Teaching Hospital (CWTH) in Medical City, Baghdad, we have worked tirelessly over more than twenty years to deliver the best pediatric cancer care possible in very challenging circumstances. Our intention, whenever possible, is holistic care of the child. Sometimes this is by design – a special project or program. But for the most part the approach to care beyond the standard accepted medical/scientific aspects – psychosocial and palliative care, our understanding of what is most effective for our patients as individuals and members of communities in Iraq is a function of who we are historically, culturally, socially and spiritually. This is generally true of all countries and cultures, in the view of medical anthropology. It needs to be factored into our consideration of palliative care.

* Address for correspondence: salmahadad@yahoo.com

Our goal in this chapter is to share a narrative of holistic care in challenging circumstances. We hope it will expand and contribute to our collective understanding of palliative care as it is interpreted and implemented across cultures, using the concept and practice of holistic health care in Iraq as an example.

A Brief History

Iraq has suffered a great deal over the last decades. Wars, economic sanctions, violence and instability over many years have taken an enormous toll. Many if not most of the systems, institutions and government structures that support a modern industrial country have been damaged or broken. Everything – from the education and health care system to the health-sustaining infrastructure of water purification and the electric grid, along with the transportation system – has been negatively affected. Every person has been affected in one way or another. They may have lost a relative or close friend. They may have lost their job, or their house, or their health. As pediatric oncologists, we feel we have lost a good deal of our institutional and professional capacity to treat the young patients who come to us with serious, life-threatening cancers.

Iraqis have been living with the life-threatening "diseases" of violence, chaos and instability. The overall health of the population, which WHO defines as "...a state of complete physical, mental and social well-being and not merely the absence of disease or infirmity," has suffered. Our sense of well-being, our capacity to enjoy life and believe in a better future, has been compromised. Many people have lost hope. On some level the country would benefit from a program of palliative care to support us as we try to recover and rebuild, reconstruct our institutions, our communities, and our civic, professional and personal lives.

There is little concept in Iraq about the philosophy of palliative care as it is defined by WHO and implemented around the world. Even among medical personnel and other professionals, palliative care is simply seen as the care of terminal patients with advanced disease. Outside the medical community, the Iraqi public lacks a clear understanding about chronic diseases in general and cancer specifically. People suffering from chronic disease are seen as a burden to the community, with a stigma attached to those with cancer. Investigating the theory and philosophy, or investing scarce resources in palliative care is, then, a totally strange concept. Many doctors understand the value, but we are constrained by more urgent priorities: the lack of building capacity, comprehensive cancer care centres, and multidisciplinary teams to implement palliative care programs.

Iraq had one of the best health-care systems in the Middle East before 1990: a system of primary, secondary and tertiary care facilities that provided free, good-quality services. [2] This changed dramatically after 1990. UN Sanctions and wars and the aftermath of violence, political, economic and social instability created a health care crisis in the country. Overall health – especially the health of children and other vulnerable groups – declined. The U5MR – "…the single most significant indicator of the state of a nation's children…increased from 50 to 130 deaths per thousand live births in the decade 1990-2000. [3] It was a perfect storm: Iraqi's overall health and well-being was declining at the same time that the capacity of the health care system was in collapse at every level.

There were some changes, some improvements after the 2003 regime change, but we are still far below the expected standard. Hospital and private laboratories are still functioning without national or international quality control. For the most part, things have been slow to change and difficult, given the ongoing instability and violence. Doctors and other health care professionals continued to leave the country especially during 2006, in response to the increased violence and sectarian tension. Our current health care system is still extremely compromised. Basically, we are providing almost the same level of services we provided thirty years ago.

The enormous challenges of the last decades make our work going forward difficult. Researchers confirm what we already know from our personal and professional experience: people living in societies ruptured by war and natural disaster face greater levels of emotional distress, yet these are the very societies in need of productive, healthy citizens.

About Children's Welfare Teaching Hospital

CWTH is a tertiary hospital with 240 beds; the oncology unit has a capacity for 30-40 beds, but the number of actual inpatients is 60-80. The hospital is managed by the Iraqi government and the staffs are governmental employees. Services are free but somewhat limited. Prior to 2003, patients were referred and came to this unit from all parts of Iraq. That has changed, however, with the construction of new pediatric cancer units in Kurdistan. In addition, it is difficult for referred patients and their families to travel to and from the hospital because of the ongoing lack of security.

We treat all childhood cancers except brain tumors; there is no radiotherapy center or multidisciplinary care team in Medical City to assist in the management of these kinds of tumors. In addition, there is no space to accommodate such a program. We have an average of 300 newly malignant cases per year, with an annual range of 235-398 for the last twelve years. The average registered mortality rate over the last ten years ranged between 10%-20%. Two-thirds of these occurred during induction as a result of the lack of optimum supportive care.

When a family reaches our center, they are either referred for further management after being told about the diagnosis, or they are undiagnosed and referred for diagnosis, or they are referred without being told about the disease, or, lastly, they come for a consultation and diagnosis without referral, as their case was mismanaged elsewhere.

A child's cancer diagnosis is shocking for a family in any circumstance. It is perhaps even more difficult to face in a post-war society, when life already includes so many significant challenges. The child, at the time of diagnosis at our hospital, is tired, exhausted from the disease and its complications. The child may be suffering from iatrogenic complications as a result of earlier, improper treatment or mismanagement of their disease. The families are often exhausted from their interactions with other doctors and facilities. They are shocked when they hear that the scientific and medical equipment and tools needed for the proper diagnosis and treatment of their child's illness are either not available or of questionable standard. The services are free but many things are missing and ultimately the costs for the patients are much more than they expect, whether for surgical intervention or lab tests or medicines or frequent visits to private clinics. On top of all these concrete concerns, parents suffer a great deal knowing their child has cancer, and knowing it can be fatal. They worry that revealing information about their child's illness will affect their relationships with other family members and with members of their community – teachers at school and neighbours at home.

Palliative care programs, as they exist in other places, would start here, with a well-trained team to help from the moment of diagnosis. In Iraq, however, these difficult moments are the responsibility of the doctors. We do our best to create a positive connection with the child and family, but at the same time we are already worrying about practical matters that will affect us and the child: about providing a bed for the newly diagnosed patient in the unit, and the need for more medicines which are often not available or are inconsistently supplied. We must discuss the issue of visitation by extended family members. Our policy does not allow this, which often angers parents to the extent of considering refusing the treatment option.

Doctors are the ones who must explain the rules and regulations. They are the ones who must help parents face their fears about their child and their anxieties about other aspects of their lives that will be affected by the child's illness. The family would like us to solve all of the problems the illness creates. They want us to treat the child; provide all the needed drugs; decrease pain and suffering; find a solution for the loss of the father's and/or mother's daily wages, and give official leave for parents to be absent from jobs; explain all aspects of the disease to the extended family members who might be influencing the family to refuse the idea of treatment by chemotherapy; and lastly, provide financial support to poor families. Our burden is this: as all doctors, we care deeply about these children and families, yet we find, for reasons beyond our control, that we cannot give them the level of help and the care they need in these moments, or indeed in the weeks or months that follow the diagnosis.

We can spend 30-60 minutes with the family at the time of diagnosis, explaining treatment options and giving a prognosis according to our survival rates data. Sometimes we must work to convince the family of the importance of treatment and explain that the disease can be cured, and that it is not necessarily fatal. After that, unfortunately, there is very little time to talk with the child except during medical treatments and/or procedures. During a patient's stay, doctors must secure the chemotherapeutics, antibiotics and necessary supportive treatments. They must ensure the proper medical therapies with the pharmacy, which has no active role in dispensing the medicines; they depend on the doctor's advice. There is little or no support staff at the hospital, no secretaries to help with administrative work such as scheduling, copying, phone calls and other basics.

Neither is there time to talk with siblings who might visit. The situation is difficult because parents don't want, or don't have a way --they don't know how-- to talk with their sick child or with the other children about cancer. They themselves lack a good understanding of the disease. Without a well-trained multidisciplinary team or without even one specialist to help us, and without time or a private space, there is no way to answer questions or educate the family about living with chronic disease, no way to sooth the anxieties and fears of the patient or the family.

The doctors and to a lesser extent nursing staff will manage the child over the course of treatment. There is a chronic shortage of doctors and college-trained nurses in this specialty. There is no multidisciplinary team to help deliver holistic care to patients. There are no social workers, teachers, spiritual advisors who might improve the psychological state of the child or family, or nurture their spiritual strength, and no one who might distract them with meaningful activities.

The system in Iraq requires a companion to stay with the child throughout their stay at the hospital. This is always a female relative – a mother, grandmother or aunt in most cases. Fathers are not allowed to stay, although many remain nearby, sleeping outside in the hospital garden. The benefit for children is that they continue to be in the care of a family member, and the mother is relieved to be with her child. The father, however, is often unhappy with being separated from them. Yet, having both parents on site creates other pressures: someone must be found to care of siblings left at home, and jobs and wages can be lost as the family attends to what is often a long-term health crisis.

But they are with us, and in the end, parents help fill some of the gaps created by the lack of staff and services at the hospital. For instance, a father can bring food to his wife who may not be getting meals through the hospital food services, or he can bring extra food for a child who is on steroids and has a voracious appetite. Fathers are asked to run important errands: bringing blood and blood products from the blood bank; taking blood samples to the lab, which is in a different building, a ten minute rapid walking distance from the hospital unit; carrying personal correspondence and requests for consultations - such as surgical consultations – to doctors at other hospitals who do not respond to phone calls; and taking blood samples to private labs if we cannot process the blood in Medical City. Perhaps engaging fathers and mothers in the care of their child gives them some solace and a sense of partnership with the medical team. Oftentimes it helps us develop more positive relationships. But most importantly, it is good to have them on-site in case there is an emergency with their child.

To see the fathers sleeping in the garden at night, even in winter, is something terrible. They have no access to shelter or parent houses – no bed, bath or food-preparation facilities. And they live like this, sometimes for weeks at a time, if the child is in critical condition. Yet, even this seeming tragedy has some advantages, which we will discuss later in the chapter.

Medical Care

Two-thirds of the pediatric patients who come to CWTH are in an advanced stage of disease. The median total diagnosis delay is 55 days (range 3 days- 36 months) and the median physician delay is 43 days, which is more than double the longest doctor delays mentioned in the literature, although the patient's delay in seeking diagnosis/treatment is comparable to that mentioned elsewhere. This late diagnosis, along with iatrogenic complications – steroid pre-treatment in acute lymphoblastic leukemia patients misdiagnosed as rheumatoid arthritis or acute Idiopathic thrombocytopenic purpura, masking the cancer diagnosis and inducing partial remission; an aggressive intestinal resection for intestinal lymphoma; enucleating the eye just to take a biopsy; a ruptured renal tumor as a result of an inexperienced surgery – can make for a poor prognosis.

Nurses in our unit face a challenging situation: they put in many hours of work with more patients in serious or critical condition than their peers in other units. The absence of a central catheter, and using only peripheral veins in children, puts more burden on nurses as they spend a significant amount of time trying to find a small vein for the cannula. In addition, lack of proper equipment to use infusion pumps makes the work in the oncology unit a very difficult task.

The situation makes it difficult for us to attract enough experienced and well-qualified nurses, who are in short supply in Iraq anyway. Our nurses are mostly secondary school graduates; only 25% are college graduates. Many of them lack proficiency in English, the official language of medicine in Iraq. They have not received basic education or training in nursing and medical fundamentals. There is a need for more and better training and educational opportunities for nurses. We have tried to take advantage of various international training opportunities, but the language, education and training gap has made it difficult; our nurses find themselves at too great a disadvantage.

For several years we had a crisis in the number of nurses, averaging a 1:20 nurse/patient ratio in the morning to 1:30-40 at night. Just in the last 2 years we achieved a relatively good nurse/patient ratio in the unit: 1:15-20 at night and 1:5 in the morning. In many cases what our nurses lack in basic education and practice is offset by a more-than-usual passion about the patients. We know that this counts for a lot in terms of quality of life in the hospital for these children and parents. And, the caring attention and hard work of the nurses eases the burden of care for the doctors. We recognize, nevertheless, that the unit needs a team of college-educated nurses whose specialty is pediatric oncology.

Hospitals in Iraq do not have a system of triage, which contributes to the burden on physicians. Before 2003, patients with land-line telephones could call specialists at their home if there was an emergency. The number of calls was limited, but still, it was a burden on the physicians, as most of the parents didn't know what constituted a medical emergency that would warrant a call to a doctor's home. The magnitude of burden on physicians increased after 2003, as mobile phones became accessible and the parents started to call at any time without limitation. Although this practice is exhausting for the doctors but it helps the patients who live in far governorates and sometimes be a lifesaving measure.

In terms of drugs, opioids have been used in hospitals in limited amounts for many years, mainly for post-operative patients, burns, and those with myocardial infarctions. The primary opioid was pethidine. The medical establishment in Iraq, as in other countries, worried about drug addiction and the improper and over-prescription of narcotics by health professionals. As a result, the supply of morphine was disrupted and the dispensing of these drugs is still restricted.

The primary available drugs at CWTH are propoxyphene, codeine and acetaminophen. In 2013, morphine became available in our unit but only to inpatients, as it is in an injectable, not oral, form. Doctors must submit special forms to be signed by the hospital manager; for each request only one ampoule can be dispensed. Another drug was introduced recently: fentanyl 8.4 mg per transdermal patch. However there are, as yet, no clear regulations for dispensing these drugs. Because of the restrictions and limitations mentioned above, drugs are reserved for patients who are in the advanced or end stages of disease such as unresectable tumours or severe pain from deep venous thrombosis. They are not prescribed for those who have pain from peripheral cannulation, mucositis or extravasations.

There is an enormous difference in the amount and use of pain-relieving drugs available to patients in low- and middle-income countries as compared to those in high-income countries: 54 mg vs. 97,400 mgs. "High income countries account for less than 15% of the world population, yet more than 94% of global morphine consumption. [4]…In the case of strong opioid analgesics, and considering a wide spectrum of types and causes of pain, including cancer, 83% of the world's population (5.5 billion people) live in countries with low to nonexistent access, 4% has moderate access, and only 7% has adequate access. [5]"

When children become critically ill and in need of end-of-life care, their families often bring them to CWTH, where they were first diagnosed and treated, even if they live far from Baghdad. There are no community nurses in Iraq to offer at-home health care services such as providing pain-killers or oxygen. Regional hospitals often refuse to manage a child with cancer because they lack the necessary expertise in these diseases; if they do agree to take the child, the quality of care is unsatisfactory. Thus, families bring their child back to CWTH, where they know the staff and know they will receive better care. Nevertheless, as the child reaches the last minutes of life, there are no facilities for resuscitation and there is no intensive care unit. All the patients die in their room in the unit. Doctors try to be with the dying child and the family, to stay with them for a while at the time of death. But sometimes, due to understaffing, this is not possible. The primary physician may be busy with other patients. In these situations there are, unfortunately, no other staff people available to stand in for the doctor.

Members of the extended family who are not usually allowed to visit or permitted to stay are now allowed into the room to be together with the dying child. If the child dies at the hospital, the family usually prefers to keep him or her in the room until the discharge has been arranged. For cultural and emotional reasons, they do not want the child's body refrigerated, even if it takes some time for discharge. Because we have more than one patient in a room, this creates an extremely difficult situation for the other child or children, and the mothers, in that room, as they are faced with the reality of death and a vision of their own possibly similar destiny.

In some cases, families may choose to take their child back home as he or she nears death. Despite the difficulties, travel with a sick child can be easier than transporting the child's body, which can be expensive and emotionally draining, with many obstacles and check-points along the way.

After a death, there is no time for communication with the family during bereavement, although in a few cases we may call them on the telephone. Occasionally the family will come back to see us, bringing other relatives. This gives us an opportunity to remember and talk about the deceased child, to offer our thoughts to the parents and help them process their loss. But in most cases the hospital is a sad memory, and parents and others family members avoid contact as much as possible.

Supplementing Medical Care: Psychosocial Intervention, Mental Health and Palliative Care

Science and medicine have a place in Iraqi history dating back to Sumer civilization in southern Mesopotamia in 2000 B.C. Mental health was recognized and acknowledged early on as an important part of a person's overall health. "Psychiatric hospital care in Iraq began as early as the late eighth century with Islamic hospitals, which incorporated Galenic medicine, spirituality, mysticism and music therapies in treating persons with mental illness". [6]

In his essay, *Insanity in Byzantine and Islamic Medicine,* Michael Dols writes at length about Islamic medicine, hospitals and mental health. "It is misleading, first of all to call these institutions 'hospitals,' as I have done because of the term's modern connotations. The medieval hospital was basically a civilian charitable institution, which more closely resembled a present-day convalescent or nursing home.... They were carefully planned, containing inpatient and outpatient departments with separate wards for male and female patients. Special wards or halls were devoted to surgery, eye diseases, bone setting, and internal maladies which roughly corresponded to the specializations of the medical profession. The most remarkable aspect of the Islamic hospitals was the inclusion of a section for the mentally ill.... In which Islamic doctors were able to interpret their Galenic heritage quite literally and to consider insanity as a mundane affliction like all other illnesses." [7]

We cite this history because such understanding of the interrelatedness of physical health with social well-being, mental health and emotional health continues to influence our thinking to this day, even if we are very far removed from that time and unable as doctors in our own time to influence institutional and/or governmental support for programs that reflect this understanding.

On some level, as is clear by what has been written previously in this chapter, there are many other pressing priorities to be attended to. Nonetheless, in our own practice, in our attitude toward patients and their families, we try to do whatever we can to provide emotional and psychosocial support in addition to medical care. As a small example, when a patient is admitted, a photo is taken for our records. But in addition, we use the photo to create a card which we give as a gift to the child and his or her family. We are also vigilant about taking photographs of the children at celebrations or special events in the unit. These photographs create a positive and normalizing narrative – a documentation of a child doing what all children do. It helps create a sense of hope and optimism about the future, not just for the patient but for all of us involved in caring for the child.

One year, we initiated a support group for families – for the mothers who stay with the child, and the fathers who stay overnight outside the hospital. Every week, we spent an hour or an hour and a half with them. Sessions would start with the restatement of an old philosophy: Doctor-patient-disease is three legs of a triangle. If the patient joins the doctor, they will overcome the disease but if the patient joins the disease, then they will overcome the doctor's efforts. During these sessions we were able to talk about cancer and the challenges doctors face trying to overcome the disease in Iraq. We talked about problems people face living with and providing care for a child with cancer. We talked about the importance of caregivers working (and living) in harmony on behalf of the sick child. We answered questions, and parents were able to share their thoughts with others in a similar situation. Everyone found these sessions worthwhile, but we were forced to abandon them because of the burden of our medical activities. It is a good example of a valuable project that cannot be sustained because of understaffing in the unit and a lack of qualified, trained people to help.

We didn't have a play/activity room before 2004, as we needed the space to accommodate more patients, and in addition, art supplies and other materials were not available at that time because of the UN embargo on Iraq. When we could find paper and crayons – sometimes visitors brought them – we invited children to draw pictures in their room, and we would hang them on the walls of the unit. We recognize the importance of art as an expressive medium and also as a way for a child to both engage with and escape from fears and anxieties associated with their illness and hospitalization.

In 2001 we began a project with a US-based organization, the Iraqi Children's Art Exchange (ICAE). They brought art supplies and children's art – greetings and good wishes – from the US. Children at the hospital made drawings in response, destined for children in the US. In addition to providing art materials and an incentive to create art, the exchange project helped lessen our feelings of isolation from the outside world, especially before 2003. Only in 2004 was the play/activity room in the cancer unit created, but it was closed in 2008, as was the whole hospital, for renovation, which has not been done till this day. We were obliged to leave the hospital building which housed us, and we transferred to a nearby hospital in the same complex.

In 2010 we tried to set up a mobile art/activity project in the unit. Supplies and equipment were donated through ICAE, and they hired a young woman to supervise the children's activities. We had small tables and chairs that could be set up wherever there happened to be extra room. Everyone was well-intentioned, but the project was not successful. Its problems pointed to the many weaknesses in our health and education system that make these important child-centered projects unworkable. First, we could not find people in Iraq who are trained to work with children and families in a hospital setting. Secondly, the supervision and coordination of the project, and of the project coordinator, fell to the doctors in the unit, who had no time, or training really, for such activities. We realized after some months that we couldn't undertake these formal programs in the unit until we have adequate financial resources to support the program, a specially designated space in the unit, and trained people to implement such programs successfully. We can and we do, however, continue with informal art projects with the children. Children's art is supported and encouraged through our collaboration with the Japanese NGO JIM-NET, the Japan-Iraq Medical Network. We have also participated for two successive years in the annual drawing competition sponsored by Karim Rida Said Foundation.

A very successful activity for our patients outside of the hospital is Dynamo Camp [8], "a place where children suffering from serious illness can just be children." We have been participating in Dynamo Camp, in Florence Italy for a number of years. We have sent more than 100 children to the camp, accompanied by oncology fellows and nurses who also benefit from experiencing this program first hand. It is a learning experience for them, and also a respite. Sometimes we forget that the hospital staff also needs opportunities to renew their energy and strength.

We are part of our culture in Iraq which views the child as a creature who has no right to decide things for him/her or to do most things alone. A child is and should be dependent on the parents, of course. However, with time, when we talk with the child directly and inform him/her about certain facts which give real promise, the child begins to communicate directly with us, becoming more interactive, with a stronger personality. Children ask questions, and after few months, whatever the age of the child, there is a meaningful relationship that develops with the doctors which enables direct conversation and discussion about many things. Sometimes this extends to email, direct phone calls, or text messages. We feel that these children appear to be older than their peers, with a more mature personality and better self-esteem. We see this particularly in patients who finish treatment and have the chance to go to Dynamo Camp; they react independently from the first step of the trip to the last.

In the end, we must do the best we can in our particular time and in our particular situation in Iraq. Sometimes, when we have a moment to think, we see that what seems like a negative has positive aspects on which we can build. For instance, it is very difficult for fathers to have to stay outside the hospital. Some mothers need and want the support of their husbands, and some children prefer their father, or miss him desperately when he is not around. It is terrible to see them living outside, without shelter. Yet, the fathers, spending hour after hour with each other, form their own kind of "therapy" or support group. They exchange stories and information. Fathers who have been at the hospital a longer time can explain many things to help newly arrived fathers cope with their situation – about how best to help those inside, and about the disease they are encountering. They can also offer each other emotional support and concrete ideas and solutions to commonly faced problems, such as losing a job because of their child's illness. Moreover, because we depend on them for important errands, a certain positive bond can develop between doctors and fathers – a sense of shared commitment and responsibility for the well-being of the child. The father is an important figure in a family, someone who is expected to protect, support, sustain and nourish the family. It is difficult when they cannot control what is happening to their child or to their family. Being at the hospital and helping with errands seems like a small thing, but it is nonetheless something that gives them some agency and sense of purpose.

Another example of a positive emerging from a negative: as UN sanctions took hold, people began experiencing financial problems and started to move in together. Sometimes a household would reach 17-22 members, who began to depend on each other for financial, emotional and social support. This created strong new family bonds which helped sustain them in hard times. Moving back together was also significant for the general health of the community, beyond the family. It is important for individuals and groups within a community to have ways to meet their needs, especially, perhaps, in the chaos of war and its aftermath when structures and social systems outside of family and home disappear. From a medical perspective, large families living together helped create a reliable source of blood for children when there was no blood available at the blood bank. Moreover, the parent could stay in the hospital, leaving the children in the big family house & providing financial support. After death, being in a large family helps buffer grief and provides support in the bereavement period.

Iraqis are traditionally very social people with large, caring extended families. When a child is sick, large numbers of relatives come to visit the child and the parents, even in times when security was very bad. The oncology unit policy strictly restricts visitors and we have to enforce these rules. Yet, the demonstration of caring, wanting to be together, and sharing the troubles of the family would have a very positive psychological effect on the family and on the child. If extended families were allowed to visit and to be present as the child nears the end stage of life, or dies, the parents would benefit greatly by such support, knowing that they are not alone and are surrounded by many people whom they love and who love them in return. Their presence and concern has a positive and soothing impact on the affected family, deeper, perhaps, and more profound than what a professional person working in palliative care at a hospital could expect to achieve.

We do not have professional chaplains to provide pediatric palliative care in our setting. Instead, as most of our patients are Muslims, the parents during hospitalization usually start to observe rituals such as reading the Koran or listening to religious lectures on TV, as in Muslim culture death is viewed as an act of God which is not to be questioned by humans. Muslims believe that all children are innocent and that after death their souls ascend directly to paradise. The birth of a child is regarded as a gift from God, who can take back his gift whenever he wishes. Adolescent patients reflect on these principles and often start to read the Koran and renew their belief. Faith in God and religious rituals increase in intensity at or near the time of death, to the extent that some families can accept the death as the universal destiny of all humans. They keep faith in this belief and thank the staff and leave in a peaceful way.

The National Council for Hospice and Specialist Palliative Care Services (1997) defines psychosocial care as "...concerned with the psychological and emotional wellbeing of the patient and their family/carers..." [9] Doctors, nurses and other caregivers must be considered, because along with parents and the patient they constitute a community of people inevitably affected by the disease. This is especially important for us in Iraq, where medical staff faces chronic burn-out and exhaustion.

In the beginning of 2003, collaboration with an Italian team of doctors from Rome University changed our lives and theirs, providing us with much-needed social, psychological and professional support to carry on in our challenging circumstances. Communicating for two hours weekly by video conference linkage a reprieve from the severe stress of our daily activities. We find collegiality and valuable professional opportunities to address critical medical and scientific issues. Our patient outcomes, in some cases, have improved, which contributes to our confidence and our capacity to care for patients. Despite all obstacles, we find ourselves improving. This collaboration/psychosocial intervention have been the single most significant aspect of improving cancer care in our unit. It supports the holistic goal of palliative care.

CONCLUSION

Doctors in Iraq, suffering from the cumulative effects of a series of long-term crises, find us in need of help. Our team at CWTH has both reached out to, and been open to, offers of international help and collaboration for the last two decades. Through our own efforts, combined with those of partners, we are developing, and in some cases implementing, appropriate goals and a vision of holistic care – including palliative care – for our patients, for hospitals, and for the Iraqi health-care system overall.

Still, there is no actual work on palliative care in our country, and it does not appear that we will have a real program in the near future. The most practical option for training is to offer short courses in palliative care and award a certificate of attendance. It is simply not possible to develop or implement a university degree program in palliative care on a national level at this time in Iraq. Palliative care, like any human developmental milestones, needs time and has a cephalo-caudal progression. We began to understand this developmental process – like an infant who needs to understand everything slowly and in the appropriate way – through the excellent workshops arranged by MECC.

Most Iraqi medical schools are undergoing a transition to an integrated medical curriculum, and some have already implemented the new program. This raises the possibility of adding courses on palliative care in all specialties as part of updating the medical curriculum. For this to happen, the national academic medical community will need to exert some effort to increase awareness about the importance of palliative care programs and convince the decision-makers to introduce them. It is too early to think of palliative care in Iraq, because the country is in a state of chaos, with limitations and hardship in all areas of health and education services. We need to respect human rights to receive standard conventional medical care. Then we can convince the decision-makers and experts in the field of medicine that palliative care is an urgent necessity to be applied as part of the optimization of medical services, especially for patients with chronic diseases.

REFERENCES

[1] Knaul, Felicia Marie, Frank, Julio and Schulman, Lawrence for the Global Task Force on Expanded Access to Cancer Care and Control in Developing Countries. *Closing the Cancer Divide: A Blueprint to Expand Access in Low and Middle Income Countries.* (Boston: Harvard Global Equity Initiative), November 2011.

[2] Diaz Juan and Garfield, Richard, *Health and Nutrition.* Iraq Watching Briefs, (WHO, 2003)

[3] UNICEF. Official Summary *The State of the World's Children,* 2002.

[4] Knaul FM, Adami HO, Adebamowo C, et al. The global cancer divide: an equity imperative. In: Knaul FM, Gralow JR, Atun R, Bhadelia A (Eds.) for the Global Task Force on Expanded Access to Cancer Care and Control in Developing Countries. Closing the Cancer Divide: An Equity Imperative. Boston, MA: Harvard Global Equity Initiative, 2012; 29-70.

[5] Seya MJ, Gelders SFAM, Achara OU, Milani B, Scholten WK. A first comparison between the consumption of and the need for opioid analgesics at country, regional, and global levels. *Journal of Pain & Palliative Care Pharmacotherapy* 2011; 25:6-18.

[6] Hamid HI, Everett A. Developing Iraq's Mental Health Policy.PSYCHIATRIC SERVICES ♦ ps.psychiatryonline.org ♦ October 2007 Vol. 58 No. 10.

[7] M. Dols. Insanity in Byzantine and Islamic Medicine. Dumbarton Oaks Papers. Vol. 38, Symposium on Byzantine Medicine (1984), pp. 135-148.

[8] Dynamo camp; we don't know how to cite it

[9] What do we mean by 'psychosocial'? A discussion paper on use of the concept within palliative care. The National Council for Palliative Care Mar. 2000. Available from: http://wwwncpcorguk/publications/archiveshtml [Last cited on 2010 Jun 22].

In: Palliative Care to the Cancer Patient
Editor: Michael Silbermann

ISBN: 978-1-63117-709-5

Chapter 4

PALLIATIVE CARE IN THE ISLAMIC REPUBLIC OF IRAN

Maryam Rassouli, Ph.D., R.N.[1,*] and Moosa Sajjadi, R.N.[2]
[1]Shahid Beheshti University of Medical Sciences, Teheran, Islamic Republic of Iran
[2]Gonabad University of Medical Sciences, Gonabad, Islamic Republic of Iran

INTRODUCTION: NECESSITY AND IMPORTANCE OF PALLIATIVE CARE IN IRAN

According to the World Health Organization, palliative care has been defined as "an approach that improves the quality of life of patients and their families facing the problem associated with life-threatening illness, through the prevention and relief of suffering by means of early identification and impeccable assessment and treatment of pain and other problems, physical, psychosocial and spiritual." [1]

The growing elderly population, an emphasis on people's quality of life, and the enhancement of social welfare standards has led to the provision of services, palliative care, and the institutionalization of establishments that provide these services in many advanced countries.[2] According to the World Health Organization, over half the countries in the world are trying to prevent cancer, and provide treatment and care for cancer patients. The organization's latest study, presented in its February 2013 meeting on World Cancer Day, was a warning to the many countries that do not presently have a cancer control plan, which involves prevention, early diagnosis, treatment, and care. There is an urgent need for help to reduce cancer mortality, provide suitable long-term treatment and care to prevent pain and human suffering, and support the socio-economic development of countries. [3]

Cancer is the third leading cause of death in Iran, claiming more than 30,000 lives annually.[2] Given the growing elderly population of the country, increased life expectancy, industrialization, and increasing environmental contaminants, it is expected that the incidence of cancer will double within the next two decades. According to the World Health

* Corresponding author: Email: rassouli.m@gmail.com.

Organization's forecast, the incidence of cancer in Iran will reach 85,653 cases, and its mortality will reach 62,897, by the year 2020. It is hoped that proper scientific planning to prevent the incidence of controllable and preventable cancers will help lower this trend. [4]

In 2009, of the total number of 74,067 registered cancer cases, 41,169 cases [55.58%] were males and 32,898 cases [44.41%] were females. Thus, the relative gender ratio of cancer incidence that year was 125, which means for every 100 female patients, there were 125 male patients. Breast cancer in women ranked first, peaking at age 50-55. The five most common cancers in women were breast, skin, colon, rectum, stomach, and esophagus, respectively, and the five most common cancers in men were skin, stomach, prostate, bladder, colon and rectum, respectively. The five most common cancers in Iran irrespective of gender were skin, breast, stomach, colon, rectum, and bladder [Table 1]. Generally, the incidence rate of cancers increases with age, peaking at around 80-84 years of age, and decreases after age 85, which could be due to lower patient referrals and lack of access to diagnostic means for the elderly.[5]

The need for providing supportive and palliative care is explained in the Development of a Comprehensive National Program for Palliative and Supportive Cancer Care Project, based on three perspectives: human rights, people's satisfaction, and reduced health expenses. Its conclusion is that in palliative care units, a reduction in unnecessary diagnostic-treatment procedures and a better understanding of the needs of patients with incurable diseases lead to reduced health costs, along with increased patient satisfaction. Furthermore, it emphasizes that palliative care is one of the basic principles in the control of cancer.[6] However, the present status of palliative care services in Iran presents a different picture. In Iran, care services for patients with incurable diseases, especially when they are in end-of-life stages, are provided by the patient's family members at home. Even though all hospitals admit such patients and provide them with services, the concept of palliative care is totally new, and services provided for these patients are very limited. In effect, these patients can be admitted to hospitals and receive routine services and care just like other patients. [7]

Table 1. The ten most common cancers in Iran (2009)

Cancer type	N	%
Skin	9,114	12.3
Breast	7,822	10.6
Stomach	6,886	9.3
Colon and anal canal	6,210	8.4
Bladder	4,601	6.2
Prostate	3,856	5.2
Leukemia	3,461	4.7
Esophagus	3,297	4.5
Lung, bronchus and trachea	2,992	4.0
Non-Hodgkin lymphoma	2,345	3.2
Others	23,483	31.7
Total	74,067	100

Adopted from annual reports of cancer cases
(available at: http://www.ircancer.ir/Default.aspx?tabid=95#.)

Given the growing increase of cancer in Iran, and the importance of improving the health and quality of life for these patients and for their families, palliative care of cancer patients is particularly important. This issue has attracted the attention of relevant authorities in recent years.

PRESENT STATUS OF PROVIDING PALLIATIVE CARE FOR CANCER PATIENTS

Providing hospice and palliative care, especially when the morbidity and mortality of cancer is high and there is a need for specialized supportive care, pain management and control of symptoms, is one of the main requirements of a health care system. [8] Yet, in contrast to the existence of a primary health care system in Iran, there is still no plan to provide specialist palliative care services; the health care services do not provide special palliative care services associated with end-of-life for patients and their families. In such a care system, it can be assumed that cancer patients who require palliative care have no access to the facilities they need. Patients and their families are in stress as they seek a means of pain relief, as health-care providers often refrain from or are unable to provide appropriate medication at the right time. [9]

Rather, the website of the Iranian Palliative Care Association encourages families to provide end-of-life care for their patients at home, with one of its aims the reduction of unnecessary costs of hospitalization and medical tests for such patients. This approach accords with Iranian cultural beliefs and the wish to die among family members and loved ones. In such circumstances, the duty of care falls on first-degree family members (spouse, children, and siblings), who are responsible for the financial, practical, and logistic aspects of care. Women look after the patient's nursing care and feeding, while giving hope to the patient. Usually, an older member of the family, preferably the oldest son, is viewed as the head or leader of the support team. [7]

Death is a central concept in Islam, and 98% of Iranians are Muslims. In Persian cultural terms, death is well expressed in the celebrated narrative poem from *Masnavi* by the 13th century Persian Sufi saint and poet Rumi, in which death is regarded as a rebirth in the cycle of life. It describes the human embryo changing from a spiritless body to vegetative life, then to animal life, and eventually to human life. [10] In Iranian Islamic folklore, death is the time to be accountable to God and to be responsible for what one has done in this world, which causes death and dying to be a frightening experience. Moreover, in Iranian culture there is a difference between a good death and a bad one: death with pain is a bad death, and death in peace with no pain is considered a good death [7]. In Islam, death is viewed as a transition between two parts of one continuous life: for the faithful, death is comfortable, and for sinners, death is a very hard experience. [11] A painful death is considered atonement for sins committed in this world. This perception of death leads to prayer and acts that help the dying person avoid a bad death, such as placing the Quran by the patient's bedside to ease the pains of dying even if the patient might be unconscious. While death is seen as inevitable, it is rarely seen as normal, but rather as horrific and tragic. This view of death, if not in complete contrast to death with palliative care, is certainly different from it. [7] Viewed from the perspective of palliative care, by comparison, death can be described as: "We all die, and although this reality is as much a part of life as birth, thinking about it is not easy." [12]

To cope with stresses induced by disease and the prospect of death, most people turn to religion to elevate the patient's mental state. Such an approach is highlighted by the Iranian Palliative Care Association, which views religious counseling as one of the objectives of palliative care in order to raise the patient's and family members' spirits. Accordingly, what raises Iranian patients' hopes in most circumstances includes pilgrimages to Mecca and other religious sites, sacrificing animals to cure the patient, praying and taking part in religious ceremonies, and helping people in need to satisfy God so as to heal the patient. [7] In short, one of the most important needs of cancer patients in Iran is their spiritual needs [13], so that incorporating this aspect in palliative care programs seems a necessity.

Palliative care is based on a holistic approach that considers patients' and their families' physical, mental, social, and spiritual dimensions. For optimal implementation of palliative care, health care providers should have an appropriate understanding of patients' symptoms [2], as the range of symptoms in patients with incurable diseases, particularly cancer, is highly varied and includes pain, nausea, vomiting, constipation, weakness, anorexia, depression, dyspnea, etc. [10].

Although public opinion in Iran insists on palliative care of cancer patients in their own homes, still, there is no research evidence that would show the inclinations and preferences of cancer patients with regard to palliative care, although the establishment of special palliative care centers in the second and third levels of the health care system in Iran has been strongly recommended. [9] There are few studies in the area of patients' end-of-life needs and the importance of holistic care in the control of pain and physical symptoms, as well as attention to patients' mental, spiritual, and social needs. In Iran, healthcare providers do not possess adequate training in spiritual care for end-of-life patients, and the majority are unable to provide spiritual support or conduct a conversation about death with patients. [11]

Currently, cancer patients in Iran receive medical services they require, such as diagnostic and treatment courses, in public and private hospitals and in day care clinics. After each treatment course, patients are discharged with simple and brief guidance until the next treatment course. Usually, these patients do not receive necessary care and information such as nursing care, consultations with doctors, and care associated with their social, mental, physical or spiritual needs. There are a number of scattered charitable or community centers across the country that provide palliative care in Iran [2]. Although such charitable organizations are few, they provide effective cooperation in this area, assisting palliative medicine centers at the Tehran Cancer Institute and the Said-Al-Shohada palliative medicine center in Isfahan by providing palliative care directly. The Mahak Institute of palliative and treatment services for cancer children and the Sepas Organization of psycho-social support of cancer patients are examples of these organizations. Efforts in the cancer-related palliative care program have been made to facilitate the establishment of palliative and supportive medicine units in the country, especially in selected hospitals in the provinces of Gilan, Golestan, Ardebil, and Zanjan. [14]

There is only one public hospital in Iran that provides palliative care for cancer patients admitted to the emergency ward. Approximately a third or more of the patients admitted to the emergency ward are in advanced or end-of-life stages. For this number of patients, there are only 10 vials of morphine for all their daily requirements. Moreover, patients in the emergency ward normally have to wait for days for the management of their symptoms (usually pain and respiratory distress) or for terminal care. [15]

Opioids are the most widely used drugs for pain relief in advanced cancer patients. In Iran, the most frequent reasons for administration of these drugs in women are cancers of the breast, colorectal, lung, stomach, and primary and metastatic bone problems, and in men, cancers of the stomach, lung, colorectal, prostate, and primary and metastatic bone problems. [16] Patients procure the required opioids from the Office of Addictive Drugs. The most frequently used drugs for patients' pain relief include morphine, methadone, opium and codeine phosphate. In Iran, opioid drugs do not have sufficient diversity, and the official medical channels of prescription and procurement are inadequate for many doctors and unfamiliar to almost all patients. The use of existing and prescribed drugs does not accord with specific guidelines and standards, and drugs are administered according to the individual doctor's experience and patients' needs. Consequently, inappropriate use, including abuse, inaccurate dosage, inappropriate administrative path, inappropriate frequency, lack of recognition of and inadequate dealing with drug side-effects, ignoring drug interactions, and other problems are frequently observed. The development of standard treatment guidelines by the medical committees of the leading universities, with the assistance of the Ministry of Health, can be effective in providing better services for pain control and palliative care of the patients. [16]

History of Palliative Care in Iran

Given the nature of cancer, the aim of establishing cancer associations in advanced countries was to control the disease comprehensively in a multidisciplinary teamwork. Accordingly, and collectively, the establishment of Iranian Cancer Association was proposed to the Commission of Scientific Societies in the Ministry of Health and Medical Education, and, after approval, this multidisciplinary scientific society, comprising specialists in the field of cancer including radiotherapy, oncology, surgery, pathology, radiology, pediatrics and adult hematology oncology, and basic sciences, began its activities in 2003.

The following programs, among others, have been initiated by the association: holding 8 congresses annually in the field of cancer macro-policies, launching an official Iranian Cancer Association Website, conducting numerous research projects, developing countrywide cancer treatment guidelines, implementing and publishing cancer audits, publishing books on cancer specialties, communication with health policy makers, and ongoing communication with cancer-related NGOs. [3]

The Shahid Beheshti University of Medical Sciences Cancer Research Center held the first (2008) and second (2009) National Congresses on Cancer Supportive and Palliative Care, and in 2010 held the first International Congress, stimulating a qualitative and quantitative growth in research articles. The aim was to convince decision makers in this field to take the supportive and palliative care of cancer patients seriously, and to draw specialists' attention to the need for supportive and palliative care, which was somewhat successful and had a positive effect as well. [17]

The Iranian Cancer Research Network became operational in September 2006 with the aim of promoting indigenous cancer research, and coordinating the various research, operational, and service sectors of the country in this field. The network's scope of activity included all the health system's research, comprising all of the country's scientific centers active in the field of cancer. Every research center working in the field of cancer can be a member of this network [18]. According to the constitution of research networks approved by the Ministry of Health, in addition to the university research centers, other organizations, individuals, and entities can join in the formation of research networks and contribute to them. Some of the centers that are members of this network include the Hematology and Oncology Research Center, Shahid Beheshti University Cancer Research Center, Tehran University Cancer Research Center, Nuclear Medicine Research Center, Breast Cancer Research Center, Oncology Studies Research Center, Gastroenterology Cancers Research Center, Nursing and Midwifery Care Research Center, and several others. [19]

One of the most valuable activities of the Iranian Cancer Research Network in palliative care is a project titled Development of Cancer Patients' Palliative Care Services Plan in Iran, currently being conducted with the support of the Cancer Department of the Ministry of Health and the cooperation of member research centers and scientific societies in the Iranian Cancer Research Network. The plan for the development of a comprehensive national program of supportive and palliative cancer care was initiated by a letter sent on June 14th, 2011, by the health and medical deputies of the Ministry of Health to the president of the Iranian Cancer Research Network, stressing the importance of palliative medicine as one of the components of the comprehensive cancer control plan, and an essential need in the country's treatment management. The Cancer Research Center was requested to take the necessary steps to compile palliative medicine service plans based on operational and scientific evidence. [20]

Accordingly, an assessment of the current status of palliative care is being developed. Additional information about this project is available at www.palliative.ir. Given the need for palliative care, the Cancer Research Center has already begun research projects in this area, including: Design and Development of Curriculum of Inter-disciplinary Education of Palliative Care of Cancer Patients, and: Comparison of Performance of Palliative Medicine Center of Tehran University of the Medical Sciences Cancer Institute with Standards of Selective Middle Eastern Countries, and Presenting a Model for Iran. [14]

A draft of this program has been presented in a comprehensive format covering all aspects of palliative care in detail in four chapters. The first chapter deals with basic concepts of the palliative care system and the need for attention to, and provision of palliative care in terms of human rights, people's satisfaction, and reducing costs. The second chapter discusses the values and ethical principles of the palliative care system. The third chapter discusses recommended objectives and strategies based on the status of the health care system in Iran. Lastly, the fourth chapter describes the development of processes and structures of the supportive and palliative care system. In order to make the program comprehensive, a variety of existing structures throughout the world which provide palliative care services have been explored, such as Hospital Palliative Care Units (HPCU), Hospital Palliative Care Counseling Teams (HPCT), hospices, community care, care at home, and day-care clinics. Palliative care and support processes are presented. These processes include control of the patient's pain and physical symptoms, and spiritual, psychological, social, and cultural care, along with support of the patient's family and caregivers, each discussed in primary, secondary, and tertiary health care. The path of providing palliative and support care is explained as a six-stage process, from contact with the patient until after death. Support processes responsible for providing infrastructures to implement the palliative care system, such as governmental policy-making regarding the system, provision and management of financial and human resources, manpower training, information management, and management of facilities and equipment, etc., are presented in full.

Iran's status in terms of world palliative care (2011) has been classified as group 3a, on a par with countries such as Egypt (compared to 2006, Iran has climbed up a step from group 2 to 3a). The status of palliative care in countries in this group is scattered and not well supported; budgets are highly dependent on the financial support of a single source (such as the government); NGO's are not involved very much; palliative care services are often based on home care; and the ratio of service centers to population is very low [21, 22]. Moreover, one of the main challenges to pain management in palliative care programs is restricted access to morphine. [14]

State of Human Resources and Palliative Care Education in Iran

Proper planning in relation to end-of-life care for patients with incurable diseases, especially cancer, is an understood requirement in the health care system in Iran, but requires education, improvement in doctors' communication skills, the provision of palliative care services, the development of multidisciplinary tasking, and the provision of proper insurance services. [23]

Nurses in palliative care teams are usually the first care providers to evaluate the patient's condition and determine the type of his/her pains and needs. They tend to spend more time with patients and can help in related decisions. Nurses need to project empathy, honesty, acceptance, and trustworthiness, as their positive attitude toward incurable patients, and this type of care, is highly important to help them carry out their duties. Attitude is important in performance and behavior. In Iran, very few studies have been conducted on the attitudes of nurses and nursing students toward care for dying patients. The results indicate that their attitude is not positive. [24, 25], and in fact reveal that attitudes of nurses toward palliative care are relatively negative or at best neutral. [26] Nurses in Iran have a low level of information and knowledge about palliative care [27], this attitude is somewhat associated with nurses' education level and the ward they work in, so that nurses working in oncology ward have more negative attitude. [22]

In a study by Ghanbari & Baghfalaki (2009) to determine research priorities in the field of cancer as viewed by nurses, the first five priorities of the participating nurses were found to be: assessing the socio-economic effects and psychological effects of the diagnosis of cancer on the family; oral care; nutritional needs; and strategies to address continuing hospital care at home Notably, despite the recognition of palliative care in the hospital and at home as an important priority, the nurse's role in palliative care was ranked as the 14th priority (out of a total of 20 priorities). Thus, in the opinion of the study subjects (nurses participating in the International Congress on Cancer held that year), providing palliative care for cancer patients did not require determining or explaining the nurse's role in the care team, or else, the participating nurses were not familiar with the concept of palliative care and its requirements at all. [28]

End-of-life care and palliative care are still new subjects in Iran. The curriculum for Bachelor of Nursing, which is a four-year course in Iran, offers no particular academic unit, or any clinical training in palliative care, even though subjects related to death and dying are provided in other courses. There are also no palliative care centers or hospices such as those in the Western countries at all. Yet, hospitals are expected to provide palliative care for people in the end-of-life stages. [29]

In many countries, general practitioners (GPs) have the main responsibility for providing medical care, especially palliative care for patients. In Iran, given the development of the general practitioner's role in the form of family doctors, it seems that they will assume the principle role in this area. Yet, there is no official training in palliative care during the general medical education course in Iran. [2] The results of a study (Asadi-Lari et al., 2009) indicate that only 12% of Iran's general practitioners have an excellent or very good knowledge of palliative care, and more than half have poor or no knowledge in this area. Only 22% of the participating doctors were aware of the WHO pain control guidelines or were fully conversant with the management of patients' physical symptoms. More than half admitted having a poor knowledge of pain control in relation to the principles of end-of-life and palliative care. Apparently, the deficiency in doctors' awareness of palliative care can be attributed to medical education in Iran, which is symptomatic rather than holistic. [2]

Furthermore, despite the existence of the WHO guidelines in the area of pain management and the treatment of cancer patients, their pain is still not well-managed. One of the most important obstacles in these patients' pain control is the doctors' lack of knowledge. A study by Eftekhar et al. (2007) found that despite the positive attitude of doctors toward pain control for cancer patients, and their awareness of the importance of pain management for these patients, half the doctors did not treat their patients' pain, pointing to a lack of pain control specialists and a lack of personnel knowledge of pain management as the most important obstacles to proper pain management. Most participating doctors in the study asserted that they were dissatisfied with the pain management training given during their medical education. [30]

One of the courses designed and developed to enhance the awareness and performance of doctors in the area of palliative care is the Graduate Specialist Education Program of Palliative Medicine Fellowship, which was approved in February 2008 by the Iranian Council of Graduate Medical Education Office of the Ministry of Health and Medical Education. The course, which lasts 15-18 months, focuses on enhancing quality of life to the maximum possible level through the control of symptoms and signs using specialized medications, as well as spiritual, psychological, and social support. The course aims to heighten the medical, practical and research capabilities of doctors responsible for the care of patients with progressive and incurable diseases. [31]

The development of an inter-disciplinary approach to provide training in the palliative field was introduced at an initial meeting in March 2011 by experts in medicine, nursing, pharmacy, nutrition, psychology, rehabilitation, law, medical education, and the clergy, who presented their views on the development of an inter-disciplinary education curriculum. This was followed by a proposal presented in April 2012 with the aim of designing and developing the first inter-disciplinary education curriculum in the country for training in the palliative care of cancer patients at the Nursing and Midwifery Research Center of Isfahan University of Medical Sciences. The objectives of the project included assessing the status and needs of palliative care of cancer patients, determining priorities of inter-disciplinary palliative care needs in cancer patients, defining the duties of participants in the education program, and developing the goals of inter-disciplinary education in the palliative care of cancer patients. Twenty active members of care teams were interviewed and over 50 cancer patient files were reviewed to study their physical, mental, social, and spiritual problems. This data was collected and classified in seven domains, and a questionnaire focusing on the educational priorities of a palliative care inter-disciplinary short course was designed. Separate progress reports in each of the seven areas of the project were presented (March 2012), namely physical needs, spiritual care, ethical considerations, communication, mental health, legal considerations, and education of the patient and the family. [32]

PALLIATIVE CARE OBSTACLES AND FUTURE PROSPECTS

Several obstacles have been identified in providing palliative care in the Middle Eastern countries, including Iran, some of which are as follows:

- Insufficient government support of providing palliative care in the health system
- Problems associated with restricted access to opioids (opioids phobia) together with insufficient training in the use of these drugs
- Lack of appropriate training
- Limited resources, especially financial resources [8, 33].

Moreover, in the experts' opinion, there are several innate obstacles to providing palliative care that require more attention in order to facilitate such care. For instance, medical personnel have traditional attitudes toward the management of incurable diseases that are difficult to change. Additionally, there are no clear and specific medical rules to protect personnel from legal actions brought against them when they are not prepared to provide unnecessary and wasteful treatment to satisfy the patient's family or their unrealistic expectations. Furthermore, the extant care providers' knowledge in the area of palliative care and its philosophy, management of symptoms, and how to provide palliative care is poor, and there are very few specially trained caregivers engaged in providing palliative care for cancer patients. Lastly, the high mortality rate of cancer is widely viewed as an indicator of the care system's inefficiency, even for patients with advanced and incurable cancers. [15]

Few studies have been conducted on palliative care in Iran. Cancer research centers, medical schools, education departments and nursing schools, on the one hand, and financial institutions, pharmaceutical companies, and policy makers on the other, are needed to support research in palliative care so that better quality of life can be provided for patients with incurable diseases. [9]

Another important obstacle to the development of palliative care in Iranian society is cultural and social norms that cause doctors to refrain from telling the truth to patients, leading to numerous moral dilemmas in relation to end-of-life care for cancer patients. [23] Informing cancer patients is a complicated issue that is influenced by many factors such as culture, family, the condition of the patient, economic factors, and beliefs. In some cases, patients have no desire to receive such information. A study by Vahdaninia & Montazeri (2003) shows that a large percentage of participating doctors do not convey the true diagnosis of the disease to their patients, with the primary obstacle being the family's request not to reveal the diagnosis to their patient. [34]

Possible obstacles to training staff may also be one of the challenges which may not be simply possible despite the importance of holding continuous training courses to improve care. Educating doctors may be possible through fellowship courses, medical conferences, and on-line training, but educating nurses can be difficult. Many nurses working in oncology wards face restrictions in participating in education programs offered by sponsoring institutions due to family problems and little knowledge of English, while enrolling in on-line education programs is not possible due to work schedules or lack of access to a computer or the Internet at home. [35]

The structure of service-providing centers for cancer patients may also be an obstacle. Centers that cancer patients visit provide medical services only, and have not been designed, or are not suitable for providing supportive and palliative care services. [23]

More basically, one of the most important challenges in providing palliative care is patients' payment and suitable insurance coverage. With appropriate insurance coverage and government financial support, patients could have more suitable medical services, and doctors would be under less stress. [23]

Future Prospects for Palliative Care in Iran

In light of palliative care progress indicators, it is expected that palliative care in Iran will experience progress in the future. In the 2006 ranking, Iran was placed in the second group of countries, which are countries that are building capacity for palliative care [22]. Given the steps taken in this area, Iran's ranking was improved, and in the 2011 ranking, was elevated to 3a group [21]. It is hoped that as a result of activities that have begun in this area, more progress can be witnessed in palliative care in Iran.

It seems that an awareness of the need for palliative care, at least on the part of health care professionals, has been created. Accordingly, experts and interested parties, while convening and participating in international congresses, have attempted to create international connections with other palliative care-providing organizations. As for local progress, attempts have been made to attract support from the government and the Ministry of Health, and to design and implement palliative-related studies. Possibly, with the draft of the Development of a Comprehensive National Program for Supportive and Palliative Care project bearing fruit, the status of palliative care in Iran will evolve and improve suitably.

Based on the existing status of palliative care in Iran, the following recommendations for the development of palliative care in the country are:

- Viewing palliative care as a necessity at the national level of the healthcare system, which must be adopted urgently
- Education about the principles and the philosophy of palliative care as a subject in all medical and specialized courses, particularly in emergency medicine, must be offered
- Creating and institutionalizing palliative care services in the community as a priority

- Assigning a specific unit to oncology in all emergency wards for specialized attention to these patients' needs
- Regular visits to patients in the emergency ward by a palliative care team with an oncology specialist, for better control of symptoms, decision- making and future planning
- Referral of advanced cancer patients to palliative care ward after discharge from the emergency ward [15].

Accordingly, in finalizing the draft operational program of palliative medicine recommendations provided by experts regarding the cancer control program in the Islamic Republic of Iran, the following aspects were included: the development of home care, training health specialists, and free access to adequate amounts of morphine or analgesic drugs; necessary education for the management of patients in this stage (including pain, symptom control, and psychological support) by health care providers (such as doctors at all levels, nurses, and medical service assistants); ensuring that palliative care provided at home meets minimum standards; revision of supportive and palliative care guidelines that are more than 5 years old. [3]

CONCLUSION

In the past two years, attention to palliative care has increased significantly as a result of the National Cancer Research Network and its related centers becoming operational with the support of the Ministry of Health. However, such care is provided in only a few scattered centers, and most patients with cancer are deprived of palliative care. Given the increase of programs to implement and develop palliative care in Iran, it seems that such care will witness significant development across the country. Meanwhile, there is a long way to go to achieve a favorable situation, requiring collective effort and multidimensional support.

REFERENCES

[1] World Health Organization.WHO definition of palliative care. Available at: http://www.who.int/cancer/palliative/definition/en./Accessed Nov 8, 2013.

[2] Asadi-Lari, M; Madjd, Z; Afkari, ME; Goushegir, A; Baradaran, HR. The concept of palliative care practice among Iranian General Practitioners. *Iranian Journal of Cancer Prevention*, 2009, 2(3), 111-116.

[3] Cancer Reseach Network. Iran's national cancer research network newsletter, Number 2, March 2013. [Persian]. Available at: http://login.research.ac.ir /Repository/UploadSenderSubSystem /80d32e1f-b771-4582-b95d-bf3f1cf5bed9.pdf. Accessed November 8, 2013.

[4] Iran's Cancer Registry System [Persian]. Avilable at: http://www.ircancer.ir/Default. aspx?tabid=95#. Accessed November 8, 2013.

[5] Iran's Cancer Registry System. Country Reports on cancer (2009) [Persian]. Available at: http://www.ircancer.ir/default.aspx?tabid=88&ArticleId=350. Accessed November 8, 2013.

[6] Cancer Research Center. Development of a comprehensive national program for palliative and supportive cancer care project [Persian]. Available at: http://crc.tums.ac.ir/Default.aspx?tabid=519. Accessed November 8, 2013.

[7] Abedi M. Palliative Care within the Iranian Context: Re-defining Palliative Care, Deploying Spirituality as a Support Measure and Need for Cultural Sensitivity. Available at: http://wwwinter-disciplinarynet/wp-content/uploads/2012/02/abedisp paperpdf.2012. Accessed November 8, 2013.

[8] Bingley, A; Clark, D. A comparative review of palliative care development in six countries represented by the Middle East Cancer Consortium (MECC). *Journal of pain and symptom management*, 2009, 37(3), 287-296.

[9] Asadi-Lari, M; Madjd, Z; Akbari, M. The need for palliative care services in Iran; an introductory commentary. *Iranian Journal of Cancer Prevention*, 2008, 1(1), 1-5.

[10] Zahedi, F; Larijani, B; Tavakoly Bazzaz, J. End of life ethical Issues and Islamic views. *Iran J Allergy Asthma Immunol*, 2007, 6(Supplement 5), 5-15.

[11] Asadi-Lari, M; Goushegir, SA; Madjd, Z; Latifi, NA. Spiritual care at the end of life in the Islamic context, a systematic review. *Iranian Journal of Cancer Prevention*, 2008, 1(2), 63-67.

[12] Davies, E; Higginson, IJ. The solid facts: Palliative Care. Available at: http://www.euro. who.int/__data/assets/pdf_file/0003/98418/E82931.pdf: OMS; 2004. Accessed November 8, 2013.

[13] Rahnama, M; Khoshknab, M; Maddah, SS; Ahmadi, F. Iranian cancer patients' perception of spirituality: a qualitative content analysis study. *BMC nursing*, 2012, 11(1), 11-19.

[14] Cancer Research Center. Development of a comprehensive national program for palliative and supportive cancer care project [Persian]. Available at: http://crc.tums.ac.ir /Default.aspx?alias=crc.tums.ac.ir/palliative. Accessed November 8, 2013.

[15] Tahmasebi, M. Palliative Care for Cancer Patients in the Emergency Department in Iran. 13th World Congress of the European Association for Palliative Care. 2013, [Poster]

[16] Mohagheghi, MA; Sedighi, Z. Pain Control in Cancer Patients by Opiate Use. *Tehran University Medical Journal*, 2003, 61(2), 95-102 [Persian].

[17] Shahid Beheshti University of Medical Sciences.Cancer Research Center [Persian]. Avaialable at: http://crc.sbmu.ac.ir/?siteid=148&pageid=9757&siteid=148. Accessed November 8, 2013.

[18] Cancer Research Center.Cancer Institute of Iran [Persian]. Avalable at: http://crc.tums.ac.ir/?tabid=112. Accessed November 8, 2013.

[19] Cancer Rsearch Network [Persian]. Available at: http://cancernet.research.ac.ir/Forms/NetworkMemberArkan.aspx. Accessed November 8, 2013.

[20] Cancer Research Center. Development of a comprehensive national program for palliative and supportive cancer care project [Persian]. Available at: http://crc.tums.ac.ir/ Default.aspx?tabid=550. Accessed November 8, 2013.

[21] Lynch, T; Connor, S; Clark, D. Mapping levels of palliative care development: a global update. Journal of pain and symptom management. 2013, 45(6), 1094-1106.

[22] Wright, M; Wood, J; Lynch, T; Clark, D. Mapping levels of palliative care development: a global view. *Journal of pain and symptom management*, 2008, 35(5), 469-485.

[23] Mobasher, M; Nakhaee, N; Tahmasebi, M; Zahedi, F; Larijani, B. Ethical issues in the end of life care for cancer patients in Iran. *Iranian journal of public health*, 2013, 42(2), 188-196.

[24] Iranmanesh, S; Dargahi, H; Abbaszadeh, A. Attitudes of Iranian nurses toward caring for dying patients. *Palliative & supportive care*, 2008, 6(4), 363-369.

[25] Iranmanesh, S; Savenstedt, S; Abbaszadeh, A. Student nurses' attitudes towards death and dying in south-east Iran. *International journal of palliative nursing*, 2008, 14(5), 214-219.

[26] Razban, F; Iranmanesh, S; Rafiei, H. Nurses' attitudes toward palliative care in south-east Iran. *International journal of palliative nursing*, 2013, 19(8), 403-410.

[27] Iranmanesh, S; Razban, F; Tirgari, B; Zahra, G. Nurses' knowledge about palliative care in Southeast Iran. *Palliative & supportive care*, 2013, 1-8.

[28] Ghanbari Khanghah, A; Baghfalaki, M. Nurses'perspectives of nursing research priorities about cancer patients. *Iran Journal f Nursing (IJN)*, 2009, 22(57), 1-11.

[29] Cheraghi, MA; Payne, S; Salsali, M. Spiritual aspects of end-of-life care for Muslim patients: experiences from Iran. *International journal of palliative nursing*, 2005, 11(9), 468-474.

[30] Eftekhar, Z; Mohaghegh, MA; Yarandi, F; Eghtesadi-Araghi, P; Moosavi-Jarahi, A; Gilani, MM; et al. Knowledge and attitudes of physicians in Iran with regard to chronic cancer pain. Asian Pacific journal of cancer prevention: *APJCP*, 2007, 8(3), 383-386.

[31] Specialized courses in palliative care in Iran. Iranian Council of Graduate Medical Education. Ministery of Health. [Persian]. Available at: http://cgme.behdasht.gov.ir/uploads/264_920_CurriculumFlo_TebeTaskini.pdf. Accessed November 8, 2013.

[32] Design and develop the interdisciplinary education curriculum of palliative care for cancer patients.Cancer Research Center [Persian]. Available at: http://crc.tums.ac.ir/Portals/6/Files/Progress%20Report%20For%20MHME%20website_2.pdf . Accessed November 8, 2013.

[33] Mamishi, N; Behroozishad, F; Mohagheghi, MA; Eftekhar, Z; Shahabi, Z. The study of nurses' knowledge and attitudes regarding cancer pain management. *Hayat*, 2006, 12(2), 23-32 [Persian].

[34] Vahdaninia, M; Montazeri, A. Giving information to cancer patients from viewpoint of medical and health specialists. *Payesh*, 2003, 2(4), 259-65 [Persian].

[35] Day, SW; Segovia, L; Viveros, P; Alqudimat, MR; Rivera, GK. The Latin American Center for Pediatric Oncology Nursing Education: development, implementation, and accomplishments. *Cancer nursing*, 2013, 36(5), 340-345.

In: Palliative Care to the Cancer Patient
Editor: Michael Silbermann

ISBN: 978-1-63117-709-5

Chapter 5

ISLAMIC CULTURE IN THE MIDDLE EAST: A GLIMPSE INTO ILLNESS AND DEATH

Lea Baider[1,*], Ph.D. and Gili Goldzweig[2], Ph.D.
[1]Assuta Medical Center, Tel Aviv, Israel
[2]Tel Aviv-Yaffo Academic College, Tel Aviv, Israel

INTRODUCTION

Islam: Paradigms of Culture

> Islam is like a river in that it takes its color from the cultural bed through which it flows.

Culture is the mechanism through which people learn how to be in the world – how to behave, and how to infuse their existence with meaning. Interpretation of culture provides the context for living under normative conditions, in geographic settings, and across life events. Culture underlies priorities in healthcare services as one of the foundations for wellbeing, survival, human interactions, quality of life and care (Schim, et al. 2011).

Triandis (2007), describes culture as a construct that is still being defined and debated in academic literature and professional disciplines, but there is emerging consensus on several variables: 1) culture emerges in interactions between humans and environments; 2) culture consists of shared elements; and 3) culture is transmitted across time periods and generations.

Dimensions of cultural variables form a background to human interaction across age, health and illness and come to the foreground when people face the realities of imminent mortality. Issues of tradition, rituals, family values, and the meaning of life and death become increasingly relevant within the context of illness and health. It is then that patients, families, and physicians negotiate the complexity of care within the perception of the reality of death and dying (Doorenbos, et al. 2008).

* Address for correspondence: baider@cc.huji.ac.il.

Although much of the extant work on cultural diversity in healthcare has focused on issues of race, ethnicity, social disparities and religion, the perspective should be broadened to acknowledge differences and similarities between and within groups. Age, gender, systems of belief, socioeconomic status, and education are important factors when working with concepts of culture and health.

Individual backgrounds, experiences, and levels of exposure to societal cultural patterns vary widely geographically, and change over time, place, and socio-political realities. Understanding ways in which social groups and families tend to differ in dimensions of illness and health allows for ways to think together about similar trends rather than extreme diversity.

Cross-cultural encounters in healthcare present a challenge in the face of entrenched privileges that accrue by virtue of education, income, gender, and race/ethnicity. Acknowledging the profound and pervasive effects of the aforementioned cultural factors, and working toward their mitigation could be essential for solving problems related to equal access to healthcare on the macro level (Schim, et al. 2010).

Middle East: Shifting Boundaries

There are currently more than 1.6 billion Muslims living in all parts of the world and representing nearly 25% of the world's population (www.pewforum.org), with the global Muslim population projected to increase to more than 2.2 billion by 2030. About 75% of the world's Muslims live in the 49 Muslim Majority Countries, while approximately 25% live in non-Muslim majority countries in the developing world (Kaniklides, 2012)).

There are no natural borders to delineate boundaries in the Middle East. Syria, Egypt, Lebanon, Iran, Sudan, Jordan, Turkey, and North Africa all contend with border disputes. Middle Eastern society has been in a state of flux for more than a century as it responds to technological and social advances and retools its identity, all the while experiencing political and ideological tension as a multiplicity of forces compete for its future.

In a world characterized by significant cultural, economic, and social complexities, theoreticians and researchers have noted a fault line or sphere of incongruence that divides Western and Islamic cultures and civilizations (Lewis, 2002). Western and Islamic societies have different value systems and definitions of normative behavior. They differ in their degree of emphasis on individualist versus collectivist values; their championing of traditional values versus "modernist" systems of belief about family care; and their degree of tolerance of individual needs versus social needs and pluralism (Cohen, A.B. 2010).

There is pronounced conflict caused by the clash between modernity and tradition, manifested in the struggle between traditional Islam and the modern world. Islam is viewed not simply as a religion, but as a cultural identity and heritage (L. Hazleton, 2009).

Islam, the youngest of the three monotheistic faiths, shares its basic doctrines about God, the need for prophets to guide humanity, and the final Day of Judgment with Judaism and Christianity. Muhammad proclaimed the message about the unity of God and the need to build an ethical order on earth as a fulfillment of one's submission (literal translations of *islam*) to the will of God. Muslims believe that God revealed this message in the Qur'an, presented to Mohammad by Archangel Gabriel. The Qur'an and Muhammad's exemplary life (*sunnah*), constitute the foundations for Muslims' religious life.

Quandaries in Health Policy: Cancer

"Blessed are the hearts that can bend; they shall never be broken…" (A. Camus)

In Islam, life is viewed as a time of preparation for the hereafter, while death is viewed as the beginning of a different form of life referred to as *Al-Barzakh* (the interval between death and resurrection). A spiritual caregiver, or a person of wisdom, will usually remind a dying person of the great generosity of Allah and will encourage him/her to look forward to Allah's blessings and forgiveness.

The Prophet said, "None of you should die without having good expectations in Allah." He also visited a young man who was dying and asked him, "How do you feel?" The man replied, "By Allah, O Messenger of Allah, I have hope in Allah and I fear my sins." The Messenger said: "These two qualities do not dwell together in a person's heart in this situation (of dying) but Allah will grant him what he hopes, and save him from what he fears."

In Muslim countries, religious scholars – the *ulema* – are not actively involved in deliberations to formulate priorities in health policy according to the moral and legal limits provided by Islamic scriptural sources. New medical and health procedures are often imported without due respect for the religious, social, and individual norms of the population. Furthermore, such technologies and health policies may contravene people's rights to adhere to their cultural beliefs and practices.

Projections indicate that the Middle East will see some of the highest increases in cancer incidence in the decades to come, with an increase of approximately 181% in cancer mortality over the next 15 years, roughly by 2019 given the time of the projection. In Middle Eastern countries, cancer is typically diagnosed at a more advanced stage of disease. In Palestine, 42% of cases were reported at stage III and 18% were stage IV, for a total of 60% non-early cancers (Dey, S., Soliman, AS, 2010).

The largest increases in numbers of cancer cases and deaths in the Middle East occur in low- and middle-income societies with inferior education, where more than 80% of the world's population resides, and where the increase in average age and changes in exposure to cancer risk factors are most pronounced. Within this population cancers are diagnosed at a later, less curable stage, and there is limited capacity for cancer treatment. Consequently, cancers are more likely to result in suffering and death (Saca-Hazboun, et al. 2012).

Muslim families contribute significantly to the decision-making process in all health matters. Parents, spouses, and elder children, in descending order, tend to be the decision makers, as opposed to autonomous individuals as in the Western milieu.

Muslim women tend to neglect themselves. They take care of their children, husbands and parents. They take care of every family member, but their concern about their own health is at the bottom of their priority list (Mehta, et al. 2013).

Seventy-five percent of women with early stage breast cancer are from higher socioeconomic groups and are better educated. Approximately 90% of these women receive adequate treatment resulting in overall survival of about 75% at 10 years. In contrast, 50% of the women who present with advanced disease are from lower socioeconomic and educational backgrounds. Of these economically-challenged women, only 44% receive adequate treatment resulting in a ten-year survival rate of 50%. Literacy levels and ignorance play a major role in determining the prognosis (Mehta, 2013)).

The stigma attached to breast cancer in Muslim countries, especially in lower socioeconomic groups and among poorly educated women, is a significant barrier (Bener, et al. 2010). This leads to a reluctance to seek medical care, and to a tendency among women to exhaust alternative treatment options before seeking appropriate medical help, both of which lead to delayed diagnosis and give the cancer more time to advance (Hag, et al. 2010).

Therefore, it is essential that healthcare policies appreciate the differences in values, attitudes, beliefs, and behavioral norms related to illness and the dying process, that are held by various cultural and ethnic groups (Giger, et al. 2007).

With respect to modern medical and health policies and their social implementation, Muslim legal scholars are under pressure to respond to the questions – moral and legal – pertaining to healthcare and terminally ill patients (Silbermann, et al. 2011; Silbermann, M., Hassan, EA: Cultural Perspectives in Cancer Care: Impact of Islamic Traditions and Practices in Middle Eastern countries. J. Pediatric Hematology Oncology. 2011, 33: 81-86).

Policy Recommendations

- Specific strategies and health policies that are greatly improving cancer screening in Egypt, Jordan, Saudi Arabia, the United Emirates, and Iraq and should be more widely extended
- Cultural and educational challenges in Middle Eastern Islam should be addressed so as to expand health education to the entire population, particularly the less-educated
- Breast cancer screening should be urgently leveraged to draw attention to general women's health and women's health promotion and health education
- Male family members should be targeted for enlistment in the cause of cancer education
- Anti-smoking campaigns and programs to encourage giving up smoking among elderly patients should be an integral part of policy

Pursuit of Loyalties: Family in Islam

> "What causes the rain to fall and smoke to evaporate? Why does the white snow kill the colorful flowers? Why does anybody become ill? Why am I the one who is dying?"
>
> (Muslim patient)

In trying to understand a culture and its ways of structuring its particular society, much can be learned from addressing the manner in which family systems, communication, and coping are channeled toward illness and death.

For Islam, the debate concerning knowledge and consent with respect to illness and healthcare revolves around family norms based on the Qur'an. The family as the basic unit is responsible for decisions about treatment and disclosure. Such cultures value non-malfeasance (doing no harm) and protect patients from any emotional and physical harm caused by directly addressing illness and end-of-life care (Searight, et al. 2007).

Whether or not a medical team can prolong life by introducing invasive treatments without causing further harm is a joint decision made by all associated with the patient's family, and not with the patient. In some instances the matter is even referred to the religious leaders, who provide prescriptive rulings for the families' consideration (Abyad, A. 2009).

Muslim families believe that sending a relative to a hospital or hospice without curative intent may be a form of shirking the responsibility to care for family members at the end of life.

In a research study patients stated that they preferred to die at home or in a holy place such as a mosque or in Mecca or Medina, but this may reflect religious idealism rather than practicality. Care for the dying has been seen as a family responsibility with illness and death being managed at home (Tayeb, 2010).

Characteristics of the Family in Islam

- Honor (self-respect/self-esteem) and religious beliefs– expectation of equal treatment regardless of wealth, position, or rank within the family system
- Imposed rules or decisions sanctioned by religious norms and social family traditions
- Unquestionable loyalty to the extended family and the religious community, and absolute solidarity and obedience to male authority
- Family as the basis for self, social, and religious identity
- The individual identity *is* "the family"

In the Western world, individual autonomy, truth, and open communication are the core of the dominant bioethical cancer framework (Surbone, A., Baider, L. 2013). The perception of autonomy and openness as empowering and providing a sense of control, tends to be blind to the fact that the decision-making process of the individual is involved in a complex relationship with his/her social surroundings. In Islam, families prefer to live with uncertainty about the fate of one of its members rather than confront an accurate prediction or 'death threat.'

The total involvement of the family in Islamic culture is natural in the context of the long-held values of respect for unconditional solidarity in accordance with the normative religious-cultural tradition. The family is identified as a social entity whose being, integrity and cohesion are only understood within the dynamic of the family and not within its individual members (Baider, 2007).

With respect to the life expectancy of a relative, Muslim families are usually skeptical about definitive responses from healthcare professionals. They are likely to be more comfortable with less definitive answers and even with responses like "this is in Allah's (God's) hands, and we can never predict this accurately." Muslims believe that the longevity of every person is only known to Allah who predetermined the exact time of death (Kagawa-Singer, 2010).

More than 250 Muslims in Saudi Arabia (where family is central to the local culture) were interviewed about what constitutes a "good death," starting with the elements identified in Western communities. The authors found that participants identified elements in three main domains: 1. Faith and belief; 2. Self-esteem and image as perceived by family; and 3. Satisfaction about family security after the death of the patient. Several successful attempts have been made to incorporate these outcomes and other Muslim-centered elements into medical-nursing training in palliative and end-of-life care.

Feasible Path for Change: Palliative Care

> "Looking at the diverse approaches to illness and death, we learn not only about the diversity of beliefs, we also learn about ourselves…" (Joris de Bres, 2005)

The following paragraph is part of a taped "interview" with a patient that was conducted with the permission of the patient and her family (the interview was translated from Hebrew into English).

Amaal, a 36-year-oldwoman, was a married mother of four who had never worked outside her home. She lived in her husband's parents' house with other family members in an Arab village in northern Israel, near the border with Lebanon.

Amaal was diagnosed with metastatic breast cancer with brain, bone and liver metastases. During the last month of her life she spent most of her time in bed due to pain and weakness. Her family was opposed to giving her strong opiates so all she received were fluid infusions that contained some 20 mg. of valium, administered by a nurse from a neighboring Arab village with the family's consent.

I met Amaal twice when she came to the hospital for consultations about her anemia and anorexia. She heard her prognosis from the physician and was aware of the terminal nature of her illness but had never cried nor complained. Amaal was always surrounded by relatives and never left alone. I traveled to their home to see her a few days prior to her death.

Amaal was in bed in a room facing Mecca. There was no door, just a heavy curtain hanging at the entrance. About ten male family members were seated, praying silently. Women were crying loudly among additional tapestries and hanging rugs.

Aamal was whispering, apparently daydreaming:

> "…I spoke with my angels… many angels await me in their paradise of Allah… from there, as in a reflection in a mirror, I see my children… how they play, how they grow… I feel so ashamed of my illness… I bring shame to my husband's family… it is as if Allah wants to test my fidelity to Him… But He chose me! I prayed and starved my body of any pleasures… but the illness grew inside me, without my noticing… I didn't want to think about it… I didn't want to bring shame to my family… I confess all my sins… Perhaps I must be punished for my thoughts... dreams… fantasies… But Allah will forgive me. I dream of angels waiting for me in a radiant light of warmth and love… And my soul is joyful, rising to the stars of my new life…"

Could this be described as denial? Could it be a denial of the pain and the grief? Could it be self-consciousness or a possible split personality among identities as a mother, a wife, and a dying person? Perhaps Amaal experienced total acceptance of and submission to her illness within her system of beliefs. Perhaps the displacement of her illness was a paradoxical form of hope within her religious culture.

Amaal came for consultation when she was already at an advanced stage of her illness, at which point palliation and pain control were the most appropriate medical care. Amaal's strong belief furnished her with meaning, a sense of purpose, a desire to repent, and the willingness to accept death as a part of life.

Could Western medical thought condone such passive and submissive acceptance? Perhaps religious and cultural quandaries could guide our psychological approach and temper it with open compassion, increased flexibility and unrestricted acceptance.

The Qur'an offers a sober reminder that there are times when people need to recognize their limits and trust nature to take its course (Qur'an 39:42). Life is sacred because God is its origin and its destiny. Death does not happen except by God's will, as dictated in the Qur'an. Islam believes in the hereafter, where final judgment will take place and people will be adjudicated to Heaven or Hell based on their lawful or unlawful deeds, respectively (Al-Hilali, 1994).

While illness and disease may be regarded as a test from Allah they carry tidings of forgiveness and mercy (Al-Jibaly, 2000). The Muslim world view of health and illness incorporates the notion of accepting illness and death with patience, meditation and prayers and accepting that illness, suffering and dying are part of life and a test from Allah.

Rassool (2009) highlights that in Islam, illness is part of the continuum of being, and prayer is salvation. Nevertheless, Islamic teachings encourage Muslims to seek treatment when they fall ill. The Prophet said, "Seek treatment, because Allah did not send down a sickness but has sent down a medication for it – known to those who know it and not known to others – except for death." In terms of treatment options, Muslim patients resort to the Qur'an, spiritual healing, traditional healing practices, and modern medicine. The spiritual healing practices include recitation of verses of the Noble Qur'an and specific Prophetic supplications (Al-Jauziyah, 1999).

Some Muslim scholars tend to be stricter about withdrawing rather than withholding treatment, even when both are considered medically futile. This outlook may be attributed partly to the relative emotional ease of treatment withholding as opposed to withdrawal. Nonetheless, this view may also be explained by reference to the Islamic jurisprudence principle "certainty cannot be overridden by uncertainty," as it is certain (100% probability) that withdrawing a treatment will deprive a patient of any potential benefit associated with it, whereas it is uncertain (less than 100% probability) that maintaining that particular treatment will cause harm (Al-Shanqiti, 1998).

As patients, families, and communities grapple with the realities of human mortality, terminal illness comes into focus in ways that heighten the relevance of cultural and religious concerns. As families interact with patients dealing with life-limiting conditions, issues of care across cultural boundaries become critically important. Integrating palliative care and enhancing patient and family health skills requires nuanced understanding of the cultural contexts for those who provide care and those who receive it (Silberman, 2012).

Palliative care programs focus on interdisciplinary collaboration to provide comfort for the patient and family within their unique cultural contexts. However, even within hospice programs, there continue to be problems with providing care in ways that respect cultural diversity and maximize availability, accessibility, and acceptability of services (AHRQ, 2010).

As hospice care is increasingly available for terminally ill patients the care of dying Muslims may be a challenge to predominantly Western culture. One of the pre-eminent goals of palliative medicine and hospice is to approach the patient and family from their personal cultural and religious perspective (Sarhill, 2009) (Chung, 2003).

Harford, et al. (2013) holds that individuals facing life-threatening illnesses of any kind in any setting would benefit from palliative care. However, the vast majority of the world's palliative care services exist in high-income countries that represent less than 20% of the world's population.

One of the palliative care premises in our analysis concerned the use of opioid analgesics. Of course, palliative care involves much more than pain relief. Indeed, cancer patients at an advanced stage of the illness experience a range of symptoms that require medical management. Cancer patients tend to experience multiple symptoms including what has been termed 'symptom clusters' i.e., two or more symptoms that present together. Symptom clustering has also been documented in Muslim patients in Kuwait (Alshemmari, et al., 2011) (Cleary, et al. 2013).

Some Muslims may perceive suffering as a means of atoning for one's sins, and to the extent that this interpretation exists among Muslim patients, it may contribute to low opioid usage among the less-educated. It should be noted that clearly not all Muslims adhere to this idea, and the linkage of suffering and atonement is not unique to Islam but is also a belief held by some Christians (Ar-Atiyyat, 2010). It is likely that there will be distinctive combinations of barriers that vary from country to country even among the poorly educated and so local research would be most appropriate. Once the barriers are better understood, educational efforts aimed at overcoming them can be designed, evaluated and implemented.

Moreover, the barriers to the rational use of opioid analgesics vary, depending on location, but certain barriers are common. Barriers to accessing oral morphine include excessively strict national drug laws and regulations, fear of addiction, poorly developed healthcare systems and lack of knowledge at all levels including healthcare providers. To address and reduce these barriers, changes will be needed not only in laws and policies but also in knowledge, attitudes, and behaviors of medical practitioners as well as among patients and their families and their social milieu (Cleary, 2013) (Anderson, 2010).

Concepts Influencing Terminal Care in Islam

- Culture and cultural norms, including those of concealment
- Communication according to needs and awareness
- Integration and involvement of family and male relatives in any health decision
- Traditional beliefs and religion as a basis for care
- Respect for the degree of fatalistic perception
- Respect for denial
- Misperceptions about the adverse effects of screening procedures, such as pain, discomfort, fear and anxiety
- Illness as stigma
- Access to quality healthcare during the process of death and dying

Palliative Care

Could we formulate rational, deductive principles for health policy that would speak for the entire spectrum of religious and ethical norms of Islam? This paradigm should have relevant implications for health policies, which must set justifiable, legal and religious standards for healthcare (Mobeireek, et al. 2008).

Moreover, there is a clear need for more adequately trained healthcare professionals who possess the knowledge and skills to become leaders in a new policy area of palliative care (Surbone, A., Baider, L., and Kagawa-Singer, M.A., 2010).

Alongside major demographic shifts and globalization there is an increasing need for cultural integration in healthcare policy and palliative care. Cultural pluralism, in life as in medicine, enriches our lives while also representing a moral and ethical quandary when medical values and religious norms diverge. Respect, compassion and tolerance are the virtues required to practice terminal and palliative healthcare processes in multicultural societies. They can be learned through cultural competence – knowledge and awareness about different needs and modes of care in a diversity of value systems that enable health professionals to overcome cultural barriers. Ensuring that such cultural competence, tempered with compassion, flexibility and sensitivity, permeates healthcare systems should be our goal and our challenge for the future.

References

Abyad, A. (2009). Health care services for palliative care in the Middle East. *Middle East Journal, 12,* 1-4.

AHRQ, Agency for Healthcare Research and Quality (2010). National Healthcare Disparities. Rockville, M.D. Department of Health and Human Services.

Al-Atiyyat, N.H. (2010). Culture diversity and cancer pain. *Journal of Hospice and Palliative Nursing, 11.*154-163.

Al-Hilali, M.T., Khan, M.M. (1994). *Interpretation of the Meanings of the Noble Qur'an in the English Language.* Riyadh, Saudi Arabia: Dar-us-Salam.

Al-Jauziyah, I. (1999). *Healing with the Medicine of the Prophet (pbuh).* Riyadh, Saudi Arabia; Dar-us-Salam: Abdul Rab J, trans.

Al-Jibaly, M. (2000). *The Inevitable Journey Part 1: Sickness: Regulations and Exhortations.* Texas: Al-Kittab & As-Sunnah Publishing.

Al-Shanqiti, M.M. (1998). *Rules of Surgical Operations and its Consequences.* Taif, Saudi Arabia: Al-Siddiq, 324.

Alshemmanary, S., Ezzat, H., Samir, Z., Sajnani, K. and Alsirafy, S. (2011). Symptoms burden in hospitalized cancer patients in Kuwait and the need for palliative care. *American Journal of Hospice and Palliative Medicine, 27,* 446-449.

Anderson, BO. (2010). Understanding social obstacles to early breast cancer detection is critical to improving breast cancer outcome in low- and middle-resource countries. *Cancer, Oct 1; 116(19),* 4436-9.

Baider, L. (2007). Cancer in different cultural contexts: how is the family affected? *EONS Newsletter, 17,* 18-19.

Bener A, Alwash R, Miller CJ (2010). Knowledge, attitudes and practices related to palliative care among Arab women. *Journal of Cancer Education, 16,* 215-220.

Chung, Y. (2003). Remembering spiritual care. *International Journal of Palliative Nursing, 6,* 4-13.

Cleary, J., Silbermann, M., Scholten, W., Radbruch, L., Torode, J., Cherny, N.I. (2013). Formulary availability and regulatory barriers to accessibility of opioids for cancer pain in the Middle East: a report from the Global Opioid Policy Initiative (GOPI). (Supplement 11). *Annals of Oncology*. (in press).

Cleary, J., Silbermann, M., Scholten, W., Radbruch, L., Torode, J., Cherny, N.I. (2013). Formulary availability and regulatory barriers to accessibility of opioids for cancer pain in the Middle East: a report from the Global Opioid Policy Initiative (GOPI). (Supplement 11). *Annals of Oncology*. (in press).

Cohen, A.B. (2010). Many forms of culture. *American Psychologist, 64,* 194-204.

Dey, S., Soliman, AS, (2010). Cancer in the global health era: opportunities for the Middle East and Asia. *Asia Pac Journal of Public Health, Jul; 22* (3 suppl): 75S-82S.

Doorenbos, A.Z., Given, B., Given, C.W., Verbitsky, N. (2008). Symptoms experience in the last year of life, among individuals with cancer. *Journal of Pain and Symptoms Management, 32,* 403-412.

Giger, J.N., Davidhizar, R.E., Fordham, P. (2007). Multi-cultural and multi-ethnic considerations developing cultural competence. *Journal of Cultural Diversity, 13,* 3-9.

Hag,N., Hag, M.M. Abida Hague (2010). Breast cancer incidence and risk reduction with reference to Muslim countries. *JIMA Journal of Islam Medical Ass., 45,* 18-27.

Harford, J. B, Aljawi, D.M. (2013). The need for more and better palliative care for Muslim patients. *Journal of Palliative and Supportive Care, 11,* 1-4.

Hazleton, L.(2009). *After the Prophet.* New York: Doubleday, London.

Kagawa-Singer M., Valdez D., Yu M. et al. (2010). Cancer, culture and health disparities: time to chart a new course? *CA: Cancer Journal of Clinicians, 60,* 12-39.

Kaniklides, C. (2012). Cancer, culture and cooperation in the Middle East. *European Association for Cancer Research* – EACR – Cancer in the Middle East. Internal Publication.

Lewis B. (2002). *Western impact and Middle Eastern response.* New York: Oxford University Press.

Mehta, T., Al-Enezi, S. (2013). Arab Health Round Table: Cancer in the Middle East. Conference in Dubai. Internal Publication.

Ibid.

Mobeireek, A.F., Al-Kassimi, F., Al-Zahrani, K., Al-Shimemeri, A., et al. (2008). Information disclosure and decision-making: the Middle East versus the Far East and the West. *Journal of Medical Ethics, 34,* 225-229.

Rassool, G. (2009). The crescent and Islam. *Journal of Advanced Nursing, 32,* 1476-84.

Saca-Hazboun, H., Glennon, CA. (2012). Cultural influences on health care in Palestine. *Clinical Journal of Oncol Nurs, June; 15(3),* 281-6.

Sarhill, N., Le Grand, S., Islambouli, R., Davis, M.P., Walsh, D. (2009). The terminally ill Muslim: death and dying from the Muslim perspective. *American Journal of Hospice and Palliative Care, 18,* 251-255.

Schim, S.M., Benkert, R., Bell, S.E., Walker, D., Danford, C. (2010). Social Justice: added metaparadigm concept for urban health. *Public Health, 18,* 103-110.

Schim, S.M., Doorenbos, A.Z. (2011). A three-dimensional model of cultural congruence. *Journal of Social Work, 6,* 256-270.

Searight HR, Gafford J. (2007).Cultural diversity at the end of life. *American Family Physicians, 72,* 515-522.

Silberman, M., Amount, M., Dahaer, M. (2012). Palliative cancer care in the Middle Eastern countries: accomplishment and challenges. *Ann. of Oncology, 23,* (Supplement 3), 15-25.

Silberman, M., Hassan, EA (2011). Cultural Perspectives in Cancer Care: Impact of Islamic Traditions and Practices in Middle Eastern countries. *J. Pediatric Hematology Oncology, 33,* 81-86.

Surbone, A., Baider, L. (2013). Personal values and cultural diversity. *Journal of Medicine and the Person* in press (online).

Surbone, A., Baider, L., and Kagawa-Singer, M.A. (2010). Cultural competence in the practice of patient-family centered oncology. *Journal of Geriatric Oncology, 1,* 45-47.

Tayeb, M.A., Al-Zamel, E., Fareed, M.M. and Abouellail, H.A. (2010). A good death: perspectives of Muslim patients and health care providers. *Ann. Saudi Med., 30,*215-221.

Triandis, H.C. (2007). *Culture and Psychology in Kitayana, S., Cohen, D. (Ed.) Handbook of Cultural Psychology.* New York: Guildford Press. Pp. 59-76.

In: Palliative Care to the Cancer Patient
Editor: Michael Silbermann
ISBN: 978-1-63117-709-5

Chapter 6

PEDIATRIC PALLIATIVE CARE IN ISRAEL

Sergey Postovsky, M.D. and Myriam Weyl-Ben-Arush, M.D.
Department of Pediatric Hematology Oncology, Meyer Children's Hospital, Rambam Health Care Campus, The Bruce Rappaport Faculty of Medicine, Technion-Institute of Technology, Haifa, Israel

INTRODUCTION

Every year between 400-450 new cases of cancer among children between the ages of 0 to 18 years are registered in Israel. The delicate intricacies involved in supporting children suffering from terminal cancer and their grief-stricken families call for specialized services by a well balanced team of inter-disciplinary professionals trained in palliative care. In most of the Israeli institutions, the team includes the following professionals: palliative care pediatric oncologist, clinical nurse, social worker, clinical psychologist, art and music therapist. Place of death of pediatric cancer patients in Israel varies according to the local facilities. The staff education includes short courses in palliative medicine designed for medical students, nurses and pediatric oncologists fellows.

The presence of qualified medical and psychosocial personnel representing people of different walks of life allows a better provision of optimal palliative care for children with cancer. Practically every medical and psychosocial staff of pediatric oncology departments has representatives of every religious and ethnic communities existing in Israel, speaking Hebrew, Arabic, Russian, and other languages. Several associations support palliative programs, these organizations are members of the European Association for Palliative Care (EAPC) and take an active part in its regular activities. It is our intention to cultivate academic and scientific activities in the field of palliative medicine in pediatric oncology through interdisciplinary research and development initiatives. Israeli palliative services are promoted for the benefit of individuals and their families during the difficult periods of living with the disease, dying from it and grieving.

EPIDEMIOLOGY

The data on childhood cancer in Israel in the years 1998 to 2007 were obtained from the Israeli National Cancer Registry (INCR) [1]. Between 1998 and 2007, 4255 new cases of cancer among children below the age of 20 years in Israel were analyzed retrospectively. An age-adjusted incidence rate of 172.4 per million for children aged 0 to 19 years and 153.4 per million for children aged 0 to 14 years was reported.

The 5-year survival rates ranged between 77.9% and 83.9% when comparing the different age groups. Adolescents had the highest 5-year survival rates and the 5-9-year age group had the lowest. Infants' 5-year survival rate was 78.9%. Table 1 show the incidence and survival rates in Israel according to the main diagnoses and ethnicity in comparison to the numbers seen in the SEER databases. The 5-year survival rate was 72.8% for the Arabic population compared to 83.2% for the Jewish population (P<0.001). In leukemia, lymphoma, CNS tumors, and bone tumors, Jewish children had higher survival rates especially (P<0.05) (Figure 1).

No significant differences were observed in comparison with the data analyzed in Europe and the United States. A lower incidence of cancer was found in Arab Israeli children and the adolescent populations compared with the Jewish population, with a geographically increased incidence in the center of Israel compared with Judea and Samaria, the south and the north of the country (Figure 2). No evident cause was found to explain the difference in survival between the Jewish and Arab children.

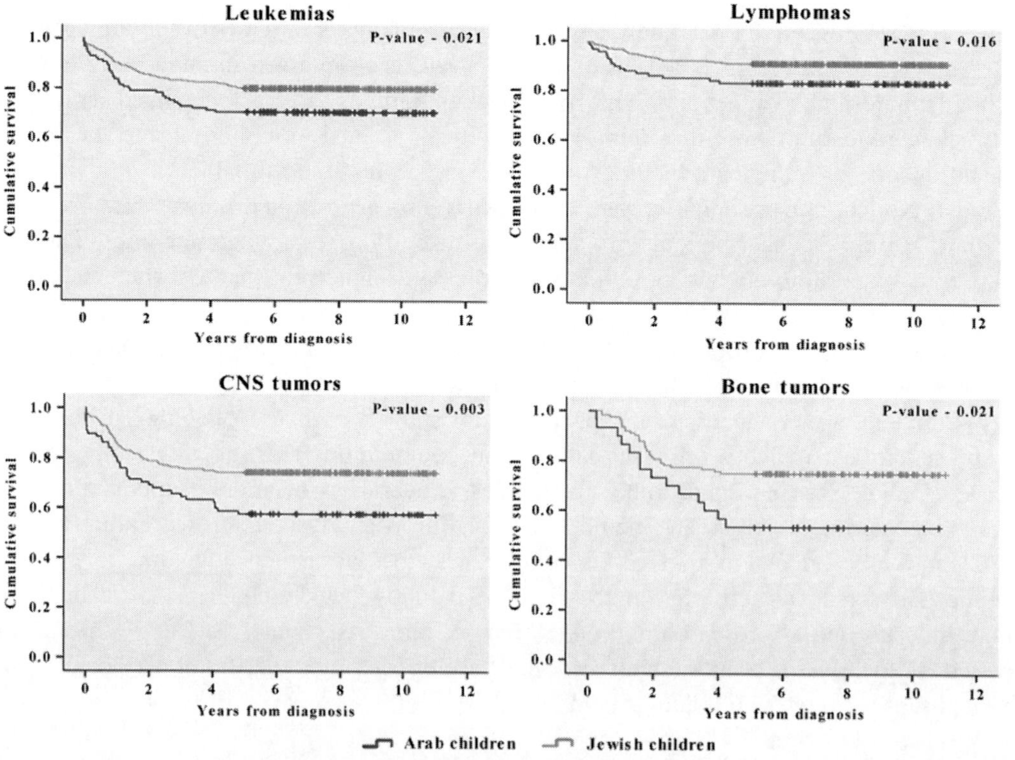

Figure 1. Survival rates of childhood cancer diagnosed in Israel, 1998-2003, in diagnostic groups by ethnicity with statistical significance (P < 0.05).

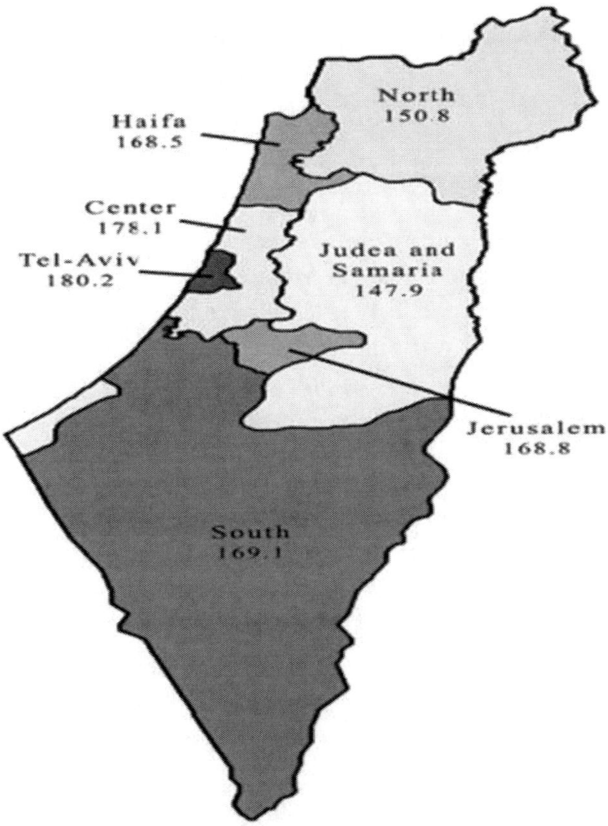

Figure 2. Distribution of pediatric cancer according to geographical districts of the State of Israel.

Table 1. Years survival rates in Israel according to the ICCC3 groups and ethnicity compared to the SEER project in USA

Diagnosis – ICCC3	Israel			Seer 1999-2006
	Total	Jews	Arabs	
Total	73.0%	76.2%	63.1%	79.8%
I Leukemias	67.8%	71.3%	58.7%	78.4%
II Lymphomas	83.8%	87.8%	71.5%	88.4%
III CNS neoplasms	83.8%	87.8%	71.5%	71.6%
IV Neuroblastomas	65.6%	64.9%	67.3%	72.6%
V Retinoblastoma	92.3%	94.1%	88.9%	97.6%
VI Renal tumors	83.7%	84.6%	81.5%	87.7%
VII Hepatic tumors	34.6%	42.9%	25.0%	62.0%
VIII Malignant bone tumors	61.3%	65.6%	45.0%	68.5%
IX Soft tissue sarcomas	70.3%	72.0%	64.8%	70.7%
X Germ-cell neoplasms	91.9%	92.0%	91.3%	89.6%
XI Other epithelial neoplasms	89.1%	90.0%	85.0%	91.3%
XII Other and unspecified malignant neoplasms	63.6%	77.8%	46.7%	

PALLIATIVE CARE FOR CHILDREN IN ISRAEL

Palliative care for oncological children in Israel is provided in several ways. First and most important, it is conducted in departments of pediatric oncology/hematology within large hospitals under the auspices of the Ministry of Health [2].

There are six major pediatric oncology centers in Israel located within large university-affiliated hospitals (Rambam Health Care Campus in Haifa in the north, Soroka Medical Center in Beer Sheba in the south, Hadassah Medical Center in Jerusalem, and Chaim Sheba Medical Center at Tel Hashomer, Schneider Children's Medical Center in Petach Tikva, and Sourasky Medical Center in Tel Aviv in the center). Within each of these centers, there is staff dedicated to the management of children who need palliative care. Such a team is usually comprised of a physician, registered nurse, clinical psychologist and social worker who routinely occupy their positions in the department of pediatric oncology/hematology and have special knowledge in the field of pediatric palliative care. Many of the physicians and nurses of these teams have gained their knowledge and experience by attending various courses in palliative care existing within different frames of learning and continuous education. Pediatric oncology treatment is also provided in other, smaller medical centers. The number of children treated in these hospitals is usually significantly smaller and necessary supportive and, if needed, palliative care is provided within general pediatric departments where these patients are usually hospitalized. In such circumstances, palliative care is provided by local medical and psychosocial staff existing in these departments of general pediatrics [2].

Given the modern approach to palliative care as an integral part of supportive care, the principles of such care should be applied by the members of the above-mentioned teams, from the very first steps of managing a child's cancer and not necessarily only in patients with incurable disease. With such a broad definition of palliative care being taken into account, it is now clear that each and every child receiving oncological treatment in a pediatric oncology/hematology department becomes a subject for intervention by the pediatric palliative care team. Obviously, when death is approaching, the function of such a team becomes even more vital [3].

The aim of pediatric palliative care teams (PPCT) working within the frame of pediatric oncology/hematology departments is directed at timely and sensitive discussion of such aspects of management as implementation of Do Not Resuscitate orders, possible provision of fluids and parenteral nutrition, initiation of palliative sedation, and management of depression [4-7].

The palliative care team consisting of medical and psychosocial staff plays a vital role in conveying comprehensive and timely management of all these problems and providing all necessary assistance for parents and other involved in the last weeks, days, and hours of the child’s life. The palliative care team cannot avert approaching death, but it is responsible for making it as peaceful and as free of suffering as possible. This is achieved by vigorous control of all physical symptoms in the dying child and by paying close attention to all existential, emotional, and social demands of both the child and his relatives [4, 8].

According to the modern concept of palliative medicine, proper care is not completed with the death of the child. In an absolute majority of instances, the members of the palliative team connect to the parents after the child's death to ensure the "normal" rehabilitation process of family members and frequently perform at-home visits even beyond usual working hours [4, 5].

In especially difficult to manage cases such as those with intractable pain or respiratory problems caused by the accumulation of fluids in the pleural space, members of the PPCT receive help from other specialists and services existing in the hospital, e.g., anesthesiology, pain clinic, chest surgeons, etc. Such tight cooperation of many specialists facilitates more comprehensive and successful management of pediatric palliative patients at the end of their lives.

Obviously, there are many aspects of the PPCT's activities that should be improved. First, there is a significant lack of communication between the PPCT and the outpatient pediatric palliative cervices existing within the framework of the health funds. Second, the lack of proper funding enabling effective functioning of these teams practically precludes the performance of regular home visits to needed patients by members of the PPCT. This, in turn, leads to increased frequency of hospitalization in situations where these hospital admissions could have been avoided [9-12].

During the course of treatment, the pediatric cancer patient receives remedial help and home tutoring to help him/her make up material missed during long absences from school. The home tutoring comes from two sources: one from the Ministry of Education which sends a teacher to the home to help make up school work; and the second comes from the Israel Cancer Society which provides student tutoring for 6 weekly hours to the sick child. The tutoring is given in the patient's home on a one-to-one basis. This aid continues as long as the patient feels well enough to cooperate and is able to benefit from it. It allows for a feeling of normalcy, hope and continuity in his life. As his medical condition deteriorates, it is often necessary to reduce the remedial help until it is eventually discontinued. This decision is usually taken by mutual agreement between the home tutor and the child's parents [13].

Place of Death of Pediatric Cancer Patients in Israel

Despite obvious advantages to keeping the child at home during the final phase of his/her life, still too few pediatric cancer patients die at home. There are several explanations as to why the overwhelming majority of children spend their last days of life in hospital. First, the complexity and severity of symptoms and the burden of suffering is too great to be managed successfully in the home setting. Many pediatric patients with terminal cancer suffer from widespread metastatic disease either in the bones (neuroblastoma) or lungs (sarcoma), while others with incurable brain tumors have locally advanced or disseminated within CNS disease. Because of the wide-spread or locally advanced nature of their tumors, most such patients suffer from significant pain and/or respiratory difficulties. These symptoms are very difficult or even impossible to control at home without applying palliative sedation as a method of last resort at the end of life. Unfortunately, internal regulations existing within various health funds does not allow the implementation of palliative sedation in the home setting for these children. Second, despite the fact that almost all the health funds have some form of unit specialized in providing palliative care for adult patients with terminal cancer, the medical staff of these units do not have a sufficient level of expertise in the field of pediatric palliative care. And, finally, keeping the dying child at home frequently poses significant physical, emotional and financial strain on parents and other family members. Sometimes young siblings of a dying child become exposed to the profound suffering experienced by their loved brother or sister and this experience may bear the potential of psychological damage for these young children. Many parents decide in favor of a hospital for their dying child in order to spare their other children from this exposure [4, 14, 15]. In addition, such a decision taken by parents facilitates other factors, such as easy accessibility of pediatric oncology departments with well-established relationships between the dying child and his parents on one side and departmental medical and psychosocial staff on the other.

Taking all the above into account, we can suggest the following steps directed at the improvement of providing palliative care at the end of life for pediatric cancer patients at home. First, creation of conditions which will allow medical and psychosocial staff from the hospital to provide this kind of care at the child's home. Alternatively, education of existing medical and psychosocial staff of the health funds to provide them with the necessary knowledge and skills for successful palliative care of pediatric patients. And, last but not least, effective communication between the hospital and the health fund teams should provide a professional platform for effective collaboration with the ultimate aim directed at providing the best possible care at home for these patients and their families.

In order to solve or at least alleviate the problem of dying at home, the Chaim Sheba Medical Center in Tel Hashomer created a Palliative Care Unit (PCU) that is fully integrated into the Pediatric Hematology Oncology Department [16]. The majority (59%) of patients admitted after the PCU establishment were hospitalized in the PCU, including 49% of the good prognosis patients and 91% of the poor prognosis patients. Poor prognosis patients were hospitalized in the PCU earlier and with a higher frequency compared to children with curable disease. After the PCU opening, there was a significant decline in the percentage of patients who died in the general pediatrics ward, hematology-oncology ward, and at home, from 40%, 26% and 28% to 4%, 8%, and 16%, respectively. Creation of this unit has resulted in exposure of the majority of children with cancer to palliative care. For poor prognosis patients, palliative care is introduced early enough to allow a gradual transition from symptom control after diagnosis to end of life care. Unfortunately, some administrative problems which have risen in the Department of Pediatric Oncology at Sheba Medical Center have hampered the further development of this interesting and promising program.

In those cases where the family decides to take their child home, palliative care units of the health funds provide the child with the necessary amount of narcotics, analgesics and other drugs. Within the home palliative care setting, the child may receive fluids and nutrition administered either enterally or parenterally, as the absolute majority of pediatric cancer patients have some kind of central venous line inserted during the course of his/her disease and treatment. It is important to stress that there are no limitations in the use of narcotics and other drugs directed at alleviating the suffering of a dying child in Israel. The unlimited availability of opioids for medical purposes both in in- and out-patient settings represents a major benefit for all palliative patients, including children. The only criterion the treating physician uses when administering these drugs to a child dying from cancer is the clinical efficacy and toxicity of the prescribed medication. Although there is no financial reimbursement for providing consultative services during off-work hours, practically all pediatric oncologists provide their mobile phone numbers to the families of dying children so as to be available at any given moment, along with a direct and unobstructed telephone connection to the corresponding pediatric oncology departments on a 24/7/365 basis. This direct and easy availability of experienced senior departmental personnel for such families sometimes allows the parents of dying children to more successfully cope with the many different problems arising during the final stage of a child's life and facilitates keeping these patients at home for longer periods of time and sometimes even until the very moment of death.

EDUCATION IN PEDIATRIC PALLIATIVE CARE

1. Since 2013, there has been a recognized residency in palliative care. As a part of their curriculum, medical residents enrolled in palliative care programs should spend some time in the pediatric oncology/hematology departments. The time allotted for this rotation should ideally allow residents to acquire basic knowledge and necessary experience in managing pediatric oncology patients at the end of their lives.
2. Several faculties of medicine of various universities offer short courses in palliative medicine designed for 6th year students. These courses are not obligatory and only interested students take them as part of their curriculum. For example, 6th year students at the Rappaport Faculty of Medicine at Technion-Institute of Technology in Haifa may choose a course of one week's duration. Within the time-frame of this course, students attend the Department of Pediatric Oncology/Hematology at Rambam Health Care Campus (two academic hours only) where they have an opportunity to meet the pediatric oncologist who is responsible for palliative care in the department and discuss with him various aspects of the management of children with advanced and incurable cancer.
3. On the Faculty of Medicine of Technion in Haifa, the only certified thananologist in Israel regularly conducts seminars on such topics as death and grievance. Aspects that are relevant for pediatric palliative care are also discussed in this forum.
4. After graduation and during their residency in pediatric oncology/hematology departments, young doctors are regularly exposed to the various aspects of palliative care. They routinely care for children with incurable cancer at the end of life under the close supervision and guidance of a pediatric oncologist who is experienced in the field. Pediatric oncology residents are expected to continuously improve their knowledge and skills in palliative care by attending and conducting such academic activities as journal club departmental meetings, and attending and taking an active part in "breaking bad news" sessions together with senior physicians. As a part of their education in palliative medicine, pediatric oncology residents routinely care for patients with pain, vomiting, seizures and other noxious symptoms encountered during the course of their illness and especially when death is approaching. They take a part in the discussion of indications for starting palliative sedation for such patients and in conducting it. In summary, regular exposure to various aspects of palliative care occurring in everyday practice during their residency in the department of pediatric oncology/hematology allows pediatric oncology residents to attain the necessary level of knowledge and experience to successfully manage various difficult situations which they will encounter in their future practice while caring for children dying from cancer. Upon completion of their residency and in order to become

licensed in Israel as a pediatric oncologist/hematologist, every doctor has to pass a two-part exam (written and oral). Some of the questions on the written exam deal with various aspects of pediatric palliative care in the everyday practice of the pediatric oncologist/hematologist, thus allowing assessing his/her competency in this field.

5. After successful completion of their residency, pediatric oncologists continue their education in the field of palliative care. There is a possibility to gain experience from internationally renowned specialists from abroad through visiting them at their places of work in big hospitals with a high patient load. During the last decades, at least three pediatric oncologists visited Children's Hospital in Boston, MA, for further education. The Israel Society of Pediatric Hematology Oncology also organizes regular palliative care meetings where pediatric oncologists and other medical professionals have an opportunity to discuss their problems and exchange the results of their work and research with other colleagues. Frequently, renowned specialists from abroad are invited to such conferences as guest speakers.
6. A training program for medical and psychosocial staff involved in the palliative care of children was supported by the UJA-Federation of New York at Ben Gurion University in Beer Sheba. The aim of this program was the creation of an interdisciplinary team for further improvement in palliative care and education. The members of this training program included pediatric oncology physicians, nurses, psychologists and social workers (about 40 participants). Four seminars were organized with the help of invited specialists from abroad to prepare a standard teaching program. Upon completion, the members of this project went to all the main medical institutions in Israel to further educate local medical communities. Unfortunately, the program was stopped for financial reasons.
7. In January 2014, the Israel Ministry of Health and the Israeli Scientific Council will start a two year fellowship in palliative care designated to prepare specialists working both in pediatric and adult oncology. All pediatricians willing to accomplish this fellowship will have to spend the required amount of time in pediatric oncology departments.

Ethnic, Religious and Socio-Economic Characteristics of Families Involved in Palliative Care

According to the United Nations Human Development Index (HDI), Israel is ranked 22/177 countries worldwide (value 0.908) [17]. This places Israel in the group of countries with high human development. According to Israeli law, access to medical care in state-funded hospitals is equal for any patient, irrespective of racial, ethnic, religious or social background.

Israel is a small but very heterogeneous state. People living in Israel represent various religious denominations with different ethnic and cultural backgrounds. Children living in Israel obtain their education through both secular and religious school systems. Cultural, ethnic and religious traditions existing within their local communities and families exert significant influence on their formation as citizens of the State of Israel. Advanced planning of end-of-life issues by medical personnel involved in the management of a child with incurable cancer infers close collaboration with the child's parents and often other members of the family. The decision-making process regarding various aspects of such sensitive and emotionally laden topics as the approaching death of someone's son or daughter is not straightforward and is always very complicated [3, 4]. Many aspects of the child's management, both from the doctor's and the parents' perspective, may be seen differently, and many factors may potentially influence the decisions that are to be made in the child's best interests. Every person is a unique biological, psychological, and social creature. Every decision made is influenced by a variety of factors, many of them connected to cultural, religious, social, and educational backgrounds [18, 19]. It becomes especially important when a child is diagnosed with cancer and especially when it becomes clear that there are no more realistic prospects for his/her survival. The presence of qualified medical and psychosocial personnel representing people of different walks of life allows a better provision of optimal palliative care for children with cancer. Practically every medical and psychosocial staff of pediatric oncology departments has representatives of every religious and ethnic communities existing in Israel, speaking Hebrew, Arabic, Russian, and other languages.

Taking into account the religious, ethnical and socio-economical characteristics of dying children's families may be a valuable factor for providing "tailored" palliative care for these children. Thus, for example, according to the study performed in the Department of Pediatric Oncology/Hematology at Rambam Health Care Campus, the process of decision-making on DNR orders was influenced by the level of the parents' formal education and by the monthly family income level (socio-economic status), and not by religious background. It was interesting to see that religious affiliation itself, with the exception of Druze, did not play a significant role in the decision-making process regarding whether to accept or deny a DNR order. In that aspect, the relatively small group of Druze parents stands apart. Despite a common language with the Muslim and Christian Arab populations residing in Israel, the Druze population has very distinctive cultural and religious characteristics. One of the main beliefs of the Druze religion is Determinism. Druze believe that destiny is predetermined by God and that they do not have the right to change their fate. Another key feature of the Druze religion is a belief in reincarnation. Druze do not mourn the dead, for they believe that, once a person dies, his/her soul goes immediately to the body of a baby born that minute. It is likely that the Druze's strong religious beliefs directly influence the decisions concerning the end-of life issues of their children [19].

In addition to Israeli children who received oncological treatment in the departments of pediatric oncology, during last two decades we have witnessed a significant increase in the number of children from abroad (predominantly from the countries of the former Soviet Union) actively seeking medical help in our country. These children frequently have advanced cancer at the time of their arrival in Israel and, after updating their diagnoses and degree of tumor spread, many are found to be not curable. Despite the grave ultimate prognosis, the parents of these children frequently opt to stay in Israeli for further treatment notwithstanding the small if any chances for ultimate survival. In such circumstances, the palliative care for these children is provided by the members of the PPCT of corresponding departments of pediatric oncology. In addition to the enormous stress imposed by the very fact of the incurability of their children, the parents experience many other profound problems stemming from cultural, linguistic, financial and other difficulties. Not always is there adequate psychosocial support provided for these families, since cultural and language barriers are not easily overcome due to the deficit of Russian-speaking clinical psychologists and social workers. There is no financial reimbursement and, therefore, there are no incentives (besides purely altruistic) for the psychologist and social worker to be involved in the management of such patients, even if the language barrier is solved with the help of translators. Thus, at present, all if any psychosocial support of pediatric palliative oncology patients from abroad is conducted absolutely voluntarily.

Children from the Palestinian Authority represent another group of non-Israeli citizens receiving medical help in the departments of pediatric oncology. There are fewer obstacles in providing palliative care for such children in comparison with children from the Russian Federation and other former Soviet countries. First, the parents of these children usually have less financial problems as their treatment is subsidized by the Palestinian Authority and they do not have to pay for the treatment from their own pockets. Second, the relative proximity of almost every Israeli hospital to the territory of the Palestinian Authority makes it relatively easy for the child and parents to get back to their homes when the medical condition allows. Such a close connection with home may significantly alleviate psychological stress for the Palestinian child with cancer receiving treatment in Israel. When death approaches and there is no more anticancer treatment, many Palestinian families choose to return to their native cities and villages where the child spends his/her last weeks and days in familiar surroundings. In such instances, members of the medical and psychosocial staff in the departments of pediatric oncology communicate with their Palestinian colleagues, be it either in the West Bank or Gaza. Frequently and when needed, Palestinian oncology patients are provided with the necessary analgesics and other drugs to ensure their arrival at the local hospital without exaggeration of their symptoms caused by their transportation. This communication is facilitated by the fact that, in some pediatric oncology departments in Israel (as for example at Rambam Health Care Campus in Haifa), there is a specially allocated social worker who is a native Arabic-speaking specialist dedicated to providing social support for this group of patients.

Organization of Support for Palliative Care Initiatives

In Israel, several associations support palliative programs:

1) The Israel Association of Palliative Care (Tmicha) was created in 1993 to promote the development of services and education by conducting annual professional conferences.
2) The Israel Palliative Medical Society was established in 1996 as a branch of the Israel Medical Association.

Both these organizations are members of the European Association for Palliative Care (EAPC) and take an active part in its regular activities.

The development of various services in palliative care are supported by several Israeli voluntary associations, such as the Israel Cancer Association, Larger than Life, Amoutat Haim, and others, as well as foreign associations (International Children Cancer Foundation (ICCF) and the Middle East Cancer Consortium (MECC).

Conclusion

Despite the significant success that has been achieved in the treatment of pediatric cancer in Israel, palliative care still lags behind the required level. In Israel, pediatric palliative care services need to be further developed. This requires significant financial support from various governmental bodies to provide much needed help in establishing a material basis for the creation of dedicated units and further education of medical and psychosocial staff. Despite the obvious obstacles, however, we have witnessed certain and sometimes significant progress in Israel in this field of medicine in recent years. Palliative services are developed for the benefit of individuals and their families during the difficult periods of living with the disease, dying from it and grieving.

Conflict of Interest

The authors have no conflict of interest to declare.

References

[1] Rabinowicz R, Barchana M, Liphshiz I, Futerman B, Linn S, Weyl-Ben-Arush M. Cancer Incidence and survival among children and adolescents in Israel during the years 1998 to 2007. *J. Pediatr. Hematol. Oncol.* 2012; 6:421-429.

[2] Ben-Arush MW. Current status of palliative care in Israel: a pediatric oncologist's perspective. *J. Pediatr. Hematol. Oncol.* 2011; 33 Suppl 1:S56-9.

[3] Waldman E, Wolfe J. Palliative care for children with cancer. *Nat. Rev. Clin. Oncol.* 2013; 10:100-107.

[4] Postovsky S, Ben Arush MW. Care of a child dying of cancer: the role of the palliative care team in pediatric oncology. *Pediatr. Hematol. Oncol.* 2004; 21:67-76.

[5] Duncan J, Spengler E, Wolfe J. Providing pediatric palliative care: PACT in action. *MCN Am. J. Matern. Child Nurs.* 2007;32: 279-87.

[6] Postovsky S, Moaed B, Krivoy E, Ofir R, Ben Arush MW. Practice of palliative sedation in children with brain tumors and sarcomas at the end of life. Pediatr. *Hematol. Oncol.* 2007; 24:409-415.

[7] Postovsky S, Levenzon A, Ofir R, Ben Arush MW. "Do not resuscitate" orders among children with solid tumors at the end of life. *Pediatr. Hematol. Oncol.* 2004; 21:661-668.

[8] Tadmor CS, Postovsky S, Elhasid R, Ben Barak A, Arush MB. Policies designed to enhance the quality of life of children with cancer at the end-of-life. *Pediatr. Hematol. Oncol.* 2003; 20:43-54.

[9] Carroll JM, Santucci G, Kang TI, Feudtner C. Partners in pediatric palliative care: a program to enhance collaboration between hospital and community palliative care services. *Am. J. Hosp. Palliat. Care.* 2007; 24: 191-5.

[10] Knapp CA, Madden VL, Curtis CM, Sloyer PJ, Huang IC, Thompson LA, Shenkman EA.Partners in care: together for kids: Florida's model of pediatric palliative care. *J. Palliat. Med.* 2008; 11: 1212-20.

[11] Schmidt P, Otto M, Hechler T, Metzing S, Wolfe J, Zernikow B. Did increased availability of pediatric palliative care lead to improved palliative care outcomes in children with cancer? *J. Palliat. Med.* 2013; 16:1034-1039.

[12] Wolfe J, Friebert S, Hilden J.Caring for children with advanced cancer integrating palliative care. *Pediatr. Clin. North Am.* 2002; 49: 1043-62.

[13] Bouffet E, Zucchinelli V, Costanzo P, Blanchard P.Schooling as a part of palliative care in paediatric oncology. *Palliat. Med.* 1997;11: 133-9.

[14] Bluebond-Langner M, Beecham E, Candy B, Langner R, Jones L. Preferred place of death for children and young people with life-limiting and life-threatening conditions: a systematic review of the literature and recommendations for future inquiry and policy. *Palliat. Med.* 2013;27: 705-13.

[15] Hechler T, Blankenburg M, Friedrichsdorf SJ, Garske D, Hübner B, Menke A, Wamsler C, Wolfe J, Zernikow B. Parents' perspective on symptoms, quality of life, characteristics of death and end-of-life decisions for children dying from cancer. *Klin. Pediatr.* 2008; 220: 166-74.

[16] Golan H, Bielorai B, Grebler D, Izraeli S, Rechavi G, Toren A. Integration of a palliative and terminal care center into a comprehensive pediatric oncology department. *Pediatr. Blood Cancer* 2008; 50:949-955.

[17] Bentur N, Emanuel LL, Cherney N. Progress in palliative care in Israel: comparative mapping and next steps. *Isr. J. Health Policy Res.* 2012; 1: 9.

[18] Schultz M, Baddarni K, Bar-Sela G. Reflections on palliative care from the Jewish and Islamic tradition. *Evid. Based Complement Alternat. Med.* 2012; 2012:693092.

[19] Hileli I, Weyl Ben Arush M, Hakim F, Postovsky S. Association between religious and socio-economic background of parents of children with solid tumors and DNR orders. *Pediatr. Blood Cancer* 2014; 61: 265-8.

In: Palliative Care to the Cancer Patient
Editor: Michael Silbermann

ISBN: 978-1-63117-709-5

Chapter 7

Integrating Complementary Medicine in Cancer Supportive Care across the Middle East: Challenges and Opportunities

Eran Ben-Arye*, M.D.
Integrative Oncology Program, The Oncology Service Lin Medical Center
Clalit Health Services, Haifa and West Galilee District,
the Bruce Rappaport Faculty of Medicine,
Technion- Israel Institute of Technology, Haifa, Israel

Prologue

Walid, a 67-year-old married man living in a Druze village in northern Israel, was admitted to the Clalit Health Services oncology service at the Lin Medical Center in Haifa, for palliative chemotherapy treatment with cisplatin and gemcitabine for advanced pancreatic cancer. Walid's oncologist nurse referred him for supportive care-oriented complementary medicine (CM) consultation provided free-of-charge to patients receiving chemotherapy within the conventional oncology department. During the initial consultation visit, the integrative physician (IP, physician with CM training) asked Walid to express his general expectations of CM care and to relate specifically to symptoms that bother him mostly and compromise his quality of life. Walid told the IP that he recently retired from his work as a journalist and experienced debilitating upper abdominal pains, flatulence, and constipation. The intensified pain caused him to refer for the hospital emergency room which was followed by the harsh diagnosis of pancreatic cancer and widespread liver metastasis. Walid's main expectations were to "know the truth about my disease", to consult the IP regarding nutritional changes he performed since diagnosis (adding turmeric, olive oil, cinnamon, anise tea to relieve constipation, and special Druze *mirla* tea for strengthening and overcoming cancer) and to reduce the anticipated chemotherapy side effects.

* Address for correspondence: eranben@netvision.net.il

Along the months that followed, the IP recommended Walid various traditional and CM treatments which were coordinated with his oncologist, nurse oncologist, psycho-oncologist, and family physician. Walid attended weekly to once every 3 weeks acupuncture sessions aiming to improve fatigue, pain, nausea, anxiety, and constipation. The treatment also included nutritional and herbal consultation regarding the use of wheatgrass juice, freshly squeezed from sprouted wheat seeds, freshly cut sage and thyme in salads, grinded black cumin seeds, honey with garlic, and a root powder of a Syrian plant (which the IP could not identify) recommended by a friend. The integrative CM treatment was complemented with Walid's participation in two 3-hour cuisine group workshops which he attended with his wife and daughter aiming to study more herbal and nutritional strategies to improve his well-being. At the 11th session the IP performed clinical assessment of Walid's well-being based on validated QOL questionnaires. Compared with the initial IP assessment, the follow-up evaluation suggested improved severity of pain, fatigue, anxiety, dyspnea, appetite, sleep and general well-being. Spiritual well-being assessment documented Walid's intensified faith, peace, and meaning which was also noticed in Walid's own words: "I feel better and sometimes I don't feel that I am having this disease; it is difficult pointing out what of all I received treatments made me *healthier* but overall I feel excellent and that what matters".

Six months following this evaluation, Walid's disease progressed and eventually chemotherapy was discontinued and palliative care was provided at home. Along the one year that commenced with the initial IP assessment, Walid attended 39 integrative sessions and received over 105 CM interventions.

TERMINOLOGY: MIDDLE-EASTERN PERSPECTIVES OF *ALTERNATIVE* VERSUS *INTEGRATIVE* CARE

Walid's story is far from representing a typical course of complementary medicine (CM) treatment provided to patients with cancer in the Middle-East. The integration of CM consultation and treatment within conventional supportive oncology care, as presented in Walid's care, is a relatively new paradigm named integrative oncology [1]. Integrative medicine (in Arabic, *al tibb al mudmaj*) calls for incorporation of CM within the conventional medical care and is provided in ongoing number of leading oncology centers across the globe (e.g., MD Anderson Cancer Center [2], Memorial Sloan-Kettering Cancer Center [3]) aiming to improve patients' well-being and ensure the safety of complementary practices, particularly concerning herbal supplement/chemotherapy interactions [4]. The integrative medicine consultation and treatment provided to Walid within the oncology department in Haifa was provided within the setting of integrative oncology program operated within the department area whereas CM-trained physicians and practitioners are working next to oncologists, nurses, and social workers [5]. The integrative process Walid experienced was expressed in various levels: referral to IP consultation was provided by the nurse oncologist; the IP assessment was documented in his medical file; tailoring of Walid's treatment plan was performed in regard to his leading concerns and symptoms supplemented with evidence-based research; risk assessment was performed regarding potential interactions of herbs with the chemotherapy Walid was treated with; and communication was initiated by the IP with the patients' oncologist and the other health care providers. Last but not least, the primary objective of the

IP was focused on improving Walid's quality of life (QOL) and well-being rather than on extending his survival by adding anti-cancer treatments. Nevertheless, this setting of integrative medicine provided within supportive cancer care is seldom recognized in most oncology centers across the Middle-East. In most cases, the use of complementary medicine (*al tibb al-mukamel*) or traditional medicine (*al tibb al-taklidi*) is dichotomized from conventional cancer care and non-conventional care is regarded as *alternative* medicine (*al tibb al-badil*). In practice, this dichotomy means that patients tend to avoid disclosure of CM use to their oncologists and health care providers and do not expect them to provide a non-judgmental consultation regarding CM efficacy and safety [6].

Prevalence of Complementary Medicine Use in Cancer across the Middle-East

The concept of traditional medicine in the Middle-East is associated with rich spectrum of historical, religious, and cultural roots embedded in the great medical schools of Egypt, Mesopotamia, ancient Greece, and Persia followed by the monotheistic input of the Judaism, Christianity, and Islam. Islamic medicine, often related as Greco-Arab medicine, is the dominant traditional school of medicine in the Middle-East, and incorporates both Greco-western and Far-eastern medical influences. In modern times, Islamic medicine with its fascinating amalgam of herbs, alchemy, mind-body-spirit and manual practices, had become secondary to conventional medicine, especially in life-threatening disease such as cancer. Nowadays, conventional oncology care is the leading medical system across the Middle-East where many of cancer care practitioners may regard traditional medicine as non-efficacious, harmful, and charlatan [7]. Yet, the prevalence of CM use among patients with cancer in the Middle-East is high and ranges from 35% in Iran [8] to 46% in Morocco [9], 51% in Israel [10], 57% in Turkey [11], 90% in Saudi-Arabia [12] and nearly 100% in Jordan [13]. Herbal medicine is the leading CM modality among patients with cancer in the Middle-East and its prevalence use ranges from 32% in Turkey [14] to 35.5% in Jordan [15], and 60.9% in the Palestinian Authority [16]. The gap between this extensive CM use among patients and cancer and perspectives of their health care practitioners is associated with high rate of non-disclosure of CM use and significantly impact doctor-patient communication. For example, in Turkey, Yildirim et al. studied women with metastatic disease and reported that 60% of CM users had not discussed CM use with their physicians or nurses [17].

Leading Integrative Oncology Research Foci in the Middle-East

In table 1, integrative oncology research themes are presented in regard to countries that lead publications in basic and clinical studies. Turkey, Israel, and Iran are the leading triad in terms of publication number (>40 publications in each country) followed by Saudi-Arabia, Morocco, Jordan, and Lebanon (>15). Uprising number of publications is recorded recently also in the Palestinian authority, Egypt, and Tunisia. Although each country has distinct research resources and interest, six prominent research foci can be identified in the region which includes Turkey, Israel, Iran, Jordan-Palestinian authority-Lebanon, Egypt-Saudi Arabia-Yemen, and Morocco-Tunisia.

Table 1. Complementary medicine (CM) research themes in oncology across the Middle-East

Country	Publication range (publication number)	Leading research themes	Researched CM modalities	Prevalence of cancer-related CM use
Egypt	>10	In-vitro research (herbs) Animal studies (herbs) Clinical studies: Honey & mucositis; Viscum Album & advanced cancer	Herbal medicine	Unpublished
Iran	>40	CM use traits Psycho-oncology & CM Ethno-pharmacological research In-vitro research (herbs) Clinical studies: Honey & mucositis; Zinc & mucositis; Ginger & nausea; HESA-A & QOL in palliative care; Praying during chemotherapy; Manual therapy & pain, fatigue; Spirituality & QOL during radiotherapy; omega-3 & neuropathy	Islamic medicine Prayer/spiritual healing Dietary supplements & herbal medicine	32, 35%
Israel	>50	CM use & Doctor-patient communication CM education in cancer care Ethics & CM regulation Psycho-oncology & CM Ethno-botanical research In-vitro research (herbs) Animal studies (herbs) Clinical studies: Wheatgrass & hematological toxicity; Viscum Album & ascites; Art therapy &fatigue, depression; Homeopathy & stomatitis : Guided Imagery & relaxation; Hypnosis & xerostomia	Herbal medicine Dietary supplements Islamic medicine TCM/acupuncture Mind-body & spirituality Anthropsophic medicine	Gynecology: 63% Pediatrics: 61% Hematology: 51% During chemo: 49% Head & neck: 6%
Jordan	>15	CM use traits & Doctor-patient communication Ethno-pharmacological research In-vitro research (herbs)	Herbal medicine Dietary supplements	Herbal use:35% Pediatrics: 65%
Lebanon	>15	In-vitro research (herbs)	Herbal medicine	Pediatrics: 15%
Morocco	>15	CM use traits In-vitro research (herbs)	Herbal medicine Islamic medicine	46%
Palestine authority	>10	Ethno-botanical research Ethno-pharmacological research	Herbal medicine	Herbal use:61%

Country	Publication range (publication number)	Leading research themes	Researched CM modalities	Prevalence of cancer-related CM use
Saudi-Arabia	>30	CM safety & quality assurance In-vitro research (herbs)	Herbal medicine	95%
Syria	1	Ethno-botanical research	Unpublished	Unpublished
Tunisia	>10	In-vitro research (herbs)	Herbal medicine	Unpublished
Turkey	>50	CM use traits Doctor-patient communication CM education in cancer care In-vitro research (herbs) Animal studies (herbs) Clinical studies: Acupressure & nausea; Post-op breathing exercises; Henna & hand-foot synd.; Kefir yogurt; Yoga & QOL; CM & radiotherapy; Relaxation & fatigue	Herbs &supplements TCM/acupuncture Mind-body Dance therapy	Pediatrics:73-77% Gynecology: 61% Overall use: 57% Advanced CA:51% During radiotherapy: 43%
Yemen	3	Ethno-pharmacological research In-vitro research (herbs)	Herbal medicine	Unpublished

In Turkey, many articles focus on the prevalence of CM use among different cohorts of patients with cancer [18,19,20,21,22,23,24,25] that also include specific populations: pediatrics (73-77% CM use) [26,27], gynecology (61%) [28], advanced cancer and palliative care (51%) [29] as well as patients during radiotherapy (43%) [30]. The spectrum of CM modalities studied in Turkey includes the use of herbs &supplements, Mind-body interventions [32], and dance therapy [33]. Some of the articles focus on CM use in regard to doctor-patient communication [34] and CM education in cancer care. Basic science research is mainly related to herbal medicine and include in-vitro [36,37,38,39] and animal studies [40,41]. Clinical research in integrative oncology is highly developed in Turkey and include studies on acupressure for improving chemotherapy-induced nausea [42,43], breathing exercises to improve post-operation outcomes [44], relaxation to improve cancer-related fatigue [45], yoga for quality of life improvement [46], and other studies on topical henna application in hand-foot syndrome [47], kefir yogurt [48], and CM in radiotherapy setting [49].

In Israel, several articles examine CM use [50] and its ramifications on doctor-patient communication [51,52,53,54] ethics and CM regulation [55,56], The research setting includes variety of malignancies (gynecology [57], pediatrics [58], hematology [59], head & neck [60], etc.) and is more focused on CM use during chemotherapy and active oncology treatment [61]. In Israeli studies, the spectrum of CM modalities is broader and resembles CM use in Europe and the US. Thus, in addition to studies on herbal [62] and traditional Islamic medicine [63,64] research covers also dietary supplements [35], traditional Chinese medicine and acupuncture [65], mind-body [66], spirituality [67], and Anthropsophic medicine [68]. Research also include topics in psycho-oncology and its relatedness to CM [5,69] as well as medical education themes on CM in cancer care [70.71]. Similar to Turkey, scientific research in Israel on CM and cancer include a rich combination of ethno-botanical research [72], in-vitro [73,74,75,76,77] and animal studies on herbs [78.79], and clinical studies in the following topics: The use of wheatgrass juice in reducing hematological toxicity of chemotherapy in advanced breast cancer [80], the Anthroposophic herb viscum Album in reducing ascites and QOL improvement in advanced cancer [81], art therapy in improving fatigue and depression [82], homeopathy and stomatitis prevention [83], guided imagery and relaxation [84], and xerostomia treatment with hypnosis [85].

In Iran, integrative oncology research focus less on the prevalence of CM use [86,87,88,89] and offer more contemplation at Islamic medicine [90], prayer/spiritual healing [91], and psycho-oncology [92,93] in addition to research on dietary and herbal supplements [94]. Ethno-pharmacological research [95] is supplemented by in-vitro herbal studies [96,97,98,99,100,101,102,103,104] but like in Turkey and Israel, clinical research is the prominent scientific arena. Clinical studies include research on mucositis treatment by honey [105] or zinc [106], ginger and improved nausea [107,108], combined herbal-marine formula (HESA-A) on QOL in palliative care [109,110,111], influence of praying during chemotherapy [112] and spirituality on QOL [113] during radiotherapy [114], manual therapy outcome in alleviating pain and fatigue [115], and omega-3 supplementation on prevalence and severity of chemotherapy-induced neuropathy [116].

Research in Jordan, the Palestinian authority (PA), and Lebanon is centered primarily in the field of herbal medicine and include studies on the extensive prevalence of herbal use by patients with cancer [117,118] (including CM use in pediatric populations that ranges between 15% to 65% in Lebanon [119] and Jordan [120]), ethno-pharmacological/botanical research (extensive studies accomplished in Jordan [121, 122] and the PA [123,124,125,126,127,128]) and impressive in-vitro herbal research [129,130] focusing on the anti-tumor effect of indigenous [131,132,133,134] and popular herbs used daily in the Arab cuisine (e.g., Origanum [135,136] and Salvia species [137,138,139]) as well as plants used on the context of traditional Islamic medicine (e.g., Nigella sativa or black cumin known in Arabic as the *seed of blessing*) [140].

Herbal-oriented research is also prominent in Egypt, Saudi Arabia, and Yemen. In these countries, basic science research is oriented in traditional Islamic herbs and folk therapies including black seed [141,142,143], honey [144], ginger [145], olive oil [146], fennel [147], fenugreek [148,149], and turmeric [150]. In contrast with the emphasis on in-vitro studies [151,152,153,154,155,156,157,158], clinical research is limited (e.g., clinical Egyptian studies on honey in relieving radio- and chemotherapy-induced mucositis [159] and Viscum Album in advanced cancer [160]) as well as research on the use and safety of CM among patients with cancer (except few studies from Saudi-Arabia) [161,162,163].

As in other Muslim countries, integrative oncology research in the Maghreb countries of North-West Africa is centered with indigenous herbal medicine. Research is oriented with French medical literature and thus publication bias may prevail in leading English-oriented database. In Morocco, several studies were published on CM use of cancer among patients afflicted with cancer [164] including in pediatric [165] and hemato-oncology [166] settings. Except one interesting study on the impact of cancer on religiosity in the context of spirituality [167], most studies in Morocco and Tunisia are centered on herbal laboratory studies [168,169,170,171,172,173,174] and await sound clinical research.

DEBATE ON THE OBJECTIVES OF INTEGRATIVE ONCOLOGY

The role of traditional and complementary medicine in the care of patients with cancer in the Middle-East is questioned by patients, clinicians, and researchers across the region. The high prevalence of CM use among patients with cancer is a cause for debate and dilemmas as well as opportunity to improve the depth of supportive care. Dilemmas on integrative oncology role and objectives include the following aspects:

a. Communication with Patients on CM Use: *To Ask or Overlook?*

Discrepancy between patients' and health care providers' perspectives on CM role in cancer care may potentially lead to patient-doctor/health provider communication gap. This gap may lead to patients' hesitation to disclose CM use and that may impair patient's care in various aspects. First, patients in the Middle-East may use CM in the context of their health belief model and affinity with traditional medicine and thus inattentiveness to their narrative may affect their compliance with conventional care. Another outcome of ineffective communication is associated with undisclosed use of herbs and supplements that can potentially interact with chemotherapy, hormonal, and biological drugs. In contrast, nun-judgmental approach of the clinician on CM themes may trigger patients to openly disclose their needs and quality of life concerns.

Shift of the clinician's perspective regarding CM from alternative to complementary and integrative is generally welcomed by patients. As there are no "alternative" patients but only alternative set of mind, clinicians and patients alike should openly discuss CM and establish consent on their expectations regarding CM. In many cases, patients may expect their health care provider not only to discuss on complementary and traditional medicine use but also to consult or refer them to professional practitioners who can provide efficacious and safe evidence-based treatment.

b. Open-Minded Skepticism: *How to Ensure Efficacy and Safety?*

Complementary to non-judgmental attitude, clinicians need to display scientific rigorous attitude based on in-vitro studies and clinical research acknowledging the limitation of published Middle-Eastern research on CM and cancer.

This attitude, named by Prof. Aviad Haramati from Georgetown University in the US as open-minded skepticism [175], is the cornerstone of ethical approach balancing efficacy and safety aspects of integrative treatment. On one hand, patients and clinicians should be aware that the proverb "natural equal safe" is far from exact [176], but at the same time acknowledge the availability of free-accessed scientific database (e.g., Pubmed) that report of the increasing research volume on CM and herbal medicine efficacy and safety in the Middle-East region.

c. Establishing Realistic Treatment Objective: *Extending Survival or Improving Quality of Life?*

Based on current scientific evidence, the major role of CM in cancer care is within supportive and palliative care rather than extending patients' survival. Although some herbs may have potential impact on survival (e.g., the herb Astragalus combined with conventional drugs in non-small cell lung cancer) [177], most integrative oncology studies focus on quality of life improvement and reduction of oncology drug side effects [178,179]. In contrast, patients in the Middle-East may use CM not only for QOL improvement but may seek a "magical remedy" that will *destroy and beat cancer* and provide cure [180]. Thus, health care providers need not only to ask their patients on CM use but to contemplate on the context of use: Do patients expect CM to cure them? Do they expect CM to improve their well-being? Disclosure of patients' expectations should be followed by a discussion on less apparent and sometimes unconscious reasons for CM use: Do you seek CM because of unanswered questions (e.g., existential fear of death) or under controlled symptoms that impair your quality of life (e.g., nausea, pain)? Followed by these questions, the health care provider may suggest establishing realistic treatment goals that resonate with patients' concerns and the need for well-being improvement. As opposed to the alternative setting of charlatans that may promise cure to the dying patients, discussion in integrative oncology setting needs to create compassion and hope that are tuned with scientific evidence and ethical integrity.

Crossing across Barriers: Establishing Collaborative Integrative Oncology Care in the Middle-East

In recent years, the Middle-East Cancer Consortium (MECC), promotes collaborative multi-national and multi-disciplinary projects to foster integrative oncology research across the Middle-East. MECC is an intergovernmental consortium established in 1996 with a mission to promote cooperation among 6 Middle-Eastern countries in caring for patients with cancer [181]. At first, collaborative team of researchers from Israel, Egypt, Turkey, PA, and Morocco reviewed research published all over the Middle-East on CM in cancer care. Historical and ethno-botanical search was performed for cancer related keywords in Middle-Eastern traditional medicine resources which traced 44 herbs in historic prescriptions. A subsequent Medline search for studies conducted in the Middle-East regarding CAM and cancer care yielded 116 articles from 12 countries. Following, potential herbs were prioritized for further. clinical research by a team of four senior oncologists specializing in gynecologic oncology, breast cancer, pediatric oncology, and hemato-oncology. Findings were presented at an MECC Workshop on Integrative Medicine in Cancer Care in the Middle-East in June 2010 in Cyprus to an extended team of participants from the Middle-East, US, Europe and other countries operating integrative oncology initiatives. These sprouts of collaboration grew into joint research initiatives (MERGIO – Middle-Eastern Research Group in Integrative Oncology) that include study performed in 16 countries on overcoming barriers to integration of complementary and traditional medicine in supportive cancer care in the Middle-East. The main objectives of these research initiatives are to provide health care practitioners and patients reliable information on integrative supportive care, to improve patient-practitioner dialogue on CM, and to enrich clinicians with efficacious and safe integrative care modalities that promote supportive and palliative care.

In conclusion, the Middle-East is the one of the ancient roots of medical care and promise substantial traditional yet innovative modalities of care that can be integrated within supportive cancer care. Case studies, such as described with Walid, the 67-year-old Druze patient who encountered with pancreatic cancer, are not just exotic Arabian night's stories but suggest a potential for advanced integrative care that combine past, present, and future. Traditional and complementary medicine in the Middle-East should be recognized as a regional and world treasure of knowledge and skills that may be quarried, chiseled, processed, and exposed by teams of researchers, medical educators, and clinicians that collaborate beyond mistrust and apprehensiveness. Hopefully, integrative oncology setting as provided to Walid will eventually expand across the region from Morocco in the West to Iran in the East, and from Turkey in the North to Yemen in the South.

REFERENCES

[1] Deng GE, Cassileth BR, Cohen L, Gubili J, Johnstone PA, Kumar N, Vickers A; Society for Integrative Oncology Executive Committee, Abrams D, Rosenthal D, Sagar S, Tripathy D.Integrative Oncology Practice Guidelines. *J. Soc. Integr. Oncol.* 2007;5(2):65-84.

[2] Frenkel M, Cohen L, Peterson N, et al: Integrative medicine consultation service in a comprehensive cancer center: findings and outcomes. *Integr. Cancer Ther.* 2010;9(3):276-83.

[3] Deng G: Integrative Cancer Care in a US Academic Cancer Centre: The Memorial Sloan-Kettering Experience. *Curr. Oncol. Suppl.* 2008;2:s108.es68-71.

[4] Ben-Arye E, Schiff E, Zollman C, Heusser P, Mountford P, Frenkel M, Bar-Sela G, Lavie O. Integrating complementary medicine in supportive cancer care models across four continents .*Med. Oncol.* 2013;30(2):511.

[5] Ben-Arye E, Schiff E, Shapira C, Frenkel M, Shalom T, Steiner M. Modeling an integrative oncology program within a community-centered oncology service in Israel. *Patient Educ. Couns.* 2012;89(3):423-9.

[6] Ben-Arye E, Attias S, Tadmor T, Schiff E. Herbs in hemato-oncological care: an evidence-based review of data on efficacy, safety, and drug interactions. *Leuk Lymphoma.* 2010;51(8):1414-23.

[7] Al-Omari A, Al-Qudimat M, Abu Hmaidan A, Zaru L. Perception and attitude of Jordanian physicians towards complementary and alternative medicine (CAM) use in oncology. *Complement Ther. Clin. Pract.* 2013;19(2):70-6.

[8] Montazeri A, Sajadian A, Ebrahimi M, Haghighat S, Harirchi I (2007) Factors predicting the use of complementary and alternative therapies among cancer patients in Iran. *Eur. J. Cancer Care* (Engl). 16(2):144-149.

[9] Brahmi SA, El M'rabet FZ, Benbrahim Z, Akesbi Y, Amine B, Nejjari C, El Mesbahi O. Complementary medicine use among Moroccan patients with cancer: a descriptive study .*Pan Afr. Med. J.* 2011;10:36.

[10] Paltiel O, Avitzour M, Peretz T, Cherny N, Kaduri L, Pfeffer RM, Wagner N, Soskolne V .Determinants of the use of complementary therapies by patients with cancer. *J. Clin. Oncol.* 2001 ;19(9):2439-48.

[11] Yildiz I, Ozguroglu M, Toptas T, Turna H, Sen F, Yildiz M. Patterns of complementary and alternative medicine use among Turkish cancer patients. *J. Palliat. Med.* 2013;16(4):383-90.

[12] Jazieh AR, Al Sudairy R, Abulkhair O, Alaskar A, Al Safi F, Sheblaq N, Young S, Issa M, Tamim H. Use of complementary and alternative medicine by patients with cancer in Saudi Arabia. *J. Altern Complement Med.* 2012;18(11):1045-9.

[13] Akhu-Zaheya LM, Alkhasawneh EM. Complementary alternative medicine use among a sample of Muslim Jordanian oncology patients. *Complement Ther. Clin. Pract.* 2012;18(2):121-6.

[14] Inanç N, Sahin H, Ciçek B, Taşc S. Use of herbs or vitamin/mineral supplements by patients with cancer in Kayseri, Turkey. *Cancer Nurs.* 2006;29(1):17-20.

[15] Afifi FU, Wazaify M, Jabr M, Treish E. The use of herbal preparations as complementary and alternative medicine (CAM) in a sample of patients with cancer in Jordan. *Complement Ther. Clin. Pract.* 2010;16(4):208-12.

[16] Ali-Shtayeh MS, Jamous RM, Jamous RM. Herbal preparation use by patients suffering from cancer in Palestine. *Complement Ther. Clin. Pract.* 2011;17(4):235-40. doi: 10.1016/j.ctcp.2011.06.002.

[17] Yildirim Y. Patterns of the use of complementary and alternative medicine in women with metastatic cancer. *Cancer Nurs.* 2010;33(3):194-200.

[18] Akyol AD, Oz B. The use of complementary and alternative medicine by patients with cancer: in Turkey. *Complement Ther. Clin. Pract.* 2011;17(4):230-4.

[19] Malak AT, Karayurt ZL, Demir E, Y Mer AS. Complementary and alternative medicine in cancer patients - analysis of influencing factors in Turkey. *Asian Pac. J. Cancer Prev.* 2009;10(6):1083-7.

[20] Can G, Erol O, Aydiner A, Topuz E. Quality of life and complementary and alternative medicine use among cancer patients in Turkey. *Eur. J. Oncol. Nurs.* 2009;13(4):287-94.

[21] Özcelik, H, Fadiloglu. [Reasons for use of complementary and alternative medicine in cancer patients]. Türk Onkoloji Dergisi, 2009;24(1):48-52.

[22] Yazar Adı: Ucan O, Pehlivan S, Ovayolu N, Sevinc A, Camci C. The use of complementary therapies in cancer patients: a questionnaire-based descriptive survey from southeastern Turkey. *Am. J. Clin. Oncol.* 2008;31(6):589-94.

[23] Er O, Mistik S, Ozkan M, Ozturk A, Altinbas M. Factors related to complementary/alternative medicine use among cancer patients in central Anatolia. *Tumori.* 2008;94(6):833-7.

[24] Yildirim Y, Tinar S, Yorgun S, Toz E, Kaya B, Sonmez S, Balsak D. The use of complementary and alternative medicine (CAM) therapies by Turkish women with gynecological cancer. *Eur. J. Gynaecol. Oncol.* 2006;27(1):81-5.

[25] Yildiz I, Ozguroglu M, Toptas T, Turna H, Sen F, Yildiz M. Patterns of complementary and alternative medicine use among Turkish cancer patients. *J. Palliat Med.* 2013;16(4):383-90.

[26] Genc RE, Senol S, Turgay AS, Kantar M. Complementary and alternative medicine used by pediatric patients with cancer in western Turkey. *Oncol. Nurs Forum.* 2009;36(3):E159-64.

[27] Karalı Y, Demirkaya M, Sevinir B. Use of complementary and alternative medicine in children with cancer: effect on survival. *Pediatr Hematol Oncol.* 2012;29(4):335-44.

[28] Nazik E, Nazik H, Api M, Kale A, Aksu M. Complementary and alternative medicine use by gynecologic oncology patients in Turkey. *Asian Pac. J. Cancer Prev.* 2012;13(1):21-5.

[29] Tarhan O, Alacacioglu A, Somali I, Sipahi H, Zencir M, Oztop I, Dirioz M, Yilmaz U. Complementary-alternative medicine among cancer patients in the western region of Turkey. *J. BUON.* 2009;14(2):265-9.

[30] Aksu MG, Bozcuk HS, Korcum AF. Effect of complementary and alternative medicine during radiotherapy on radiation toxicity. *Support Care Cancer.* 2008 ;16(4):415-9.

[31] Inanç N, Sahin H, Ciçek B, Taşc S. Use of herbs or vitamin/mineral supplements by patients with cancer in Kayseri, Turkey. *Cancer Nurs.* 2006;29(1):17-20.

[32] Ulger O, Yağli NV. Effects of yoga on the quality of life in cancer patients. *Complement Ther. Clin. Pract.* 2010;16(2):60-3.

[33] Aktas G, Ogce F. Dance as a therapy for cancer prevention. *Asian Pac. J. Cancer Prev.* 2005;6(3):408-11.

[34] Yildirim Y. Patterns of the use of complementary and alternative medicine in women with metastatic cancer. *Cancer Nurs.* 2010;33(3):194-200.

[35] Akyuz A, Dede M, Cetinturk A, Yavan T, Yenen MC, Sarici SU, Dilek S. Self-application of complementary and alternative medicine by patients with gynecologic cancer. *Gynecol. Obstet. Invest.* 2007;64(2):75-81.

[36] Unyayar A, Demirbilek M, Turkoglu M, Celik A, Mazmanci MA, Erkurt EA, Unyayar S, Cekic O, Atacag H. Evaluation of cytotoxic and mutagenic effects of Coriolus versicolor and Funalia trogii extracts on mammalian cells. *Drug Chem. Toxicol.* 2006;29(1):69-83.

[37] Ozmen A, Bauer S, Gridling M, Singhuber J, Krasteva S, Madlener S, Vo TP, Stark N, Saiko P, Fritzer-Szekeres M, Szekeres T, Askin-Celik T, Krenn L, Krupitza G. In vitro anti-neoplastic activity of the ethno-pharmaceutical plant Hypericum adenotrichum Spach endemic to Western Turkey. *Oncol. Rep.* 2009;22(4):845-52.

[38] Turan N, Akgün-Dar K, Kuruca SE, Kiliçaslan-Ayna T, Seyhan VG, Atasever B, Meriçli F, Carin M. Cytotoxic effects of leaf, stem and root extracts of Nerium oleander on leukemia cell lines and role of the p-glycoprotein in this effect. *J. Exp. Ther. Oncol.* 2006;6(1):31-8.

[39] Ozmen A, Madlener S, Bauer S, Krasteva S, Vonach C, Giessrigl B, Gridling M, Viola K, Stark N, Saiko P, Michel B, Fritzer-Szekeres M, Szekeres T, Askin-Celik T, Krenn L, Krupitza G. In vitro anti-leukemic activity of the ethno-pharmacological plant Scutellaria orientalis ssp. carica endemic to western Turkey. *Phytomedicine.* 2010;17(1):55-62.

[40] Taşkin EI, Akgün-Dar K, Kapucu A, Osanç E, Doğruman H, Eraltan H, Ulukaya E. Apoptosis-inducing effects of Morinda citrifolia L. and doxorubicin on the Ehrlich ascites tumor in Balb-c mice. *Cell Biochem. Funct.* 2009;27(8):542-6.

[41] Yazici ZM, Meric A, Midi A, Arınc YV, Kahya V, Hafız G. Reduction of cisplatin ototoxicity in rats by oral administration of pomegranate extract. *Eur. Arch. Otorhinolaryngol.* 2012;269(1):45-52.

[42] Genç A, Can G, Aydiner A. The efficiency of the acupressure in prevention of the chemotherapy-induced nausea and vomiting. *Support Care Cancer*. 2013;21(1):253-61.

[43] Taspinar A, Sirin A. Effect of acupressure on chemotherapy-induced nausea and vomiting in gynecologic cancer patients in Turkey. *Eur. J. Oncol. Nurs*. 2010;14(1):49-5.

[44] Genç A, Ikiz AO, Güneri EA, Günerli A. Effect of deep breathing exercises on oxygenation after major head and neck surgery. *Otolaryngol Head Neck Surg.* 2008;139(2):281-5.

[45] Demiralp M, Oflaz F, Komurcu S. Effects of relaxation training on sleep quality and fatigue in patients with breast cancer undergoing adjuvant chemotherapy. *J. Clin. Nurs.* 2010;19(7-8):1073-83.

[46] Ulger O, Yağli NV. Effects of yoga on the quality of life in cancer patients. *Complement Ther. Clin. Pract*. 2010;16(2):60-3.

[47] Yucel I, Guzin G. Topical henna for capecitabine induced hand-foot syndrome. *Invest New Drugs*. 2008;26(2):189-92.

[48] Can G, Topuz E, Derin D, Durna Z, Aydiner A. Effect of kefir on the quality of life of patients being treated for colorectal cancer. *Oncol. Nurs Forum*. 2009;36(6):E335-42.

[49] Aksu MG, Bozcuk HS, Korcum AF. Effect of complementary and alternative medicine during radiotherapy on radiation toxicity. *Support Care Cancer*. 2008;16(4):415-9.

[50] Pud D, Kaner E, Morag A, Ben-Ami S, Yaffe A. Use of complementary and alternative medicine among cancer patients in Israel. *Eur. J. Oncol Nurs*. 2005;9(2):124-30.

[51] Ben-Arye E, Steinmetz D, Ezzo J. Two women and cancer – The need for addressing spiritual well-being in cancer care. *Families Systems and Health*. 2007;25(1):1-9.

[52] Frenkel M, Ben-Arye E, Baldwin CD, Sierpina V. An Approach to Communicating with Patients about the Use of Nutritional Supplements in Cancer Care. *Southern Medical Journal*. 2005; 98(3):289-294.

[53] Ben-Arye E, Frenkel M. [Doctor, patient and cancer in the encounter of complementary and conventional medicine]. *The Israel Journal of Family Practice*. 2004; 14(114-115): 11-17.

[54] Popper-Giveon A, Schiff E, Ben-Arye E. I will always be with you: traditional and complementary therapists' perspectives on patient-therapist-doctor communication regarding treatment of Arab patients with cancer in Israel. *Patient Educ. Couns.* 2012;89(3):381-6.

[55] Barak F, Lugacy G, Kreitler S. Complementary medicine regulations. *Patient Educ. Couns.* 2008;73(1):166-7.

[56] Ben-Arye E, Schiff E, Golan O. Ethical issues in integrative oncology. *Hematology/Oncology Clinics of North America*. 2008;22(4):737-53.

[57] Ben-Arye E, Schiff E, Steiner M, Keshet Y, Lavie O. Attitudes of patients with gynecological and breast cancer toward integration of complementary medicine in cancer care. *Int. J. Gynecol Cancer*. 2012;22(1):146-5.

[58] Weyl Ben Arush M, Geva H, Ofir R, Mashiach T, Uziel R, Dashkovsky Z. Prevalence and characteristics of complementary medicine used by pediatric cancer patients in a

mixed western and middle-eastern population. *J. Pediatr Hematol. Oncol.* 2006;28(3):141-6.

[59] Paltiel O, Avitzour M, Peretz T, Cherny N, Kaduri L, Pfeffer RM, Wagner N, Soskolne V. Determinants of the use of complementary therapies by patients with cancer. *J. Clin. Oncol.* 2001;19(9):2439-48.

[60] Talmi YP, Yakirevitch A, Migirov L, Horowitz Z, Bedrin L, Simon Z, Pfeffer MR. Limited use of complementary and alternative medicine in Israeli head and neck cancer patients. *Laryngoscope.* 2005;115(8):1505-8.

[61] Ben-Arye E, Bar-Sela G, Frenkel M, Kuten A, Hermoni D. Is a bio-psycho-social-spiritual approach relevant to cancer treatment? A study of patients and oncology staff members on issues of complementary medicine and spirituality. *Supportive Care in Cancer.* 2006; 14(2):147-52.

[62] Ben-Arye E, Attias S, Tadmor T, Schiff E. Herbs in hemato-oncological care: an evidence-based review of data on efficacy, safety, and drug interactions. *Leuk Lymphoma.* 2010;51(8):1414-23.

[63] Zaid H, Rayan A, SaidO, Saad B. Cancer Treatment by Greco-Arab and Islamic Herbal Medicine. *The Open Nutraceuticals Journal,* 2010; 3.

[64] Popper-Giveon A, Schiff E, Ben-Arye E. We and They in the House of Healing: Debate Among Arab Complementary Medicine Practitioners on an Integrative Versus Alternative Approach to Supportive Cancer Care. *Integr. Cancer Ther.* 2013 Apr 26.

[65] Samuels N. [Acupuncture for cancer patients: why not?] *Harefuah.* 2002;141(7):608-10, 666.

[66] Baider L, Uziely B, De-Nour AK. Progressive muscle relaxation and guided imagery in cancer patients. *Gen. Hosp. Psychiatry.* 1994;16(5):340-7.

[67] Ben-Arye E, Schiff E, Vintal H, Agour O, Preis L, Steiner M. Integrating complementary medicine and supportive care: patients' perspectives toward complementary medicine and spirituality. *J. Altern Complement Med.* 2012;18(9):824-3.

[68] Bar-Sela G, Haim N. Abnoba-viscum (mistletoe extract) in metastatic colorectal carcinoma resistant to 5-fluorouracil and leucovorin-based chemotherapy. *Med. Oncol.* 2004;21(3):251-4.

[69] Gilbar O, Iron G, Goren A. Adjustment to illness of cancer patients treated by complementary therapy along with conventional therapy. *Patient Educ. Couns.* 2001;44(3):243-9.

[70] Ben-Arye E, Frenkel M, Bar-sela G, Stashefsky Margalit R, Hermoni D, Kuten A. Teaching Complementary Medicine at an Academic Oncology Department. Accepted for publication in *J. Cancer Education.* 2008;23(1):46-50.

[71] Ben-Arye E, Frenkel M. An approach to teaching physicians about CAM in the treatment of cancer. *Integr. Cancer Ther.* 2004;3(3):208-213.

[72] Said O, Khalil K, Fulder S, Azaizeh H. Ethnopharmacological survey of medicinal herbs in Israel, the Golan Heights and the West Bank region. *J. Ethnopharmacol.* 2002;83(3):251-65.

[73] Dudai N, Weinstein Y, Krup M, Rabinski T, Ofir R. Citral is a new inducer of caspase-3 in tumor cell lines. *Planta Med.* 2005;71(5):484-8.

[74] Lev-Ari S, Vexler A, Starr A, Ashkenazy-Voghera M, Greif J, Aderka D, Ben-Yosef R. Curcumin augments gemcitabine cytotoxic effect on pancreatic adenocarcinoma cell lines. *Cancer Invest*. 2007;25(6):411-8.

[75] Rubnov S, Kashman Y, Rabinowitz R, Schlesinger M, Mechoulam R. Suppressors of cancer cell proliferation from fig (Ficus carica) resin: isolation and structure elucidation. *J. Nat. Prod*. 2001;64(7):993-6.

[76] Tamir S, Eizenberg M, Somjen D, Stern N, Shelach R, Kaye A, Vaya J. Estrogenic and antiproliferative properties of glabridin from licorice in human breast cancer cells. *Cancer Res*. 2000 ;60(20):5704-9.

[77] Lansky EP, Harrison G, Froom P, Jiang WG. Pomegranate (Punica granatum) pure chemicals show possible synergistic inhibition of human PC-3 prostate cancer cell invasion across Matrigel. *Invest New Drugs*. 2005;23(2):121-2.

[78] Hochman N, Houri-Haddad Y, Koblinski J, Wahl L, Roniger M, Bar-Sinai A, Weiss EI, Hochman J. Cranberry juice constituents impair lymphoma growth and augment the generation of antilymphoma antibodies in syngeneic mice. *Nutr. Cancer*. 2008;60(4):511-7.

[79] Hong-Fen L, Waisman T, Maimon Y, Shakhar K, Rosenne E, Ben-Eliyahu S. The effects of a Chinese herb formula, anti-cancer number one (ACNO), on NK cell activity and tumor metastasis in rats. *Int. Immunopharmacol*. 2001;1(11):1947-56.

[80] Bar-Sela G, Tsalic M, Fried G, Goldberg H. Wheat grass juice may improve hematological toxicity related to chemotherapy in breast cancer patients: a pilot study. *Nutr. Cancer*. 2007;58(1):43-8.

[81] Bar-Sela G, Goldberg H, Beck D, Amit A, Kuten A. Reducing malignant ascites accumulation by repeated intraperitoneal administrations of a Viscum album extract. *Anticancer Res*. 2006;26(1B):709-13.

[82] Bar-Sela G, Atid L, Danos S, Gabay N, Epelbaum R. Art therapy improved depression and influenced fatigue levels in cancer patients on chemotherapy. *Psychooncology*. 2007;16(11):980-4.

[83] Oberbaum M, Yaniv I, Ben-Gal Y, Stein J, Ben-Zvi N, Freedman LS, Branski D. A randomized, controlled clinical trial of the homeopathic medication TRAUMEEL S in the treatment of chemotherapy-induced stomatitis in children undergoing stem cell transplantation. *Cancer*. 2001 1;92(3):684-90.

[84] Baider L, Peretz T, Hadani PE, Koch U. Psychological intervention in cancer patients: a randomized study. *Gen. Hosp. Psychiatry*. 2001;23(5):272-7.

[85] Schiff E, Mogilner GJ, Sella E, Doweck I, Hershko O, Ben-Arye E, Yarom N. Hypnosis for Post-Radiation Xerostomia in Head and Neck Cancer Patients: A Pilot Study. *Journal of Pain and Symptom Management*. 2009;37(6):1086-1092.

[86] Rezaei M, Adib-Hajbaghery M, Seyedfatemi N, Hoseini F (2008) Prayer in Iranian cancer patients undergoing chemotherapy. *Complement Ther. Clin. Pract* 14(2):90-97.

[87] Geva H, Bar-Sela G, Zhana D, Mashiach T, Robinson E. The use of complementary and alternative therapies by cancer patients in northern Israel. *Isr Med Assoc J*. 2005 7(4):243-7.

[88] Montazeri A, Sajadian A, Ebrahimi M, Akbari ME. Depression and the use of complementary medicine among breast cancer patients. *Support Care Cancer*. 2005;13(5):339-42.

[89] Montazeri A, Sajadian A, Ebrahimi M, Haghighat S, Harirchi I. Factors predicting the usc of complementary and alternative therapies among cancer patients in Iran. *Eur. J. Cancer Care* (Engl). 2007;16(2):144-9.

[90] Emami SA, Sahebkar A, Tayarani-Najaran N, Tayarani-Najaran Z. Cancer and its Treatment in Main Ancient Books of Islamic Iranian Traditional Medicine (7th to 14th Century AD. *Iran Red Crescent Me.d J.* 2012;14(12):747-57.

[91] Khorami Markani A, Yaghmaei F, Khodayari Fard M. Spirituality as experienced by Muslim oncology nurses in Iran. *Br. J. Nurs.* 2013;22(4):S22-4, S26-8.

[92] Montazeri A, Sajadian A, Ebrahimi M, Akbari ME. Depression and the use of complementary medicine among breast cancer patients. *Support Care Cancer.* 2005;13(5):339-42.

[93] Harandy TF, Ghofranipour F, Montazeri A, Anoosheh M, Bazargan M, Mohammadi E, Ahmadi F, Niknami S. Muslim breast cancer survivor spirituality: coping strategy or health seeking behavior hindrance? *Health Care Women Int.* 2010;31(1):88-98.

[94] Ahmadi A, Mohagheghi MA, Fazeli MS, Nahavandian B, Bashardoost N, Musavi Jarahi A, Gharipoor M. HESA-A: new treatment for breast cancer and choroidal metastasis. *Med. Sci. Monit.* 2005;11(6):CR300-303.

[95] Amirghofran Z, Bahmani M, Azadmehr A, Javidnia K. Anticancer effects of various Iranian native medicinal plants on human tumor cell lines. *Neoplasma*. 2006;53(5):428-33.

[96] Tavakkol-Afshari J, Brook A, Mousavi SH. Study of cytotoxic and apoptogenic properties of saffron extract in human cancer cell lines. *Food Chem. Toxicol.* 2008;46(11):3443-7..

[97] Feizzadeh B, Afshari JT, Rakhshandeh H, Rahimi A, Brook A, Doosti H. Cytotoxic effect of saffron stigma aqueous extract on human transitional cell carcinoma and mouse fibroblast. *Urol. J.* 2008;5(3):161-7.

[98] Amirghofran Z, Bahmani M, Azadmehr A, Ashouri E, Javidnia K. Antitumor activity and apoptosis induction in human cancer cell lines by Dionysia termeana. *Cancer Invest.* 2007;25(7):550-4.

[99] Varamini P, Javidnia K, Soltani M, Mehdipour AR, Ghaderi A. Cytotoxic activity and cell cycle analysis of quinoline alkaloids isolated from Haplophyllum canaliculatum Boiss. *Planta Med.* 2009;75(14):1509-16.

[100] Amirghofran Z, Bahmani M, Azadmehr A, Javidnia K. Induction of apoptosis in leukemia cell lines by Linum persicum and Euphorbia cheiradenia. *J. Cancer Res. Clin. Oncol.* 2006;132(7):427-32.

[101] Varamini P, Soltani M, Ghaderi A. Cell cycle analysis and cytotoxic potential of Ruta graveolens against human tumor cell lines. *Neoplasma.* 2009;56(6):490-3.

[102] Rajabalian S. Methanolic extract of Teucrium polium L. potentiates the cytotoxic and apoptotic effects of anticancer drugs of vincristine, vinblastine and doxorubicin against a panel of cancerous cell lines. *Exp. Oncol.* 2008 ;30(2):133-8.

[103] Amirghofran Z, Bahmani M, Azadmehr A, Javidnia K. Anticancer effects of various Iranian native medicinal plants on human tumor cell lines. *Neoplasma*. 2006;53(5):428-33.

[104] Aghbali A, Hosseini SV, Delazar A, Gharavi NK, Shahneh FZ, Orangi M, Bandehagh A, Baradaran B. Induction of apoptosis by grape seed extract (Vitis vinifera) in oral squamous cell carcinoma .*Bosn J. Basic Med. Sci.* 2013;13(3):186-91.

[105] Motallebnejad M, Akram S, Moghadamnia A, Moulana Z, Omidi S. The effect of topical application of pure honey on radiation-induced mucositis: a randomized clinical trial. *J. Contemp Dent Pract*. 2008 Mar 1;9(3):40-7.

[106] Mansouri A, Hadjibabaie M, Iravani M, Shamshiri AR, Hayatshahi A, Javadi MR, Khoee SH, Alimoghaddam K, Ghavamzadeh A. The effect of zinc sulfate in the prevention of high-dose chemotherapy-induced mucositis: a double-blind, randomized, placebo-controlled study. *Hematol. Oncol*. 2012;30(1):22-6.

[107] Yekta ZP, Ebrahimi SM, Hosseini M, Nasrabadi AN, Sedighi S, Surmaghi MH, Madani H .Ginger as a miracle against chemotherapy-induced vomiting. *Iran J. Nurs Midwifery* Res. 2012;17(5):325-9.

[108] Panahi Y, Saadat A, Sahebkar A, Hashemian F, Taghikhani M, Abolhasani E. Effect of ginger on acute and delayed chemotherapy-induced nausea and vomiting: a pilot, randomized, open-label clinical trial. *Integr. Cancer Ther*. 2012;11(3):204-11.

[109] Ahmadi A, Mohagheghi M, Karimi M, Golestanha SA, Naseri M, Faghihzadeh S, Habibi G. Therapeutic effects of HESA-A in patients with end-stage metastatic cancers. *Integr. Cancer Ther*. 2010;9(1):32-5.

[110] Ahmadi A, Mohagheghi M, Karimi M, Seyed Ali Golestanha, Naseri M. Anticancer effects of HESA-A in patients with metastatic colon cancer. *Integr. Cancer Ther*. 2009;8(1):71-4.

[111] Ahmadi A, Mohagheghi MA, Fazeli MS, Nahavandian B, Bashardoost N, Musavi Jarahi A, Gharipoor M. HESA-A: new treatment for breast cancer and choroidal metastasis. *Med. Sci. Monit*. 2005;11(6):CR300-303.

[112] Rezaei M, Adib-Hajbaghery M, Seyedfatemi N, Hoseini F. Prayer in Iranian cancer patients undergoing chemotherapy.*Complement Ther. Clin. Pract*. 2008;14(2):90-7.

[113] Bahrami M, Balouchestani E, Amini A, Eghbali M. Assessing the effect of two praying methods on the life quality of patients suffering from cancer hospitalized at Seyedo Shohada medical center of Isfahan University of Medical Sciences. *Iran J. Nurs Midwifery Res*. 2010;15(Suppl 1):296-301.

[114] Jafari N, Zamani A, Farajzadegan Z, Bahrami F, Emami H, Loghmani A. The effect of spiritual therapy for improving the quality of life of women with breast cancer: a randomized controlled trial .*Psychol. Health Med*. 2013;18(1):56-69.

[115] Aghabati N, Mohammadi E, Pour Esmaiel Z. The Effect of Therapeutic Touch on Pain and Fatigue of Cancer Patients Undergoing Chemotherapy. *Evid. Based Complement Alternat Med*. 2008. [Epub ahead of print].

[116] Ghoreishi Z, Esfahani A, Djazayeri A, Djalali M, Golestan B, Ayromlou H, Hashemzade S, Asghari Jafarabadi M, Montazeri V, Keshavarz SA, Darabi M. Omega-3 fatty acids are protective against paclitaxel-induced peripheral neuropathy: a randomized double-blind placebo controlled trial .*BMC Cancer*. 2012;12:355.

[117] Afifi FU, Wazaify M, Jabr M, Treish E. The use of herbal preparations as complementary and alternative medicine (CAM) in a sample of patients with cancer in Jordan. *Complementary Therapies in Clinical Practice*, 2010; 16(4):208-212.

[118] Ali-Shtayeh MS, Jamous RM, Jamous RM. Herbal preparation use by patients suffering from cancer in Palestine, Complementary Therapies in Clinical Practice. In press, 2011.

[119] Naja F, Alameddine M, Abboud M, Bustami D, Al Halaby R. Complementary and Alternative Medicine Use Among Pediatric Patients With Leukemia: The Case of Lebanon. *Integr. Cancer Ther.* 2010 Nov 8.

[120] Al-Qudimat MR, Rozmus CL, Farhan N. Family strategies for managing childhood cancer: using complementary and alternative medicine in Jordan. *J. Adv. Nurs.* 2011 ;67(3):591-7.

[121] Afifi-Yazar FU, Kasabri V, Abu-Dahab R. Medicinal Plants from Jordan in the Treatment of Cancer: Traditional Uses vs. In vitro and In Vivo Evaluations - Part 1. *Planta Med.* 2011;77(11):1203-9.

[122] Abuharfeil NM, Salim M, Von Kleist S. Augmentation of natural killer cell activity in vivo against tumour cells by some wild plants from Jordan. *Phytother Res.* 2001. 15:109-13.

[123] Ali-Shtayeh MS, Daoud RTE, Jamous RM. Studies on folkloric medicinal plants used by Palestinians in the Qalqilia District. *Biodiversity and Environmental Sciences Studies Series,* 2010. 5(2).

[124] Ali-Shtayeh MS, Jamous RM, Al-Shafie' JH, Elgharabah WA, Kherfan FA, Qarariah KH, Khdair IS, Soos IM, Musleh AA, Isa BA, Herzallah HM, Khlaif RB, Aiash SM, Swaiti GM, Abuzahra MA, Haj-Ali MM, Saifi NA, Azem HK, Nasrallah HA. Traditional knowledge of wild edible plants used in Palestine (Northern West Bank): a comparative study. *J. Ethnobiol. Ethnomed.* 2008. 12;4:13.

[125] Ali-Shtayeh MS, Jamous RM. Ethnobotany of Palestinian herbal medicine in the northern West Bank and Gaza Strip: review and comprehensive field study. *Biodiversity and Environmental Sciences Studies Series.* 2006;4:1-122.

[126] Ali-Shtayeh MS, Yaniv Z, Mahajna J Ethnobotanical survey in the Palestinian area: a classification of the healing potential of medicinal plants. *J. Ethnopharmacol.* 2000;73(1-2):221-32.

[127] Kaileh M, Berghe WV, Boone E, Essawi T, Haegeman G. Screening of indigenous Palestinian medicinal plants for potential anti-inflammatory and cytotoxic activity. *J. Ethnopharmacol.* 2007.113:510-6.

[128] Jaradat NA. Ethnopharmacological Survey of Natural Products in Palestine. *An-Najah Univ. J. Res.* (N. Sc.), 2005. 19: 13-67.

[129] Alali FQ, Tawaha K, El-Elimat T, Qasaymeh R, Li C, Burgess J, Nakanishi Y, Kroll DJ, Wani MC, Oberlies N H. Phytochemical studies and cytotoxicity evaluations of Colchicum tunicatum Feinbr and Colchicum hierosolymitanum feinbr (Colchicaceae): 2 native Jordanian meadow saffrons. *Natural Product research, Part a: Structure and Synthesis.* 2006; 20:558-566.

[130] Zihlif M, Afifi F, Muhtaseb R, Al-Khatib S, Abaza I, Naffa R. Screening the antiangiogenic activity of medicinal plants grown and sold in Jordan. *Planta Med.* 2012 Feb;78(3):297-301.

[131] Abu-Dahab R, Afifi F. Antiproliferative activity of selected medicinal plants of Jordan against a breast adenocarcinoma cell line (MCF7). *Scientia Pharmaceutica* (Sci. Pharm.). 2007;75:121-136.

[132] Abuharfeil NM, Maraqa A, Von Kleist S. Augmentation of natural killer cell activity in vitro against tumor cells by wild plants from Jordan. *J. Ethnopharmacol.* 2000;71(1-2):55-63.

[133] Tohme R, Al Aaraj L, Ghaddar T, Gali-Muhtasib H, Saliba NA, Darwiche N. Differential growth inhibitory effects of highly oxygenated guaianolides isolated from the Middle Eastern indigenous plant Achillea falcata in HCT-116 colorectal cancer cells. *Molecules.* 2013;18(7):8275-88.

[134] El-Najjar N, Dakdouki S, Darwiche N, El-Sabban M, Saliba NA, Gali-Muhtasib H. Anti-colon cancer effects of Salograviolide A isolated from Centaurea ainetensis. *Oncol. Rep.* 2008;19(4):897-904.

[135] Al-Kalaldeh JZ, Abu-Dahab R, Afifi FU. Volatile oil composition and antiproliferative activity of Laurus nobilis, Origanum syriacum, Origanum vulgare, and Salvia triloba against human breast adenocarcinoma cells. *Nutr. Res.* 2010;30(4):271-8.

[136] Abdel-Massih RM, Fares R, Bazzi S, El-Chami N, Baydoun E. The apoptotic and anti-proliferative activity of Origanum majorana extracts on human leukemic cell line. *Leuk Res.* 2010;34(8):1052-6.

[137] Fiore G, Nencini C, Cavallo F, Capasso A, Bader A, Giorgi G, Micheli L. In vitro antiproliferative effect of six Salvia species on human tumor cell lines. *Phytother Res.* 2006;20(8):701-703.

[138] Deeb SJ, El-Baba CO, Hassan SB, Larsson RL, Gali-Muhtasib HU. Sage components enhance cell death through nuclear factor kappa-B signaling. *Front Biosci.* (Elite Ed). 2011;3:410-20.

[139] Itani WS, El-Banna SH, Hassan SB, Larsson RL, Bazarbachi A, Gali-Muhtasib HU. Anti colon cancer components from lebanese sage (Salvia libanotica) essential oil: Mechanistic basis. *Cancer Biol. Ther.* 2008 7(11).

[140] Gali-Muhtasib H, Diab-Assaf M, Boltze C, Al-Hmaira J, Hartig R, Roessner A, Schneider-Stock R .Thymoquinone extracted from black seed triggers apoptotic cell death in human colorectal cancer cells via a p53-dependent mechanism. *Int. J. Oncol.* 2004;25(4):857-66.

[141] Hasan TN, Shafi G, Syed NA, Alfawaz MA, Alsaif MA, Munshi A, Lei KY, Alshatwi AA. Methanolic extract of Nigella sativa seed inhibits SiHa human cervical cancer cell proliferation through apoptosis. *Nat. Prod. Commun.* 2013;8(2):213-6.

[142] Salim EI, Fukushima S. Chemopreventive potential of volatile oil from black cumin (Nigella sativa L.) seeds against rat colon carcinogenesis. *Nutr. Cancer.* 2003;45(2):195-202.

[143] el-Aziz MA, Hassan HA, Mohamed MH, Meki AR, Abdel-Ghaffar SK, Hussein MR. The biochemical and morphological alterations following administration of melatonin, retinoic acid and Nigella sativa in mammary carcinoma: an animal model. *Int. J. Exp. Pathol.* 2005;86(6):383-96.

[144] Mabrouk GM, Moselhy SS, Zohny SF, Ali EM, Helal TE, Amin AA, Khalifa AA. Inhibition of methylnitrosourea (MNU) induced oxidative stress and carcinogenesis by orally administered bee honey and Nigella grains in Sprague Dawely rats. *J. Exp. Clin. Cancer Res.* 2002;21(3):341-6.

[145] Elkady AI, Abuzinadah OA, Baeshen NA, Rahmy TR. Differential control of growth, apoptotic activity, and gene expression in human breast cancer cells by extracts derived from medicinal herbs Zingiber officinale. *J. Biomed. Biotechnol.* 2012;2012:614356.

[146] Elamin MH, Daghestani MH, Omer SA, Elobeid MA, Virk P, Al-Olayan EM, Hassan ZK, Mohammed OB, Aboussekhra A. Olive oil oleuropein has anti-breast cancer

properties with higher efficiency on ER-negative cells. *Food Chem. Toxicol.* 2013;53:310-6.

[147] Esmat A Hassan , Kamilia A B. (Studies on plants with special reference to their potential use in cancer care research. Improving productivity and accumulation of principal active components in fennel plant. *Egyptian Journal of Applied Science.* 2010; 25 (6A) :187-196.

[148] Al-Daghri NM, Alokail MS, Alkharfy KM, Mohammed AK, Abd-Alrahman SH, Yakout SM, Amer OE, Krishnaswamy S. Fenugreek extract as an inducer of cellular death via autophagy in human T lymphoma Jurkat cells. *BMC Complement Altern Med.* 2012;12:202.

[149] Khoja KK, Shaf G, Hasan TN, Syed NA, Al-Khalifa AS, Al-Assaf AH, Alshatwi AA. Fenugreek, a naturally occurring edible spice, kills MCF-7 human breast cancer cells via an apoptotic pathway. *Asian Pac. J. Cancer Prev.* 2011;12(12):3299-304.

[150] Mohamad RH, El-Bastawesy AM, Zekry ZK, Al-Mehdar HA, Al-Said MG, Aly SS, Sharawy SM, El-Merzabani MM. The role of Curcuma longa against doxorubicin (adriamycin)-induced toxicity in rats. *J. Med. Food.* 2009;12(2):394-402.

[151] Mothana RA, Lindequist U, Gruenert R, Bednarski PJ. Studies of the in vitro anticancer, antimicrobial and antioxidant potentials of selected Yemeni medicinal plants from the island Soqotra. *BMC Complement Altern Med.* 2009;9:7.

[152] Mothana RA, Grünert R, Lindequist U, Bednarski PJ. Study of the anticancer potential of Yemeni plants used in folk medicine. *Pharmazie.* 2007;62(4):305-7.

[153] Mothana RA, Kriegisch S, Harms M, Wende K, Lindequist U. Assessment of selected Yemeni medicinal plants for their in vitro antimicrobial, anticancer, and antioxidant activities. *Pharm. Biol.* 2011;49(2):200-10.

[154] Mahassni SH, Al-Reemi RM. Apoptosis and necrosis of human breast cancer cells by an aqueous extract of garden cress (Lepidium sativum) seeds.*Saudi J. Biol. Sci.* 2013;20(2):131-9.

[155] El-Obeid A, Al-Harbi S, Al-Jomah N, Hassib A. Herbal melanin modulates tumor necrosis factor alpha (TNF-alpha), interleukin 6 (IL-6) and vascular endothelial growth factor (VEGF) production. *Phytomedicine.* 2006;13(5):324-33.

[156] Hawas UW, Gamal-Eldeen AM, El-Toumy SA, Meyer JJ, Hussein AA. Inhibition of the initiation stage of carcinogenesis by Salvia disermas constituents. *Z Naturforsch C.* 2009;64(11-12):831-9.

[157] El-Shemy HA, Aboul-Enein AM, Aboul-Enein MI, Issa SI, Fujita K. The effect of willow leaf extracts on human leukemic cells in vitro. *J. Biochem. Mol. Biol.* 2003;36(4):387-9.

[158] Kamilia AB, Elmakawy AI, Abdelsalam A Z E , Daewish AM. Evaluation of antimutagenic activity of lettuce leaves against genotoxicity of chlorpyifos low doses in male mice. *J. of Comunicata Scientiae.* 2010 (in press).

[159] Rashad UM, Al-Gezawy SM, El-Gezawy E, Azzaz AN. Honey as topical prophylaxis against radiochemotherapy-induced mucositis in head and neck cancer. *J. Laryngol Otol.* 2008 May 19:1-6.

[160] Mabed M, El-Helw L, Shamaa S. Phase II study of viscum fraxini-2 in patients with advanced hepatocellular carcinoma. *Br. J. Cancer.* 2004;90(1):65-9.

[161] Jazieh AR, Al Sudairy R, Abulkhair O, Alaskar A, Al Safi F, Sheblaq N, Young S, Issa M, Tamim H. Use of complementary and alternative medicine by patients with cancer in Saudi Arabia .*J. Altern Complement Med.* 2012;18(11):1045-9.

[162] Bogusz MJ, al Tufail M, Hassan H. How natural are 'natural herbal remedies'? A Saudi perspective. *Adverse Drug React Toxicol Rev.* 2002;21(4):219-29.

[163] Albedah AM. Use of Complementary and Alternative Medicine by Cancer Patients in Saudi Arabia: A Paradox in Healthcare. *J. Altern Complement Med.* 2013 Apr 26. [Epub ahead of print].

[164] Brahmi SA, El M'rabet FZ, Benbrahim Z, Akesbi Y, Amine B, Nejjari C, El Mesbahi O. Complementary medicine use among Moroccan patients with cancer: a descriptive study. *Pan Afr. Med. J.* 2011;10:36.

[165] Hessissen L, Bhour M, El Kababri M, Kili A, Nachef MN, Elkhorassani M, Khattab M. Use of alternative medicine in a Moroccan pediatric oncology unit. *J. Afr Cancer.* 2011. DOI 10.1007/s12558-011-0177-6.

[166] Tazi I, Nafil H, Sifesalam M, Bouchtia M, Mahmal L. Prevalence of complementary and alternative medicine use in patients with hematological malignancies in Marrakech, Morocco. *J. Acupunct Meridian Stud.* 2013;6(2):67-8.

[167] Errihani H, Mrabti H, Boutayeb S, El Ghissassi I, El Mesbahi O, Hammoudi M, Chergui H, Riadi A. Impact of cancer on Moslem patients in Morocco. *Psychooncology.* 2008;17(1):98-100.

[168] Merghoub N, Benbacer L, Amzazi S, Morjani H, El mzibri M. Cytotoxic effect of some Moroccan medicinal plant extracts on human cervical cell lines. *Journal of Medicinal Plants Research,* 2009; 3(12):1045-1050.

[169] Chaouki W, Leger DY, Liagre B, Beneytout JL, Hmamouchi M. Citral inhibits cell proliferation and induces apoptosis and cell cycle arrest in MCF-7 cells. *Fundam Clin. Pharmacol.* 2009;23(5):549-56.

[170] Lamchouri F, Settaf A, Cherrah Y, Hassar M, Zemzami M, Atif N, Nadori EB, Zaid A, Lyoussi B. In vitro cell-toxicity of Peganum harmala alkaloids on cancerous cell-lines. *Fitoterapia.* 2000;71(1):50-4.

[171] Abdeljebbar LH, Benjouad A, Morjani H, Merghoub N, El Haddar S, Humam M, Christen P, Hostettmann K, Bekkouche K, Amzazi S. Antiproliferative effects of withanolides from Withania adpressa. *Therapie.* 2009;64(2):121-7.

[172] Abdeljebbar LH, Benjouad A, Morjani H, Merghoub N, El Haddar S, Humam M, Christen P, Hostettmann K, Bekkouche K, Amzazi S. Kilani-Jaziri S, Neffati A, Limem I, Boubaker J, Skandrani I, Sghair MB, Bouhlel I, Bhouri W, Mariotte AM, Ghedira K, Dijoux Franca MG, Chekir-Ghedira L.Relationship correlation of antioxidant and antiproliferative capacity of Cyperus rotundus products towards K562 erythroleukemia cells. *Chem Biol Interact.* 2009;181(1):85-94.

[173] Taamalli A, Arráez-Román D, Barrajón-Catalán E, Ruiz-Torres V, Pérez-Sánchez A, Herrero M, Ibañez E, Micol V, Zarrouk M, Segura-Carretero A, Fernández-Gutiérrez A. Use of advanced techniques for the extraction of phenolic compounds from Tunisian olive leaves: phenolic composition and cytotoxicity against human breast cancer cells. *Food Chem. Toxicol.* 2012 Jun;50(6):1817-25.

[174] El Bouzidi L, Mahiou-Leddet V, Bun SS, Larhsini M, Abbad A, Markouk M, Fathi M, Boudon M, Ollivier E, Bekkouche K. Cytotoxic withanolides from the leaves of Moroccan Withania frutescens .*Pharm Biol.* 2013;51(8):1040-6.

[175] Internet site: http://www.eurekalert.org/pub_releases/2001-09/gumc-gr090401.php accessed : 2 October 2013.

[176] Yang AK, He SM, Liu L, Liu JP, Wei MQ, Zhou SF. Herbal interactions with anticancer drugs: mechanistic and clinical considerations. *Curr. Med. Chem.* 2010;17(16):1635-78.

[177] McCulloch M, See C, Shu XJ, Broffman M, Kramer A, Fan WY, Gao J, Lieb W, Shieh K, Colford JM Jr. Astragalus-based Chinese herbs and platinum-based chemotherapy for advanced non-small-cell lung cancer: meta-analysis of randomized trials. *J. Clin. Oncol.* 2006;24(3):419-30.

[178] Bokmand S, Flyger H. Acupuncture relieves menopausal discomfort in breast cancer patients: a prospective, double blinded, randomized study. *Breast.* 2013;22(3):320-3.

[179] Barton DL, Liu H, Dakhil SR, Linquist B, Sloan JA, Nichols CR, McGinn TW, Stella PJ, Seeger GR, Sood A, Loprinzi CL. Wisconsin Ginseng (Panax quinquefolius) to Improve Cancer-Related Fatigue: A Randomized, Double-Blind Trial, N07C2. *J. Natl. Cancer Inst.* 2013;105(16):1230-8.

[180] Popper-Giveon A, Schiff E, Ben-Arye E. We and They in the House of Healing: Debate Among Arab Complementary Medicine Practitioners on an Integrative Versus Alternative Approach to Supportive Cancer Care. *Integr. Cancer Ther.* 2013 Apr 26. [Epub ahead of print].

[181] Silbermann M, Dweib Khleif A, Balducci L: Healing by cancer. *J. Clin. Oncol.* 28(8):1436-1437, 2010.

In: Palliative Care to the Cancer Patient
Editor: Michael Silbermann
ISBN: 978-1-63117-709-5

Chapter 8

PALLIATIVE CARE AT THE END-OF-LIFE FOR CANCER PATIENTS IN ISRAEL: SERVICES IN THE COMMUNITY

Ron Sabar, M.D., M.B.A.*[*1], Elon Richman, B.Sc.[2], Amit Ringel, B.A.[2], Dov Rosenbaum, M.P.H.[2] and Seema Biswas, M.B.B.S., M.Sc., F.R.C.S.[3]

[1]Sabar Clinics, Israel
[2]Medical School of International Health, Ben Gurion University, Israel
[3]Ziv Medical Center, Safed, Israel

INTRODUCTION

As in much of the rest of the world, palliative care as a medical specialty is relatively new in Israel. The following chapter describes the evolution of palliative care as a medical discipline in Israel, the development of community services, cultural factors in the demand and acceptance of end-of-life care among diverse populations in Israel, and key factors in the delivery of homecare to patients in order to significantly improve their quality of life.

The aim of the chapter is to provide useful models that are innovative and cost-saving in their implementation in the development of essential services with the support of the community. We begin with an explanation of the Israeli healthcare system and the changes it has undergone in order to make palliative care provision a reality in this country.

THE ISRAELI HEALTHCARE SYSTEM

The Israeli healthcare system is essentially a socialized one where, by law, every citizen is insured and entitled to services and medication under the basic health basket, which

* Address for correspondence: ronsabar@gmail.com

typically comprises essential elective and emergency primary, secondary and tertiary care at a cost to the individual of 5% of their salary deducted as a monthly contribution to health insurance (social insurance tax). Patients who are not employed or who are unable to afford this monthly fee are entitled to these same services, paid for by the government out of the public purse. Therefore, healthcare is universally available to all citizens. The health insurance contributions to the government fund four health maintenance organizations (HMO's). Social insurance taxes are progressive, hence, the more you earn, the more you pay. Payments are per person and not per family. Access to secondary (specialist) services is based on a gatekeeper model, meaning that most services require a referral from a primary care physician.

Individuals may choose to be insured by any HMO. Their selection is usually on the basis of the proximity of services to their home or recommendations from friends and family. They may choose HMO's and switch health plans and providers once a year by simply asking to do so and paying a minimal fee (about $5 per person). In practice, very few people actually make such a transition. Different family members may join different health plans. The HMO's cannot refuse anyone, regardless of medical condition or age. They serve as both insurers and providers of care through their own primary care clinics and through the funding of hospital services. In 2012, the OECD (Organization for Economic Co-operation and Development) ranked the Israeli healthcare system fourth in the world in terms of efficiency and quality of services (after Hong Kong, Singapore and Japan).

There are four HMO's in Israel. The basket of services they provide is determined each year by an independent professional committee composed of medical specialists, experts in ethics, economics and welfare, and representatives of the Ministries of Health and Finance, as well as delegates from the general public. All HMO's are obliged to provide all services agreed for inclusion within the basket. As a result, HMO's may compete only in the quality of the services they provide, not in the combination of the actual services within the basket. This is a factor in keeping costs competitive and building in affordable choices, albeit the package of services remains uniform. All medication typically used in palliative care, palliative care services, and hospitalizations (in-patient and home hospice) are included in the basic basket, with no co-payments or limitations on use.

The majority of healthcare professionals are employees of the public healthcare system, either in hospitals or in community clinics, and almost all hospitals are publicly (government) owned. About 85% of the population holds a supplementary health insurance package which allows them to purchase services in the ever-growing private healthcare market by simply paying out of pocket to the approved providers and reclaiming the costs from their insurance. These private packages afford patients the choice of physician and hospital, important in a culture that cherishes personal choice and direct access to the clinicians involved in decisions about their health and well-being.

The overall expenditure on health in Israel has been dropping over the last decade and is now approximately 7.5% of GDP, which is much below the OECD average. Further, the ratio of private to public funding has shifted in the last two decades from 30:70 to a burdensome 40:60. Both these changes over time are largely a result of a lack of long-term budget planning by successive Israeli governments. The health budget is determined annually and is inevitably influenced by real-time priorities, making it very difficult for health policy-makers to plan ahead. In addition, there is a need for an automatic increase factor of the budget of 2%

to reflect the rate of growth in the population. The greatest public healthcare expense is in-patient care of acutely and chronically ill patients.

THE EMERGENCE OF PALLIATIVE CARE SERVICES IN ISRAEL

Modern palliative care was established in Israel by the Israel Cancer Association (ICA) in the 1970's. They launched an oncology nurse training program, teaching the basis of pain management and symptom relief [1]. A major achievement came in 1983 when the ICA opened Israel's first in-patient hospice with 19 beds for adult cancer patients in the Sheba Medical Center. This was a turning point in public awareness of palliative care and its delivery.

The development of palliative care services continued in the 1980's and 90's through public and private suppliers with a range of medical personnel, professional training and services delivered. The mainstay of care, however, remained within the domain of Internal, Family and Geriatric Medicine, with dedicated palliative care training coming mainly from a unit in Ben Gurion University of the Negev, which went on to pioneer the palliative care training program within the Family Medicine residency.

It was not until the year 2000 that the Israeli government responded to repeated demands by palliative care physicians and organizations, such as the Israeli Palliative Medical Society, Israeli Cancer Association and Israeli Medical Association, that end-of-life care be fully addressed. A committee comprising representatives of the above organizations and representatives of the Ministry of Health was founded in order to address this need, with public engagement and discussion of sensitive end-of-life issues, eventually leading to the passing of the Death and Dying Act [3] in 2005, which defines the legal terms and conditions by which a patient can give end-of-life advance directives.

ADVANCE DIRECTIVES

Advance directives allow a dying person, defined as a person with a prognosis of six months or less to live, to direct medical staff to withhold life-sustaining treatment, including, for example, cardiopulmonary resuscitation, surgery and dialysis. Notably, the directive also includes the withholding of other life-sustaining treatment such as antibiotics, enteral feeding and intravenous fluids. The only health provision patients cannot refuse in an advance directive is palliative care – symptomatic relief.

Palliative care services and plans were developed in 2009 by the director-general of the Ministry of Health in consultation with a medical professional committee, leading to standardization in coverage of home palliative care plans and hospital services [4]. Essentially, the directives state that all patients are entitled to palliative care 24 hours a day, 7 days a week, in hospitals as well as in the community, delivered by staff that must include a physician, a nurse, a social worker and a medical psychologist. The director-general has stated that these directives will become statutory in July 2013, thus allowing the HMO's and hospitals four years to develop the infrastructure required to comply with the new directives.

By the end of 2013, only 4,000 advance directives have been completed nationwide. These were filed with the Ministry of Health, a decision that has been a pitfall in all the reforms hitherto, due largely to:

1 a lack of awareness amongst the general public that advance directive forms exist;
2 medical staff failing to inquire whether patients have advance directive forms, and failing to view these forms, as they are filed in the Ministry of Health and not available at the time a patient is admitted to hospital;
3 prohibitive legal terms used in the advance directives that are unintelligible to the public and to medical personnel;
4 a failure to train physicians in the completion of advance directive forms which must be filled in by patients in the presence of a physician who then witnesses and signs the forms.

As a result, advance directives are underused and undervalued.

DEVELOPING PALLIATIVE CARE SERVICES: HMOS AND HOMECARE

As palliative care became established, homecare provision evolved, with private organizations, NGO's and then HMO's providing healthcare either directly or by contracting (out-sourcing) services [5]. This was a new factor in meeting the financial burden of service provision, as HMO's realized that out-sourcing rather than direct provision of palliative care services was more cost effective, as the costs to HMO's of delivering services directly was far in excess of smaller, more mobile companies with fewer staff and fewer procedures. A change in culture in terms of care for the terminally ill has also warranted a pragmatic stance: costs of home hospice care are dramatically lower than continuing standard oncology treatment in hospitals. This is mainly due to the reduction in direct costs related to hospitalizations, treatments, imaging and medications which are all reduced when a patient is in a home hospice setting. One would expect that the HMO's would have a huge financial incentive to shift the emphasis in end-of-life care to the community rather than to continue this in hospitals. As of today, this is still not the case. The reasons are probably due to the elaborate financial schemes between the HMO's, the Ministry of Health and public hospitals in the country. In order for a real shift in trends to occur, leading to a dramatic rise in the number of patients referred for end-of-life care in the community, there needs to be a direct financial incentive for the HMO's to do so. This plan should allow policy-makers to see the benefits and cost savings in the immediate time frame, and not just as theoretical future savings for their organizations.

Table 1 details the organizations providing palliative care services. Clalit, Israel's oldest and largest HMO, insuring and providing healthcare to over half the population, was the first to set up homecare services in the 1980's in order to provide care for patients confined to their homes through homecare units. A few of these units, comprising physicians, nurses, social workers, dieticians and physiotherapists, developed palliative care capabilities and are still operational. These units are able to offer a high level of palliative care support in the community but they cannot be considered true home-hospice units due to limited accessibility, lack of on-call 24/7 services and a lack of expertise in end-of-life medical challenges. Only a few units have developed integral home hospice services – such as the units in Beer Sheva, Haifa and Jerusalem. Together, they treat up to 90 patients at any time.

Table 1. Organizations providing public palliative care services in Israel

Organization	Description	Date established	Area covered	Number of patients treated on average per day	Illnesses treated	Age groups of patients
Clalit Home Hospice-South	HMO	1990's	Beer-Sheba, Kiryat Gat and Ashqelon	20-25	Cancer and non-cancer	Adults and children
Clalit Home Hospice- North	HMO	1998	Haifa and western Galilee	40-50	Cancer and non-cancer	Adults
Clalit Home Hospice-Jerusalem	HMO	1990's	Jerusalem	20-30	Cancer and non-cancer	Adults
Maccabi-South	HMO	2008	Beer Sheva	15-20	Cancer and non-cancer	Adults and children
Israeli Cancer Association	NGO	1990's	Tel Aviv metropolitan area	15-20	Cancer	Adults
Hadassah Mount Scopus	Public hospital	1989	Jerusalem	15-20	Cancer and non-cancer	Adults
North Galilee Home Hospice	NGO	1994	North Galilee	25-35	Cancer and non-cancer	Adults and children
Sabar Clinics	Private service provider to all four HMO's	2005	Nationwide	220-240	Cancer and non-cancer	Adults and children

The role of NGO's and volunteers in the establishment of homecare services is not to be underestimated. The Upper Galilee Home Hospice was established in 1994 with the support of dedicated volunteers. This hospice cares for two of the four HMO patients, treating approximately 30 patients at any time. The success of palliative care in Israel would not have been possible without the NGO Lillach, which lobbied for humane care of the dying and recognition that patients have the right to choose how they wish to live out their last days. This pressure on the government was crucial in pushing forward legislation towards the Death and Dying act in 2005. Moreover, provision of homecare has rested largely on volunteer organizations with novel solutions in resourcing essential equipment (including beds) at little or no cost to patients, and newer, privately owned palliative care providers.

Sabar Clinics

Sabar Clinics Home Hospice, established in 2005, is the largest and most comprehensive home hospice service in the country [6]. It is a privately owned organization that operates as an out-source service and accepts patients from only the four national HMO's. The service is provided nationwide including the Golan Heights, the West Bank and East Jerusalem, with over 220 patients receiving treatment at any time. It is the only home hospice service in the country storing all medical records as electronic files. As such, Sabar Clinics serves as proxy to state provision of end-of-life palliative care in Israel. The caseload comprises patients of all ages and Sabar Clinics has championed the provision of palliative care for patients with non-cancer illnesses as well as those with terminal cancer.

Most patients are looked after by Sabar Clinics for 19 days (some patients are referred on the day they die; some survive for well over a year). Only 10% of patients are under the care of the clinic for more than 97 days. Of deaths in patients receiving care from Sabar Clinics, 27% die within the first 7 days and 65% die within the first month. Eighty two percent of patients die at home.

The average age of patients is 68 with a standard deviation of 15 (the mode is 66). The youngest patient to date was 2 years old and the oldest patient to receive care was 100. An overwhelming majority of the patients treated have terminal cancer, with only 3% suffering from other end-stage chronic diseases.

The number of patients cared for by Sabar Clinics has increased with time: in 2011, there were 378 new patients; in 2012, there were 944 new patients; and, in 2013, there were 2,020 new patients. This increase is likely due to increased awareness of the services offered by the clinic.

Developing Palliative Care Services: Palliative Care As a Medical Specialty

The three requirements of the establishment of palliative care as a medical specialty in Israel have been the development of accredited training programs, the training of undergraduates and health professionals, and the formalization of governing bodies able to oversee training and standards in practice.

The training of doctors, initially confined to selected centers of expertise, is now nationwide. Today, all Israeli medical schools and Family Medicine residency training programs include training in palliative care. Additionally, the Israeli National Palliative Care Training Program (INPACT), established in 2006, provides postgraduate training (continual professional development) to professionals interested in palliative care. Over 1,000 healthcare professionals from all parts of the country have been trained in this program.

Following the development of a cohort of specialists and a professional governing body, palliative medicine was finally approved in 2013 as a new sub-specialty for physicians (requiring another specialization first – usually Internal or Family Medicine). To date, about twenty five physicians have been awarded the honor of being "founders" of the new specialty. During 2014 it is expected that centers will be accredited for training and the specialization program will officially begin and receive its first residents.

The palliative medicine training program is expected to comprise 24 months, 14 of which will be spent in hospice service (with a possibility of 7 months in an in-patient environment and 7 months in community hospices). The remaining 7 months are divided into 3 rotations from a choice of departments relevant to palliative care such as geriatrics, oncology, neurology or nephrology. The new specialization is expected to substantially increase awareness amongst the public of their entitlement to good palliative care, just as the recognition of pain medicine as a specialty achieved in 2010.

Nursing Specialization

The nursing division of Israel's Ministry of Health recognized palliative care as a sub-specialty (the first recognized nursing sub-specialty in Israel) in 2012. Currently, there are over 35 palliative care nurse specialists across Israel, whose duties range from coordinating palliative care programs to personally administering care. All oncology and chronic disease nurse training programs have incorporated palliative care into their curricula.

The Establishment of Deliverable Home Hospice Services

The cornerstone of palliative care is surely the prescription of opiates in doses effective for symptom relief. This, and the availability in Israeli homes of live-in-caregivers (usually foreign migrants) and low-cost sourcing of essential equipment for terminal care at home underpin the success of home hospice care in Israel.

Opioids

Opioid availability for pain management has increased in recent years, both in absolute numbers of drugs and the availability of different formulations. This is mainly due to the growing awareness of medical professionals and the general public of the concept of treating pain not just as another symptom but rather as a disease on its own [7]. This is reflected in the incorporation of pain management as an integral part of the curriculum of every medical and nursing school, the recognition of pain medicine as a new sub-specialty, and efforts made by drug companies to increase public awareness of new pain medications [8]. Currently, the range of the most commonly prescribed opioids includes morphine, oxycodone, pethidine, methadone and fentanyl. These are all available in the basic health basket, free of charge to terminally ill patients. Conversely, propoxyphene has been taken off the market in favor of tramadol because of safety profile concerns raised by the FDA (Food and Drug Administration). Pain management guidelines produced by expert panels in the Israeli Medical Association and the Ministry of Health regularly update required written documentation and reports on the administration of pain medication [9]. Opioids are defined as "controlled drugs" in the Israeli pharmacopeia, and thus can be prescribed only by a physician. Any physician (with the exception of dentists), however, can prescribe these medications; there are no limitations to a specific specialization [10]. Prescriptions must be completed correctly in numbers and words and the prescriber must be able to provide evidence of a valid medical license. As long as the prescription is written in compliance with these strict directives, there is no practical limitation on the formulations, dosage and frequency of prescriptions. Excluding the new rapid-acting fentanyl formulations, all these medications have generic options and, thus, there is no financial consideration or limitation on their use.

CANNABIS

Cannabis has been approved for medical use in Israel since the early 2000's. As in most developed countries, it is marked as a "dangerous drug" in the Israeli pharmacopeia. Indications for use are mainly patients with chronic pain refractory to other treatments and to ease symptom burden in patients with advanced cancer and AIDS [11]. A specific committee in the Ministry of Health, comprising medical and pharmaceutical professionals, legal counselors and representatives of the police, makes recommendations to the Minister of Health on all matters concerning the use of medical cannabis (as well as medical marijuana). Licenses to supply can be issued by any physician, but the requests are reviewed by a dedicated unit in the Ministry of Health. Once the license is obtained, a designated grower/distributor contacts the patient and supplies the medication in accordance with the terms of the license. Cannabis is available in Israel only as oil or flowers, either rolled up as cigarettes or for vaporizers. The use of cookies and other capsulated products has been banned. In the last two years there has been a vocal campaign coordinated by legal growers and distributors to increase awareness and access of cannabis to an ever-growing population of patients, leading to a dramatic surge in prescriptions. This rapidly shifting trend has raised many concerns about the lack of medical evidence to support its use. Concerns have also been raised about the direct grower-distributor-patient link that enables growers to directly influence the cannabis consumption of patients, which is unacceptable and illegal for conventional medications.

FOREIGN BASIC NURSING PERSONNEL

Taking care of a very ill patient at home requires first and foremost an understanding that much of the everyday nursing and basic care for the patient now falls to the family. This may be hugely prohibitive for families that do not live together or cannot afford to stay at home rather than work. Caring for a sick person at home necessitates availability 24/7 for medical and the most basic physiological needs. As yet, there is no official program in Israel to train family members to become caregivers. In an effort to provide care for old, frail or debilitated patients in their homes, the government allows the employment of overseas caregivers, mainly from the Philippines, to work as live-in aides.

Overseas caregivers are hired and trained by dedicated private agencies. Their vocational rights are long-established and enforced. Foreign aid workers must have a room of their own in the house and have a day off work every week. They are insured both with a medical and social security plan. A family member must obtain permission from the Ministry of Health and from the Ministry of Social Affairs and Social Services before receiving a license to hire a foreign aid worker. This process comes with a level of bureaucracy and delay that may render such an option irrelevant to families who need immediate assistance. In some cases the foreign aid workers become the primary caregivers to many patients. This significant help with handling basic but sometimes very difficult nursing tasks is a huge factor in assisting families to take care of a sick family member at home.

Medical Devices and Equipment

The implementation of a nationwide plan for home hospice care might have failed very early on had it not been for the two large volunteer organizations in the country (Yad Sarah and Ezer Mizion) which loan the necessary equipment to families at minimal or no cost. Loaned equipment includes fully operational hospital beds with pressure mattresses, infusion stands, wheel chairs and patient hoists and lifts. These organizations offer equipment to everyone in need regardless of age, race, religion or ability to pay. Estimated savings to the country are $320 million in hospital costs alone. According to a national survey, 1 in every 2 Israeli families has been helped by Yad Sarah. The organization relies simply on donations to meet its $23 million operating budget [12].

Equipment for the administration of medications such as oxygen, TPN (total parenteral nutrition), PCA (patient controlled analgesia) pumps and pre-made morphine solutions are all supplied by the HMO's.

Cultural Aspects of Service Provision

The three monotheistic religions in Israel hold life to be of utmost sanctity. About half the population consider themselves ultra-orthodox, religious or observant. Thus, religious beliefs must be considered in legislation and medical care for the terminally ill and dying [13]. Early on in the legislation of the Death and Dying Act, the efforts of a religious pediatrician were hugely influential in garnering the support of religious leaders and their followers. A Christian priest was also involved in policy making. Rabbis are consulted on advance directive decisions by some patients, who rely on their support in making medical choices, especially for end-of-life care [14].

Israeli law states that a patient at the legal age of consent may exercise his/her prerogative. Cultural factors, however, mitigate decisions, and medical staff are frequently obliged to discuss treatment plans with the entire family. In extreme cases the patient may be excluded altogether from the decision process by the family. A formal legal process may be exercised in cases of emergency where legal guardianship is awarded to a named family member given the power to make medical decisions on behalf of an infirm loved one. This person may exercise the orders of the Dying Persons Act by proxy with legal authorization from a court. This may not be necessary, however, and the home hospice team endeavors to be acutely aware of family considerations, the dying patients' wishes, and cultural considerations unique to each family. Many home hospice teams include a member of the local culture/religion.

EUTHANASIA

Euthanasia is illegal in Israel. There has been a legislative effort by some parliament members to promote the option of "physician assisted suicide" following the model practised in some states in the USA (Oregon, Vermont and Washington), but this option is still far from being passed in law. As cited above, a dying patient can direct the medical staff, either directly or through advance directives, to withhold life-sustaining treatment with the exclusion that continuing, ongoing treatments must not be stopped. This is relevant only to respirators. Once a patient is put on a respirator there is no legal way to stop the ongoing continuous treatment. This limitation in the law is sometimes a source of unnecessary suffering for patients and families.

CONCLUSION

Even after changes in public perception, demand and service provision, it is estimated that home and hospital palliative care services reach less than 10-15% of the people who could really benefit. There is hope among palliative care professionals that the recognition of palliative care as a specialty both for nurses and physicians will increase the number of patients receiving such care, and that training in the specialty will substantially improve the experience of patients, for example, in the completion of advance end-of-life directives. The challenge is to increase the number of patients with access to palliative care, for both cancer and non-cancer diagnoses. There is a need for medical advocacy alongside patient lobbying, utilization of the media and the creation of an environment favourable to the discussion of matters of death and dying, and the choices that people may make about how they choose to die or how they would like to see their loved ones cared for at the end of their lives. Research, regulation and quality control are essential to build on the progress made so far and to maintain standards.

REFERENCES

[1] Livneh J. Development of palliative care in Israel and the rising status of the clinical nurse specialist. *J Pediatr Hematol Oncol* 2011; 33: S157-158.

[2] Singer Y., Carmel S. Teaching end-of-life care to family medicine residents – what do they learn? *Med Teach* 2009; 31: e47-e50.

[3] Steinberg, A., Sprung, CL. The Dying Patient Act, 2005: Israeli Innovative Legislation. *Isr Med Assoc J* 2007, 9:550-552.

[4] State of Israel, *Ministry of Health: Circular of the General Administration*. No. 30/09 Issue: Operation of Palliative Care Services (Hospice) in the community, general hospitals and nursing institutions. July 12th, 2009. (Medinat Israel. Misrad Habriut. Hozer Hamenahel Haklali. Mis. 30/09 Benose: Hafalat Sherut Palliative (Hospice) Bakehilah, Bebet-Holim Klali Ubemossad siudi 12/9/2009).

[5] Bentur et al. Progress in palliative care in Israel: comparative mapping and next steps. *Israel Journal of Health Policy Research* 2012 1:9.

[6] Sabar, R. Sabar Clinics: for family health. *http://www.sabarhealth.co.il/sabar-clinics.htm* (accessed 10 January 2014).

[7] Cherny, N. Cancer pain – progress and ongoing issues in Israel. *Pain Res Manage* 2009; 14: 356-357.

[8] Cohen, M.Z., Musgrave, C.F., McGuire, D.B, et al. The cancer pain experience of Israeli adults 65 years and older: the influence of pain interference, symptom severity and knowledge, and attitudes on pain and pain control. *Support Care Cancer* 2005; 13: 708-714.

[9] Ponizovsky, A.M., Maron, E.B, Zeldin, A., Cherny, N.I. Trends in opioid analgesics consumption in Israel 2000-2008. *Eur J Clin Pharmacol* 2011; 67: 165-168.

[10] *http://www.health.gov.il/LegislationLibrary/Samim_01.pdf*

[11] *http://www.health.gov.il/Services/Citizen_Services/Pages/kanabis.aspx*

[12] *http://www.yadsarah.org.il*

[13] Barilan, Y.M. Revising the problem of Jewish bioethics: the case of terminal care. *Kennedy Inst Ethics J* 2003, 13(2):141-168.

[14] Kinzbrunner, B.M. Jewish medical ethics and end-of-life care. *Journal of Palliative Medicine* 2004, 7(4):558-573.

In: Palliative Care to the Cancer Patient
Editor: Michael Silbermann
ISBN: 978-1-63117-709-5

Chapter 9

Palliative Care in Jordan: Accomplishments and Challenges

Mohammad Al-Qadire, R.N., Ph.D.[1,2*]***, Suha Omran, R.N., D.N.Sc.***[3]
and Mona Tayyem, R.N., M.S.N.[3]
[1]Al-Bayet University, Mafraq, Jordan
[2]Al Ghad International Collages for Applied Health Sciences, Riyadh, Saudi Arabia
[3]Jordan University of Science and Technology, Irbid, Jordan

Introduction

This chapter outlines the current status and challenges of palliative care in Jordan. It begins with brief background information about Jordan, including its geographical location, population, education, culture, and healthcare system. It and then describes the available palliative care settings in the country. It also presents a complete description of pain and other symptom management currently offered for cancer patients, and discusses barriers to palliative care and pain management that can hamper patients from receiving adequate care. Lastly, current available education and training in palliative care is presented.

General Information about Jordan

Jordan is a small country located in the centre of the Middle East, surrounded by Saudi Arabia to the south and east, Iraq to the northeast, Syria to the north, and Palestine to the west (Federal Research Division, 2006). It covers an area of 92,300 square kilometres. Jordan's population was estimated at 6,508,271 in 2011 (Federal Research Division, 2006). Jordan has 12 cities, of which Amman is the largest with 2 million inhabitants (The Hashemite Kingdom of Jordan Department of Statistics, 2011), while 78 percent of all Jordanians live in urban areas (Multicultural America, 2006).

---

* Address for correspondence: mohammadqadire@gmail.com

The Jordanian population comprises 51.5% males, 94% Muslims and 6% Christians, including various denominations such as Greek Orthodox, Roman Catholic, Greek Catholic, Armenian Orthodox, Assyrian, Maronite, and assorted Protestant churches, among others (Federal Research Division, 2006). Jordan adopts the principle of religious freedom, and everyone has the right to practice religious beliefs without fear of restraint (Multicultural America, 2006). Only 2% of Jordanians are non-Arab, mainly comprising Caucasians, Chechens, Armenians, Turkmens and Gypsies. According to a US report (2006), about 33 percent of the Jordanian population is under 15 years old, 62 percent is between 15 to 64, and only about four percent are older than 65 (Federal Research Division, 2006). The average life expectancy for Jordanians is 78 years (Jordan Ministry of Health, 2008). Arabic is the official language, but English is widely understood and is used in institutions of higher education, hospitals and large companies (Federal Research Division, 2006).

EDUCATION

The Jordanian government reported literacy rates for 2003 as 90.1%. Primary and secondary education until the age of 15 is free and compulsory. The government is working on improving the output of the education system, and about 18% of the total budget is dedicated to education (Multicultural America, 2006; Federal Research Division, 2006). There are approximately 26 universities (private and public) in Jordan, and women comprise half the student body. The government is working to improve the Jordanian work force competitiveness internationally.

JORDANIAN CULTURE

The culture of Jordan is the Arabic Islamic culture, encompassing people's beliefs, rituals and values.

However, Western culture is apparent in the daily life of Jordanian people, reflected in attire, architecture and spoken language (Federal Research Division, 2006). Non-Arab minority groups in Jordan have been assimilated into the indigenous culture to the extent that it is difficult to distinguish them from natives. Jordan has a reputation for the acceptance and tolerance of others (Multicultural America, 2006). Jordanian districts have their own specific cultural characteristics, but they remain within the overall Arabic Islamic cultural sphere.

The Islamic religion and family structure are influential factors in shaping the population's beliefs. Islam is the religion of the majority of the population, and most citizens believe that illness and wellness are God's will. Religious practices are widely used to help people cope with crises. Decision-making about health issues is viewed as a social process in which all family members are involved. Similarly, the family is closely involved in the care management of the ill family member, with religious and spiritual aspects treated as important issues for patients. In the past, people died in their homes, surrounded by their families and loved ones, but nowadays people often die in hospitals and other healthcare settings while attached to life-supporting machines, surrounded by medical personnel rather than relatives. Hence, the need for palliative care is gaining momentum in Jordan.

The Healthcare System In Jordan

Jordan has a well-developed healthcare system in comparison to other countries in the region (Federal Research Division, 2006).

The prevalence of Human Acquired Immunodeficiency (HIV) is 0.1 percent, Jordan has been malaria-free since 2001, and tuberculosis has decreased by half since 1990 (Federal Research Division, 2006; Jordan Ministry of Health, 2008).

According to a Ministry of Health report (1999), about 70% of the Jordanian population is medically insured, and the government is working to increase this percentage with the aim of reaching total comprehensive medical insurance coverage (Dwayne et al., 1999). It is believed that the 70% figure has increased since this report was released 12 years ago, as many governmental steps have been taken to increase the insurance coverage. For example, two years ago children under the age of six and senior citizens were added to the medical insurance umbrella.

Generally speaking, the health care system in Jordan can be divided into two sectors: public and private (Jordan Ministry of Health, 2008).

Public Health

This sector includes:

1. Ministry of Health (MOH) hospitals and primary medical centres: these are operated by the MOH, are fully funded by the government, and are located all over the country in both cities and villages. All citizens of Jordan can be treated in these hospitals without payment.
2. Military Royal Medical services: these consist of large hospitals spread out throughout the country, operated by the leadership of the armed forces. These health services are provided to soldiers and their families. Civilians can access these services under certain circumstances.
3. University hospitals: these hospitals are affiliated with two universities (the University of Jordan and the Jordan University of Science and Technology). They are referral hospitals for complicated cases.

Private Health Sector

The private sector is operated by personal investment, and provides about 36% of available hospital beds in the country (Jordan Ministry of Health, 2008). The private sector is parallel and complementary to the public sector, is well-developed, and also serves many foreign patients who come from other countries (i.e., Iraq, Egypt, Sudan, and the Gulf region) for medical treatment.

Primary Healthcare Services in Jordan

The Ministry of Health (MOH) also provides primary care services through an extensive network of medical centres in the kingdom. These centres provide such services as general medicine, dentistry, maternity and paediatric care, and health education, as well as specialized health promotion services (e.g., smoking cessation clinics) (Jordan Ministry of Health, 2008).

MOH classifies its medical centres in three categories:

1. Comprehensive Medical Centres: providing general medical care, laboratory tests, and x-rays. In addition, dental care is available. No inpatient care.
2. Elementary Medical centres: located in small villages, providing general medical care only. Serious illnesses are referred to the comprehensive medical centre or hospital.
3. Maternity and childhood care centres: providing care for women and their babies, including follow-up care for pregnant women, vaccination, and family planning, in addition to growth and development follow-up for children.

Patients are expected to visit these centres prior to going to main hospitals. Services at these centres are available for all inhabitants in Jordan. In some cases a small fee is charged.

Cancer and Its Treatment in Jordan

Cancer in Jordan is the second largest cause of death after heart disease. Jordan has 48,300 new adult and paediatric cancer cases per year (Silbermann et al., 2012). Between 60%–70% of cancer cases are discovered at late stages (Stage III and IV) (Silbermann et al., 2012). The crude incidence rate of cancer among Jordanians was 67.1 per 100,000 (Tarawneh et al., 2007). The total number of deaths from cancer cases diagnosed in 2009 was 1,161 (24.2% of all deaths) (Tarawneh et al., 2007). The highest rate of cancer-related deaths occurred in the Amman governorate (44%), followed by Irbid (17.3%) and Zarqa (13.5%), with the lowest rate in Aqaba (1.2%) (Tarawneh et al., 2007).

Cancer can be diagnosed at primary or tertiary medical care settings. If cancer is diagnosed at a primary medical setting, the patient is usually referred to the nearest setting where cancer treatment is available and where the diagnosis is confirmed and treatment initiated. All inhabitants are eligible for free cancer treatment regardless of their medical insurance status. This includes all related expenses such as admission, all types of cancer therapy, and pain medications as well. Alternatively, patients can go directly to a private hospital if they wish to pay the cost of medical care.

Palliative Care in Jordan

Palliative care services have been introduced and integrated in healthcare systems over recent years (Stjernsward et al., 2007a; Stjernsward et al., 2007b) The essence of palliative care is to manage patients' symptoms, reduce their burden of pain, and improve their quality of life (Fallon and Hanks, 2006). This development in healthcare technology has shifted the focus from curing patients to prolonging their lives. Specialized palliative care has become an important part of healthcare systems and team work (Johnsen et al., 2009). Both physicians and nurses are a crucial component of palliative care teams (Prem et al., 2012). Overall, the need for palliative care has increased significantly (Huijer et al., 2009). However, although palliative care was introduced some decades ago, in Jordan the provision of such care is still in its infancy, is scattered, and is underdeveloped (Stjernsward et al., 2007a).

Palliative care services in Jordan are provided by two main organizations: the King Hussein Cancer Centre (KHCC), and the Al Malath Foundation for Humanistic Care. Both are based in the capital city, Amman. Their services include home-based and inpatient palliative care for adults and children.

King Hussein Cancer Center (KHCC)

The Department of Palliative Care at KHCC, a public hospital, was established in 2004 to provide palliative care for hospitalized cancer patients and palliative care training for hospital staff (mainly nurses and physicians). Palliative care is provided by a multidisciplinary care team consisting of a physician, a nurse, a social worker, a physiotherapist, a nutritionist and a spiritual healer. The department has a 30-bed capacity. However, the admission rate for this department ranges from 17- 20 cancer patients per month. It provides three main services: inpatient adult palliative care, home palliative care, and education and training. It is the only organized and planned palliative care program in the Jordanian hospitals. It provides cancer patients (adult and pediatric) and their families with the required medical, social and psychological support from diagnosis until the patient's peaceful death. The care is not limited to inpatients: outpatient services are also available. A home palliative care team conducts two weekly visits to patients in their homes. In addition, 24-hour phone service is available. An oncology nurse responds to patients' and families' queries and needs, and an on-call oncologist is also available. Regrettably, this team provides services only to patients who live in Amman. No reliable palliative care service is currently available in other cities.

Al Malath Foundation for Humanistic Care

The Al Malath Foundation for Humanistic Care, a non-governmental organization, was established in 1993 to provide palliative hospice care for patients with an end-stage disease. Its main mission is to provide patients and their family end-of-life care, and ease their peaceful death. Such care consists of medical care (mainly symptom management), psychosocial, and spiritual care. Help is also extended to grieving families after their loss. Services are provided by a multidisciplinary hospice team which includes a nurse, physician, pain management specialist, social worker, dietician, and religious cleric. Each patient is initially visited by a team member who evaluates the patient's health status and needs. A care plan is developed based on this initial assessment, with the required care provided by the appropriate member of the team. If certain supplementary training is needed (e.g., in the use of an infusion pump), the patient's family is trained in its use, remaining under supervision until the family members show competency.

A hospice nurse provides free holistic nursing care for patients. This includes a daily health assessment, intravenous care and fluid therapy, ordering and taking blood samples, patient and family education, and preparation for death acceptance. In addition, an on-call nurse is available to respond to patients' and families' ordinary or urgent needs. In addition to holistic nursing care, the foundation offers an equipment loan scheme that includes beds, wheelchairs, bathing and toilet aids, and oxygen cylinders. The foundation also offers financial help with "special last wishes," funding up to three requests or wishes, such as the cost of a special trip away, or producing a remembrance video of the patient for the family.

Unfortunately, only patients within the Amman governorate can benefit from the Al Malath Foundation's services due to limited funds and staff. However, the number of patients admitted has increased annually. An estimated 3%-10% of the admitted patients are younger than 19 years old, and half have cancer. Most patients are supported until their last days in life, while a small percentage is admitted to hospitals a week or two prior to their death upon the request of their families. In the early years of the foundation, about 60% of referrals were by nurses, but currently 77% of the patients are referred by physicians and 9%-21% of referrals are self-referred by family or friends.

There are three oncology units in the governmental hospitals in Amman, and one unit in the northern part of the country. These units can provide pain and symptom management for cancer patients. However, they lack dedicated palliative care units or teams, and only inpatient care is available. Patients who wish to die at home can have certain non-specialized care such as basic pain and symptom relief through the vast network of private and governmental hospitals, medical centres, and clinics.

PAIN AND SYMPTOM MANAGEMENT IN JORDAN

Many symptoms are reported by cancer patients, including pain, depression, distress, fatigue, decreases in functional status and changes in lifestyle (Harding et al., 2011; Akin et al., 2010; Esther Kim et al., 2009). These symptoms can be caused by cancer, its treatment, or psychological factors. Hence, the presence of such symptoms may hamper patients' response to treatment and result in treatment failure (Esther Kim et al., 2009; Fan et al., 2007; Fox & Lyon, 2007).

The symptoms profile (prevalence, burden, and impact on quality of life) needs to be addressed at both the international level (Harding et al., 2011) and the local level, in this case Jordan. Mounting interest in investigating this issue is evident from recent publications from different parts of the world (Yeh et al., 2011; Harding et al., 2011; Cheng & Lee, 2011; Kirkova, 2010; Yamagishi et al., 2009). In Jordan, studies have dealt only with single symptoms, such as depression (Mhaidat et al., 2011), or have investigated the prevalence of symptoms among a small group of cancer patients (Omran et al., 2012). Epidemiological data regarding symptoms among cancer patients are needed to bring about the improvement of care provided in developing countries such as Jordan, in view of the expectation that by 2030, 70% of the cancer burden will be borne by these countries (Harding et al., 2011). One of the most important symptoms is cancer pain.

CANCER PAIN MANAGEMENT IN JORDAN

Cancer pain is one of the most common and most difficult experiences for cancer patients and their families (Deandrea et al., 2008). An estimated 73% percent of cancer patients in Jordan reported having pain, with a high mean pain score of 7.5 (SD 2.7) (Al Qadire et al., 2013). Moreover, an estimated 31% of cancer patients with pain did not receive any treatment (Al Qadire et al., 2013). Nurses, who are in the first line of pain management, have been found to have a low level of knowledge regarding pain management, while fear of addiction is the most common misconception regarding pain medications (Al Khalaileh & Al Qadire, 2012; Abdalrahim et al., 2011; Al Qadire & Al Khalaileh, 2012).

PAIN MANAGEMENT IN CLINICAL SETTINGS: THE PROCEDURE

Theoretically, cancer patients should be asked by physicians or nurses whether they have pain or not, but in practice reporting pain depends mainly on the patient, and most healthcare providers tend to wait for the patient to report pain. If a patient has pain, a detailed form should be used to assess pain (an initial assessment form). The Jordanian hospitals use various types of pain scales, including a mix of numerical rating scales (NRS), face pain scale, and FLACC (face, legs, activity, crying and consolability) scale. These scales are suitable for adults (NRS), paediatrics (face pain scale) and the unconscious or under three-year-old patient (FLACC). Additionally, certain settings seek information such as pain location, diagnosis side-effects of pain medication, and worst pain level experienced by the patient. The form should be completed in each shift and should be kept in the patient's medical records. Most of the oncology inpatient wards used a basic mutual procedure comprising a three-step care plan: assessment, action, and re-assessment.

There seemed to be a lack of awareness about the importance of pain assessment and management. Patients sometimes wait a considerable time to receive appropriate pain medication. The sequence is that the patient calls the nurse, and the nurse calls the resident physician, who will come to assess the patient's pain. Only then will pain medication be prescribed. Thereafter, the nurse administers the drug if it is available (if not it must be ordered from the pharmacy). The time between reporting pain and the administration of the medicine can be about one hour. Most patients are not usually prescribed regular pain medication (except for specialised hospitals), with the majority given a single dose (The Hashemite Kingdom of Jordan Department of Statistics, 2004) which often leaves the patient suffering. Furthermore, often pain re-assessment is not carried out after pain relief had been given. The common practice is to give patients treatment only once pain becomes severe and intolerable. Generally, it seems that communication between patients and nurses regarding pain is poor, and the available pain management policies in the hospitals are not actually activated. This suggests that pain is treated randomly rather than systematically.

The only facility offering organized pain services is at the King Hussein Cancer Centre (KHCC) in Amman, with three core pain services: a pain program in the Department of Anaesthesiology and Pain Management, a Department of Palliative Care, and palliative care in the Department of Paediatrics. Systematic guidelines and policies organize the practice of pain management at KHCC. These services can serve as models for other hospitals in Jordan.

Other Symptoms

It may be said that the same random rather than systematic procedure in pain management in Jordan generally is used to manage other symptoms as well. However, little information is known about the non-pain symptom profile in Jordan. A few small studies were conducted on this topic recently (Mhaidat et al., 2011; Omran et al., 2012), and a large-scale study of 498 patients from three main hospitals where cancer patients are usually treated was conducted to estimate cancer-related symptom prevalence, severity and quality of life (unpublished data). The findings were that cancer-related symptoms are highly prevalent. On average, each cancer patient experienced 11 concurrent symptoms ranging from moderate to severe, and all the symptoms were found to be experienced by over 70% of the respondents. Moreover, the patients were found to have a poorer quality of life than previously reported findings from other parts of the world.

There is a pressing need in Jordan for prospective studies that evaluate the availability and adequacy of symptom management. Student and practising nurses have been found to have a low level of knowledge about pain management and palliative care (Al Qadire, 2013; Al Khalaileh & Al Qadire; 2012, Darawad & Al-Hussami, 2012). This may lead them to be more focused on treating cancer itself rather than its combined, and distressing, symptoms. Omran et al. (2012) reported that 70% of cancer patients had multiple symptoms and were in a high state of distress. This highlights the need for prospective studies to evaluate the adequacy of physicians' knowledge and ability to manage pain and other cancer-related symptoms, and would help identify their weaknesses and educational needs. Designing courses to meet these needs might also lead to introducing palliative care courses in medical school curricula.

Availability of Morphine and Benzodiazepines

Jordan was rated among the best Arab countries in the use of morphine for pain relief. Yet, morphine consumption in Jordan was 1.2mg/capita, which is lower than global average use (5.9912 mg/capita). The King Hussein Cancer Centre accounts for a major part of the consumption of opioids for pain relief.

Nevertheless, most patients with pain receive inadequate pain management. Al Qadire et al. (2013) reported in a survey that the majority of those treated (33%) receive strong opioids such as morphine but it is given as a single dose (not regularly). Most patients who receive pain medications are given these medications as stat (single) doses or as needed (PRN). Furthermore, only 14 of those patients (17%) are treated with more than one pain medication, while single drug treatment is the common practice. The most commonly used route for drug administration is the intravenous route, followed by the oral route.

Morphine is available in both its intravenous and oral preparation in Jordan (Silbermann et al., 2012). However, the problem is with its description and the regulations that govern this process. Only physicians can prescribe morphine. It is available primarily in the main hospitals but not in other medical centers (Silbermann et al., 2012). The length of morphine prescription ranges from 3 days (non-cancer outpatients) to 10 days (cancer patients). Other opioids and benzodiazepines are available but do not seem to be used effectively and are used only in small amounts (Silbermann et al., 2012).

Barriers to Palliative Care and Pain Management

A plethora of barriers hamper patients from receiving adequate palliative care and pain management. These barriers are related to healthcare providers and patients' erroneous fear of addiction, healthcare settings, and policies (Al Khalaileh & Al Qadire, 2012).

First, healthcare providers in Jordan lack adequate knowledge and training regarding pain management. Limited time is designated for pain education in the undergraduate curricula, and postgraduate pain education is limited as well. This can lead to a considerable number of misconceptions and myths regarding pain management. For example, healthcare providers (physicians and nurses mainly) erroneously believe that taking narcotics means addiction in cancer patients (Edrington et al., 2009, Finley et al., 2008, David et al., 2003, Beck, 2000). Further, nurses in Jordan have been found to have a weak knowledge of pharmacological pain treatment (e.g., correct dosage, duration of effect, drug rotation), the preferred rout of administration, and fear of addiction (Al Qadire & Al Khalaileh, 2012). Fear of addiction is a cultural fear that is prevalent among in the wider public as well as among healthcare workers. This creates a state of opioid phobia, with health professionals avoiding the prescription of opioids and patients avoiding taking them. Fear of addiction and lack of knowledge sustain healthcare providers' hesitancy to prescribe and administer morphine and other opioids for cancer patients.

Secondly, the current opioids administration policy in Jordan results in a long prescription and dispensing process. Moreover, restrictions on the length of opioid prescriptions for outpatients are implemented and are followed strictly. Therefore, healthcare providers are discouraged and are over-cautious when prescribing or administering opioids, and usually encourage patients to tolerate more pain so as to avoid dealing with opioids.

Thirdly, the dominant culture among Jordanians discourages patients, and sometimes prohibits them from receiving opioids, based on religious misconceptions. A basic Islamic principle is to submit to the will of God, and patients often endure pain for the sake of God. Enduring pain can be perceived as a source of expiation of sins and of God's reward in the afterlife. Thus, in order to be rewarded, one must tolerate pain (Forgeron et al., 2006). This belief results from a misconception of Islamic rules, as well as a confusion between narcotics and street drugs. In fact, Islam allows the use of narcotics for medical purposes, and does not require followers to suffer when treatment is available treatment. On the contrary, Islam deems it a sin to forego treatment if the treatment is available and accessible.

More broadly, there are many obstacles that hamper patients from receiving adequate palliative care, which fills a basic human need to help patients improve their quality of life during their fight against cancer. Some of the obstacles are societal, as the family views palliative care as a sign of "giving up" on the patient. This is especially so in an Islamic Arab country such as Jordan where family ties are close, to the extent that the family can deny the fact that their loved one is dying. With this, physicians may perceive referring a patient for palliative care as a failure of their medical capability and a sign of loss of prestige when explaining the true situation to patients or their families. Moreover, Muslims believe that

Allah can cure patients no matter how poor the prognosis is, and physicians thus retain a false hope that allows their patients to undergo hopeless aggressive cancer treatments.

The lack of palliative care education and training programs is a significant barrier to the development and progress of palliative care in Jordan. As a result, there is a continuous shortage of skilled practitioners capable of delivering effective palliative care for patients, which also contributes to the limited and superficial knowledge of opioids and its uses by healthcare professionals – namely low consumption of opioids for pain control, delayed referrals, poor patient-healthcare provider communication, and a lack of research on the national level.

Uneven distribution and coverage of palliative care services has been a barrier to the provision and maturation of a palliative care program in Jordan. Further, a dearth of palliative care research on the national level constitutes an additional barrier to palliative care development. One of the important issues that needs to be investigated is the availability, distribution and adequacy of palliative care in Jordan. Meanwhile, the knowledge and educational needs of healthcare providers (mainly physicians, nurses and social workers) should be examined in order to establish a comprehensive educational plan that will fill in the gaps.

Other barriers include, first, an absence of public awareness of palliative care. People are not informed about palliative care services and retains myths and misconceptions about palliative care. Second, the absence of government recognition of palliative care as an integral part of the Jordanian healthcare system, and limited finical support, prevent the development and expansion of the limited available palliative care services. Third, cultural and religious beliefs and practices may be a barrier in that cancer patients and care providers are reluctant to talk about death or hospice care. The absence of a multidisciplinary approach to palliative care services is also a barrier. Lastly, the underutilization of other professionals, such as social workers, who could help physicians and patients increase the awareness of palliative care services is an additional barrier.

Barriers to the development of palliative care in Jordan may differ in scope and context from those in other countries, yet a number of common barriers to the development of palliative care services clearly exist. A great deal of work remains to be accomplished in Jordan regarding these identified barriers.

PALLIATIVE CARE EDUCATION AND TRAINING

Palliative care education is not yet imbedded in undergraduate medical and nursing school curricula in Jordan. A single nursing postgraduate palliative care program (Masters Level) is currently available in the University of Jordan School of Nursing. In addition, there is an academic diploma program in palliative care in a private university with no connection to the National Committee on Palliative Care in the Jordanian Ministry of Health. The credibility, content and clinical training for this diploma has not yet been established or recognized. Training programs for physicians in pain medicine as a subspecialty do not exist in Jordan. Only a few physicians practice pain and symptom management, mainly in the private sector, and continuous education and in-service training in hospitals are not always available. Therefore, introducing palliative care courses on the undergraduate level, and expanding currently available postgraduate and subspecialty training is urgently needed.

Conclusion

Data on patients with cancer have been recorded for a decade. During this period, an increase in the incidence of cancer has been observed among both children and adults. The aetiology of cancer is multi-factorial, involving both environmental and genetic factors. Most Jordanian patients are diagnosed with cancer at advance stages when the disease tends to be extensive and severe. Improving the quality of care provided for cancer patients can lead to better outcomes. Hence, palliative care services provided at any point in time of the disease lead to better outcomes. Yet, palliative care has only recently been introduced in Jordan, and it is still limited, scattered, and not well integrated in the healthcare system. As a result, only a small number of cancer patients can access and benefit by palliative care, while the majority of cancer patients and their families suffer, facing cancer care on their own.

To remedy this situation the government must first adopt a national palliative care program to be implemented in all the healthcare settings in the country. Home palliative care teams should be used to encourage patients to spend their last days among their beloved family members, which might reduce the high cost of cancer treatment. Secondly, healthcare providers must be equipped with the required education and training in palliative care through scholarships, fellowships, graduate courses, workshops and conferences. This education should be designed to meet healthcare providers' needs and to hone their clinical skills and understanding of the essence of palliative care. Lastly, research in the palliative care field should be encouraged and funded to enable a continuous evaluation of our progress and to reduce the suffering of cancer patients as the ultimate goal of the healthcare system.

References

Abdalrahim, M. S., Majali, S. A., Stomberg, M. W. N. & Bergbom, I. 2011. The effect of postoperative pain management program on improving nurses' knowledge and attitudes toward pain. *Nurse education in practice,* 11, 250-255.

Akin, S., Can, G., Aydiner, A., Ozdilli, K. & Durna, Z. 2010. Quality of life, symptom experience and distress of lung cancer patients undergoing chemotherapy. *European journal of oncology nursing,* 14, 400-409.

Al Khalaileh, M. & Al Qadire, M. 2012. Barriers to cancer pain management: Jordanian nurses' perspectives. *International journal of palliative nursing,* 18, 535-540.

Al Qadire, M. 2013. Knowledge of palliative care: an online survey. *Nurse education today.*

Al Qadire, M. & Al Khalaileh, M. 2012. Jordanian nurses' knowledge and attitude regarding pain management. Pain management nursing.

Al Qadire, M., Tubaishat, A. & Aljezawi, M. 2013. Cancer pain in Jordan: prevalence and adequacy of treatment. *International journal of palliative nursing,* 19, 125-130.

Beck, S. 2000. An ethnographic study of factors influencing cancer pain management in South Africa. *Cancer nursing,* 23, 91.

Cheng, K. K. F. & Lee, D. T. F. 2011. Effects of pain, fatigue, insomnia, and mood disturbance on functional status and quality of life of elderly patients with cancer. *Critical reviews in oncology/hematology,* 78, 127-137.

Darawad, M. W. & Al-Hussami, M. 2012. Jordanian nursing students' knowledge of, attitudes towards, and compliance with infection control precautions. Nurse education today.

David, E., Deborah, J. W. & Porterfield, G. L. 2003. Barriers to cancer pain management: home-health and hospice nurses and patients. *Supportive care in cancer,* 11, 660-665.

Deandrea, S., Montanari, M., Moja, L. & Apolone, G. 2008. Prevalence of undertreatment in cancer pain. A review of published literature. *Annals of oncology,* 19, 1985-1991.

Dwayne, A., Milburn, L. & Sabri, H. 1999. Profile of the uninsured in Jordan. Available: http://www.moh.gov.jo/moh/arabic/health_researchdetails.php?researchid=150 [accessed 19 October 2010].

Edrington, J., Sun, A., Wong, C., Dodd, M., Padilla, G., Paul, S. & Miaskowski, C. 2009. Barriers to pain management in a community sample of Chinese American patients with cancer. *Journal of pain and symptom management,* 37, 665-675.

Esther Kim, J.-E., Dodd, M. J., Aouizerat, B. E., Jahan, T. & Miaskowski, C. 2009. A review of the prevalence and impact of multiple symptoms in oncology patients. *Journal of pain and symptom management,* 37, 715-736.

Fallon, M. & Hanks, G. W. C. 2006. ABC of palliative care, Wiley-Blackwell.

Fan, G., Filipczak, L. & Chow, E. 2007. Symptom clusters in cancer patients: a review of the literature. *Current oncology,* 14, 173.

Federal Research Division. 2006. Country profile: Jordan [online]. Available: http://lcweb2.loc.gov/frd/cs/profiles/jordan.pdf [accessed 17 October 2010].

Finley, G., Forgeron, P. & Arnaout, M. 2008. Action research: developing a pediatric cancer pain program in Jordan. *Journal of pain and symptom management,* 35, 447.

Forgeron, P., Finley, G. & Arnaout, M. 2006. Pediatric pain prevalence and parents' attitudes at a cancer hospital in Jordan. *Journal of pain and symptom management,* 31, 440-448.

Fox, S. W. & Lyon, D. 2007. Symptom clusters and quality of life in survivors of ovarian cancer. *Cancer nursing,* 30, 354.

Harding, R., Selman, L., Agupio, G., Dinat, N., Downing, J., Gwyther, L., Mashao, T., Mmoledi, K., Sebuyira, L. M., Ikin, B. & Higginson, I. J. 2011. The prevalence and burden of symptoms amongst cancer patients attending palliative care in two African countries. *European journal of cancer,* 47, 51-56.

Huijer, H. A., Abboud, S. & Dimassi, H. 2009. Palliative care in Lebanon: knowledge, attitudes and practices of nurses. *International journal of palliative nursing,* 15, 346-353.

Johnsen, A. T., Petersen, M. A., Pedersen, L. & Grãnvold, M. 2009. Symptoms and problems in a nationally representative sample of advanced cancer patients. *Palliative medicine,* 23, 491-501.

Jordan Ministry of Health. *2008.* Health indicators [online]. Available: http://www.moh.gov.jo/reports/headermain.jsp?firstjsp=secondaryhealthcaremenu&lang_parameter=english [accessed 19 October 2010].

Kirkova, J. D. L. M. P. A. A. T. J. 2010. Symptom severity and distress in advanced cancer. *Palliative medicine,* 24, 330-339.

Mhaidat, N. M., Ai-Sweedan, S. A., Alzoubi, K. H., Alazzam, S. I., Banihani, M. N., Yasin, M. O. B. & Massadeh, M. M. 2011. Prevalence of depression among relatives of cancer patients in Jordan: a cross-sectional survey. *Palliative and supportive care,* 9, 25-29.

Multicultural America. 2006. Countries and their cultures: Jordan [online]. Available: http://www.everyculture.com/ja-ma/jordan.html [accessed 18 October 2010].

Omran, S., Saeed, A. M. A. & Simpson, J. 2012. Symptom distress of Jordanian patients with cancer receiving chemotherapy. *International journal of nursing practice,* 18, 125-132.

Prem, V., Karvannan, H., Kumar, S. P., Karthikbabu, S., Syed, N., Sisodia, V. & Jaykumar, S. 2012. Study of nurses' knowledge about palliative care: a quantitative cross-sectional survey. *Indian journal of palliative care,* 18, 122.

Silbermann, M., Arnaout, M., Daher, M., Nestoros, S., Pitsillides, B., Charalambous, H., Gultekin, M., Fahmi, R., Mostafa, K. A. H. & Khleif, A. D. 2012. Palliative cancer care in Middle Eastern countries: accomplishments and challenges. *Annals of oncology,* 23, 15-28.

Stjernsward, J., Ferris, F. D., Khleif, S. N., Jamous, W., Treish, I. M., Milhem, M., Bushnaq, M., Al Khateib, A., Al Shtiat, M. N. & Wheeler, M. S. 2007a. Jordan palliative care initiative: a WHO demonstration project. *Journal of pain and symptom management,* 33, 628-633.

Stjernsward, J., Foley, K. M. & Ferris, F. D. 2007b. The public health strategy for palliative care. *Journal of pain and symptom management,* 33, 486-493.

Tarawneh, M., Nimri, O., Arkoob, K. & Zaghal, M. A. L. 2007. Cancer incidence in Jordan 2009.

The Hashemite Kingdom of Jordan Department of Statistics. 2004. Population & housing census 2004 [online]. Available: http://www.dos.gov.jo/sdb_pop/sdb_pop_e/index.htm [accessed 19 October 2010].

Yamagishi, A., Morita, T., Miyashita, M. & Kimura, F. 2009. Symptom prevalence and longitudinal follow-up in cancer outpatients receiving chemotherapy. *Journal of pain and symptom management,* 37, 823-830.

Yeh, E.-T., Lau, S.-C., Su, W.-J., Tsai, D.-J., Tu, Y.-Y. & Lai, Y.-L. 2011. An examination of cancer-related fatigue through proposed diagnostic criteria in a sample of cancer patients in Taiwan. *Bmc cancer,* 11, 387-387.

In: Palliative Care to the Cancer Patient
Editor: Michael Silbermann

ISBN: 978-1-63117-709-5

Chapter 10

PALLIATIVE CARE FOR CANCER PATIENTS IN LEBANON

Michel Daher, M.D.[1,*] and Ramzi R. Hajjar, M.D., A.G.S.F.[2]
[1]Faculty of Medicine, University of Balamand, Department of Surgery, and Saint Georges Hospital, Beirut, Lebanon
Vice-Chair National Committee for Palliative Care
[2]Department of Internal Medicine, American University of Beirut Medical Center, Beirut, Lebanon
Department of Internal Medicine, St. Louis University School of Medicine, St. Louis, MO, US

INTRODUCTION: CANCER IN LEBANON AND THE RATIONAL FOR PALLIATIVE CARE

Over the past century the world experienced a demographic shift that has had a profound impact on the practice of medicine and the delivery of health care. As the world population increased, life expectancy in both developed and developing countries has also increased.

Consequently, both the absolute and the relative number of older adults have grown at an unprecedented rate. This demographic shift will be felt particularly, over the next few decades, in developing countries such as Lebanon, as its relatively young population moves up the population pyramid.

In Lebanon, it is estimated that just under 10% of the population is above the age of 65 years and 1.5% above the age of 85 – a small proportion compared to Western Europe and the United States, but quite high regionally (Figure 1).

Life expectancy in Lebanon lags only slightly behind that of developed countries, and currently stands at approximately 74 years for men and 77 years for women (as little as 50 years ago, it was 60 years).

* Corresponding author: Michel Daher, M.D., F.A.C.S., Professor of Clinical Surgery, Faculty of Medicine, University of Balamand, Department of Surgery, Saint George Hospital, Beirut, Lebanon and Vice-Chair National Committee for Palliative Care in Lebanon. E-mail: mndaher@inco.com.lb.

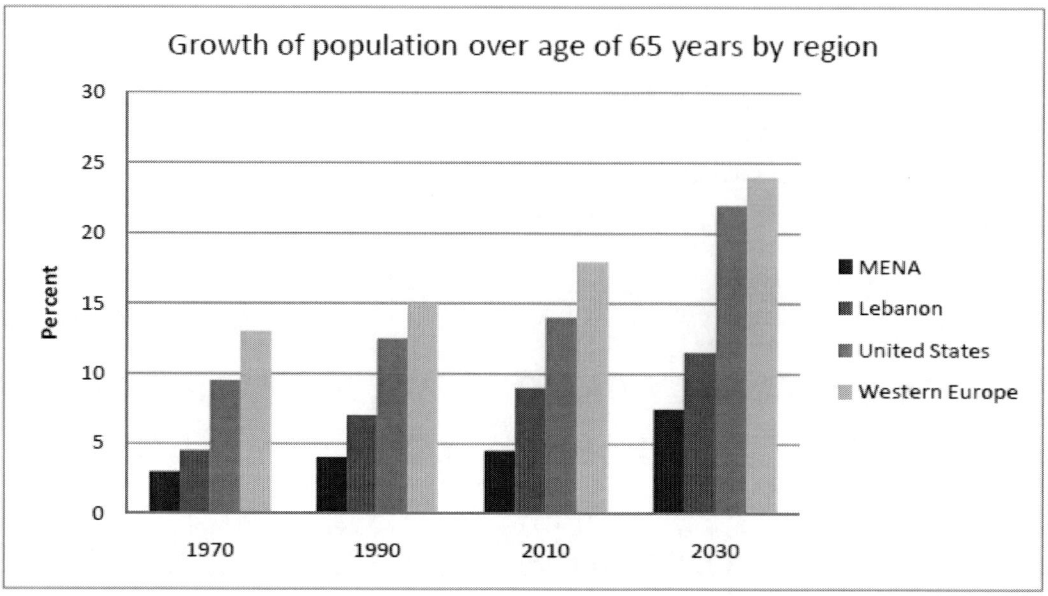

Compiled from multiple sources, and rounded to nearest half percent. [1-3] MENA: Middle East and Northern Africa.

Figure 1. Growth of population over age 65 years by region.

It is projected that in 35 years, the number of Lebanese older than 65 will double, at which time 1 in 5 residents of this small Mediterranean country – with a current population of 4.4 million – will be in the geriatric age group [1-4].

But with longevity comes chronic, costly, and serious illness, including many types of cancers, of which the Lebanese healthcare system is ill-prepared to deal with. Aside from age-related degenerative disorders, aging is a major risk factor for many types of cancers (figure 2). All-cause cancer incidence peaks at around age 70 [5].

The number of new cases of cancer in Lebanon has increased steadily over the past decade, according to the National Cancer Registry of the Ministry of Health and the World Health Organization (WHO). In 2004, almost 7200 new cases of cancer were reported in Lebanon, compared to over 9400 in the most recent report [5]. This worrisome trend is not entirely due to aging; expanded screening efforts and improved registration methods have likely contributed significantly. It is estimated that by 2030, the number of new cancer cases will approach 12,000.

Moreover, due to an indolent preventive care culture and a high prevalence of cancer-promoting behavior (such as smoking), many cancers present at an advanced stage when symptoms alert to the presence of disease and the only reasonable treatment option is palliative care. In a review of palliative care cases managed over the past two years at the American University of Beirut Medical Center (n=81), approximately 88% of cases were above the age of 65 years and 70% were for management of terminal malignancies [6]. The pattern of palliative care utilization in Lebanon is likely to change (if not the problem of late referrals) as public awareness and acceptance becomes more prevalent. In order to succeed, it will be necessary to have an integrated palliative care system in place that functions across disciplines and settings, as well as qualified personnel to lead the effort. To meet these goals, significant obstacles must be overcome today.

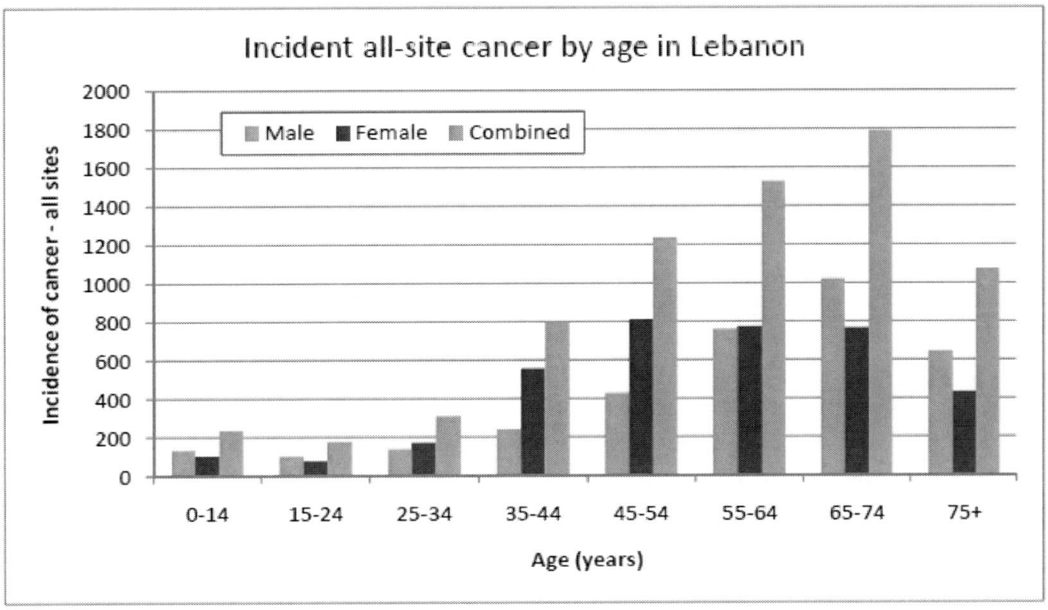

Figure 2. Incident cancer cases in Lebanon by age – 2003. All-case cancer excludes non-melanoma skin cancer.

History of Palliative Care in Lebanon

Palliative care programs, geriatric services, and long-term care facilities are in their infancy in Lebanon. Few healthcare providers have been trained in (or even exposed to) principles of palliative care. Though many nonmalignant conditions can benefit from palliative care medicine, it is practiced primarily in the realm of terminal cancer care.

Even so, by one estimate less than 10% of patients with terminal malignancies benefited from palliative care services in Lebanon today due to a deficiency of professionally trained providers, available programs, and public awareness.

Palliative care was first introduced in Lebanon in 1995 during a National Cancer Control Workshop supported by the Ministry of Health and the World Health Organization (WHO).

At that time, the pressing need for pain relief and palliative care services was identified as a high priority. In May 1999, a day-long symposium on palliative care and ethics was conducted during the Congrès d'Oncologie du Moyen-Orient, COMO IV (Middle East Oncology Congress) [7, 8]. This workshop was organized by the Lebanese Cancer Society and sponsored by the WHO. In the intervening four years between these workshops, it became clear that an interest in palliative care had taken root among certain healthcare professionals from diverse disciplines. Since then, a small but dedicated core of clinicians have championed the cause of palliative care and diligently worked towards making the dream of palliative care access for all a reality.

Pursuant to these early efforts, recommendations to the Ministry of Health and a request to the WHO for support and action were conceived. The recommendations stated that:

1) a clear national policy is needed to offer pain-free treatment;
2) an essential drug list should be established, not only for cancer chemotherapy but also for pain and other symptom management;
3) undergraduate training of nurses and physicians in palliative care should have high priority;
4) reimbursement of treating physicians for palliative care services should be sought;
5) a multidisciplinary approach to palliative care is essential for the success of the program;
6) strengthening home care agencies and social assistance programs is necessary;
7) palliative care is a right for all patients suffering from chronic and/or fatal illnesses and should be provided universally.

In May 2000, the Lebanese Pain and Palliative Care Initiative was launched under the auspices of the Lebanese Cancer Society [7, 8]. Members included physicians from various specialties, nurses, and other health professionals who work with terminal patients. The objective of this initiative was to:

- Promote the development of palliative care services and increase awareness of palliative care in academic, clinical, and social levels.
- Promote implementation of existing knowledge and expertise in palliative care, and train professionals involved in the care of patients with incurable and advanced disease.
- Promote academic studies and research.
- Support and give patronage to scientific and educational events promoting the dissemination and development of palliative care principles.
- Consolidate the efforts of professionals from various disciplines who study and practice the principles of palliative care (doctors, nurses, social workers, psychologists, volunteers and others).
- Address the ethical problems associated with the care of terminally ill patients, with special attention to local cultural context.

Good intentions alone, however, are not sufficient without means to implement them. Trained personnel, clinical experience, and leadership, were in short supply due to a culture that did not foster end-of-life care.

In 2008, a special issue on palliative care was published in the Lebanese Medical Journal (LMJ) (www.lebanesemedicaljournal.org). The LMJ is distributed to licensed physicians registered at the Lebanese Order of Physicians, thereby giving exposure of this fledgling specialty to over 10,000 members in 2008. Since then, significant strides have been achieved in education, practice, policy, and research, but a number of challenges remain which need to be addressed at the national level. Among those challenges is a persistent lack of knowledge and skills among practicing physicians, as well as inappropriate attitudes and behaviors among healthcare professionals towards end-of-life care.

A big step forward was reached on May 4, 2011 with the creation of the National Committee for Pain Relief and Palliative Care (NCPC) by the Ministry of Public Health (MPH – decree No 1/486) [9]. The NCPC is chaired by the Director of the MPH, and co-chaired by Dr. Michel Daher and Dr. Huda Huijer.

The NCPC has outlined for itself ambitious goals, and has consolidated the efforts of professionals from various disciplines and institutions committed to advancing principles of palliative care.

The efforts undertaken by this multidisciplinary committee are divided into four broad categories with specific objectives:

1 Education:
- Recommend a core curriculum for the training of healthcare professionals with emphasis on knowledge, attitudes, and skill development.
- Recommend specialization trajectories for physicians and nurses.
- Institute the importance of continuing professional education in the field as a requirement for recertification and licensure.
- Develop strategies for public education and awareness in the field of palliative care.

2 Practice:
- Develop national standards and competencies for pain relief and palliative care.
- Implement strategies to engage professionals from different disciplines in the care process such as the use of multidisciplinary care pathways.
- Recommend models for service delivery such as home care and residential care and the use of palliative care teams in hospitals.
- Develop mechanisms to empower the family and the patient to be actively involved in the care process emphasizing the importance of family and patient-centered care.

3 Research:
- Develop national research priorities for the field of pain relief and palliative care that target gaps in treatment, knowledge transfer, education, and policy.
- To recommend research methods to address the gaps in information related to pain relief and palliative care in Lebanon.

4 Public Policy:
- Promote legislation that ensures the availability, accessibility, and prescription rights of opiates.
- Recommend strategies that will ensure the practice of interdisciplinary palliative care teams in the care process.
- Develop models for cost allocation and reimbursement for pain relief and palliative care services.
- Recommend the institution of pain relief and palliative care as integral parts of the healthcare system in Lebanon.

Since its inception, the NCPC has proven effective in promoting its stated objectives. The first National Conference on Palliative Care in Lebanon took place on the International Palliative Care Day, October 13, 2012, during which the Committee was officially launched. At the conference a national strategy was outlined involving healthcare communities at large, as well as the media in order to raise public awareness. Reports prepared by the chairs of the above sub-committees were released. A second special issue of the Lebanese Medical Journal on palliative care was published in October 2013 in which the updated reports can be found (www.lebanesemedicaljournal.org).

The articles chronicle the achievements of the subcommittees thus far and outline the next steps necessary to realize the mission entrusted to the NCPC. Perhaps most encouraging, though, is the interdisciplinary cooperation and sense of purpose that emerges from these reports.

As this chapter goes to print, two additional momentous advances advocated by the Committee were realized (as will be discussed later): the recognition of palliative care by the MPH as a legitimate medical discipline, and the approval of new opioid recommendations.

Palliative care medicine in Lebanon has come a long way since its beginning at the National Cancer Control Workshop in 1995. New challenges will undoubtedly emerge. The continued shortage of qualified personnel coupled with an obstinate attitude of many physicians towards end-of-life care will only strengthen the resolve of the dedicated few who have championed the cause thus far. As palliative care enters mainstream medicine patients will soon have the means to exercise their right to a dignified death free of suffering.

Current Status of Palliative Care in the Country and in Academic Institutions

The Ministry of Public Health introduced palliative care as a patient right in the first article of the Law of 2004 on "Patients' Rights and Informed Consent" [10]. Palliative care should be considered a crucial core part of the treatment plan, implemented in parallel with curative care, and not just a final alternative when everything else fails.

In Lebanon, as elsewhere around the world, late referrals result in patients not realizing the full potential of this poorly understood specialty. Moreover, few qualified practitioners are available to meet the growing need. If palliative care services are to be offered universally in Lebanon, as dictated by patients' rights, two practical challenges must be addressed.

First, establish standards of practice for hospitals and home agencies, and second, offer postgraduate training in palliative care in order to grow the team of qualified providers. The next section will address training and education.

By current estimates, Lebanon has an annual mortality rate of 4-5/1000, or over 22000 deaths a year. There are more than 9400 new cases of cancer each year, and around 12,000 patients are in need of opiates and/or palliative care (~60% of total mortality) [11].

Nationwide, there are seven medical schools, thirteen nursing schools, over 130 medical oncologists, 15 radiotherapists, 11 geriatricians, and only two board-certified palliative care specialists (though other qualified professionals practice palliative care). Most palliative care services are provided in big cities (if available at all), leaving a large segment of the population without access to palliative care. Furthermore, over 50% of patients cannot afford palliative care services or medication, when available.

As a result, only 5-10% of patients who need palliative care receive it.

Three non-governmental organizations (NGO) provide limited palliative care services in Lebanon, though their acceptance and scope has grown considerably in recent years. "Sanad" and "Balsam" provide in-home hospice care and are committed to delivering quality end-of-life care despite constraints in personnel, funding, and societal mores. "Faire Face" group was founded in 1995 and has been providing in-hospital cancer support since 2003, among other services such as public awareness and early detection programs.

Hospital-based programs, however, are sorely lacking. The four major teaching hospitals have pain management programs and clinicians committed to palliative care, but no formal inpatient hospice programs existed until very recently.

Since March 2011, the American University of Beirut Medical Center has offered an inpatient palliative care service, under the direction of Dr. Ramzi Hajjar. Over the course of two years, 81 patients were referred for end-of-life care; most were elderly and approximately one third suffered from non-malignant conditions [6].

In late 2013, this service was developed into a comprehensive interdisciplinary inpatient program. What facilitated the growth and early success of this program was the support of the administration and their foresight regarding the role of palliative care in a tertiary-care hospital, and the unyielding efforts of Dr. Hibah Osman despite numerous challenges.

With the growing utilization of palliative care services and the introduction of new programs (early in 2014 at Hotel Dieu Hospital, UMC, and at Saint Georges Hospital, UMC), it became evident to the Practice Subcommittee of the NCPC that national standards must be established for clinicians and institutions.

In preparing a consensus statement for a national policy on the practice of palliative care in Lebanon, the subcommittee reviewed current standards from leading organizations in Europe and the United States.

Health care management systems were also reviewed. Hospital standards were based primarily on:

- A white Paper from the European Association of Palliative Care (EAPC) [12].
- National Consensus Project (NCP) Guidelines (Second edition) [13].
- Crosswalk of the Joint Commission on Accreditation of Healthcare Organizations (JCAHO) Standards and Palliative Care – Policies, procedures and assessment tools [14].

Practitioner standards of care were adopted from existing guidelines. Nursing competencies were based on guidelines from the National Hospice and Palliative Care Organization (NAPCO) [15], and the Canadian Hospice and Palliative Care Association for both Registered Nurse and Advanced Practice Nurse [16].

Physician competencies were based primarily on Center of Advance Palliative Care recommendations [17], and social workers' competencies were based on guidelines from the National Association for Social Workers (NASW) in the United States [18].

Competencies were revised to ensure that they reflected the four dimensions of palliative care (physical, social, psychological, and spiritual) and that they were appropriate in the Lebanese context. The compiled review and recommendations were summarized in the following statement:

> Research has supported the need for establishing palliative care services. Palliative care services lead to a decrease in overall hospital costs (decrease length of

stay, better care coordination), decrease in symptom intensity, increase in staff satisfaction (and thus retention), and increase in patient and family satisfaction. [19].

To that end, the subcommittee focused on setting hospital standards for palliative care and examining ways to encourage hospitals to incorporate these standards into their current systems.

The following steps were proposed to move the above recommendations forward:

1 Hospital accreditation is new to the Lebanese health care system and has played an important role in setting standards for hospitals in Lebanon. However, to date the accreditation system has focused primarily on issues of patient safety and quality improvement. The current hospital accreditation criteria are in the process of being updated and revised. The standards for Essential Palliative Care must be incorporated into the new hospital accreditation criteria to ensure that all hospitals in Lebanon are providing a basic level of palliative care to patients regardless of diagnosis or stage of the disease.
2 Palliative care standards should be publicized to allow hospital administrators to work towards attaining these goals in their own facilities. Existing palliative care programs should encourage and facilitate other centers to establishing programs and become centers of excellence that can serve as resources to health providers in the country as well as the region.
3 A palliative care curriculum should be introduced into medical and nursing schools as well as residency programs to ensure that all healthcare providers can provide a basic level of palliative care to the community.
4 Current laws restrict the prescribing of opioid analgesics to Oncologists and Pain Specialists. The recognition of palliative care as a specialty should be accompanied with the right of palliative care providers to prescribe opiates to ensure that adequate pain management is accessible to patients who need it regardless of their diagnosis or cause of their pain.
5 Adequate reimbursement for services is essential if palliative care programs are to be established. To this end, insurance reimbursement by the National Social Security Fund (NSSF) as well as private insurance companies for the provision of palliative care services should follow the recognition of the specialty.
6 Nurses play a major role in the provision and delivery of appropriate palliative care. This role should be recognized and rewarded appropriately. As the Order of Nursing moves towards establishing fields of specialty within nursing the above competencies should be used as the standards for Palliative Care Nurses.

Education and Development

Palliative care education is the first and most important step in implementing a nationwide program that is credible and effective. Until recently, little attention has been given in Lebanon to the undergraduate and postgraduate training of healthcare professionals on pain management and end-of-life care. Principles of palliative care have not been included in the state board examinations of doctors or nurses, and many healthcare professionals do not view symptom management as a goal in itself. Instead they continue to focus on curable interventions, and might view the dying process as a failure of modern medicine. Only recently have medical schools introduced geriatric instruction to their curricula. Formal training in end-of-life care continues to be overlooked by the majority of training programs.

Furthermore, the steady increase in the number of older patients and cancer patients in Lebanon has been met with a severe shortage of geriatricians and palliative care practitioners. The problem is perpetuated by the absence of fellowship training programs in either of these specialties to feed into the system. Even well-intentioned programs do not have the human resources to achieve their goal. For many reasons, too few physicians-in-training are exposed to palliative care early and often enough to experience its rewards.

Evidence of this deficit in training can be seen in the attitude of professionals towards the dying process. Most young physicians disengage in uneasy ambivalence when faced with terminal patients in whom palliative care is the only reasonable approach. In a survey of 1205 practicing Lebanese nurses and physicians, only 19.1% of physicians reported routinely informing terminally ill patients about their diagnosis though the majority of nurses and physicians (94% and 99% respectively) believed that the terminal patient *should* be informed [20, 21]. It was clear to the Education Subcommittee of the NCPC that much work was needed in this domain.

In response, the education subcommittee developed a modular curriculum for under-graduate training of medical and nursing students. It recommends that a one credit course on palliative care (21-hour modular curriculum) be integrated into undergraduate training and be a requirement by all seven faculties of medicine and eleven faculties or schools of nursing in Lebanon (Table 1).

Table 1. Proposed undergraduate national curriculum for pain and palliative care training in Lebanon

Modular Curriculum on Pain and Palliative Care. National Curriculum – Lebanon		
Course description		Duration
I	Overview of Palliative and End-of-life care	2 hr
II	Comprehensive patient assessment	2 hr
III	Communication skills and breaking bad news to patients and family	2 hr
IV	Multidisciplinary approach and team work	2 hr
V	Pain management and other common symptoms management	3 hr
VI	Psychosocial problems and their management	2 hr
VII	End-of-life care	2 hr
VIII	Ethical and legal issues	2 hr
IX	Quality of Life and Quality of Death	2 hr
X	Implementation of palliative care in Lebanon	2 hr

Furthermore, questions on pain management, palliative care, and end-of-life care must be included in all official examinations of doctors and nurses. Universities are given the flexibility to develop their own program based on staffing, scheduling, and available resources in order to reach the common objective. However, basic competencies modeled after internationally accepted standards for interprofessional education must be met. For graduating nurses, the minimum requirements include the same competencies as for physicians but with lesser emphasis on pharmacological management of pain and other symptoms, and greater focus on observing, recording, and intervening to diminish patient suffering.

With the growing gap between palliative care need and available providers, it has become clear that care for terminal patients will not be delivered primarily by fellowship-trained palliative care practitioners.

Our role is to help all those who deliver care become more adept in the principles of pain management and palliative care. At this juncture postgraduate training plays a key role.

For the few professionals who wish to pursue formal postgraduate training in palliative medicine, fellowship programs must be developed. Currently there are no postgraduate fellowship training programs in pain management, geriatrics, or palliative care in Lebanon.

On July 28, 2013, the Ministry of Public Health issued decree no 1/1048 adding palliative care medicine to the current list of specialties recognized in Lebanon. Based on this decree, a candidate must complete one year fellowship training in palliative medicine (following residency training), or a two-year postgraduate training period, in a recognized and certified program. Today, very few physicians qualify to register as palliative care specialists in Lebanon – only one is currently registered. Many more will be needed as this specialty grows.

PAIN RELIEF AND SYMPTOMS MANAGEMENT

Over the past two decades, advancements in the pharmaceutical industry brought to the market a wide spectrum of opioid products that address various pain syndromes. This has led to an increase in the medical use of opioids in patients with acute pain and terminal disease. Unfortunately, this trend was accompanied by an increase in the level of misuse, abuse and overuse across the world. In response, developed countries deployed strict policies and regulations to ensure that opioid drugs are not put to nefarious use and are shielded from other potential downside consequences.

In Lebanon, with a preexisting illicit drug abuse problem (mainly heroin), initial regulatory restrictions were taken to extreme. Although these regulations have been relaxed somewhat since 2006, underutilization of opioids continues to be problematic. Aside from regulatory constraints and limited availability, the prevailing attitude towards opioid use among patients and healthcare providers has been an obstinate hindrance. Fear of addiction or dependence is prevalent, as is the stigma of imminent (or accelerated) death associated with the use of opioids. Furthermore, many physicians under-dose or avoid opiates altogether for fear of causing harm or for lack of training. Consequently, Lebanon has a very low opioid use profile compared to nations where palliative care is well established. In 2007 opioid use in Lebanon slightly exceeded that of other Arab countries in the region (1.1 mg/capita/year versus 0.6 mg/capita/year for the MENA region, respectively), but was far short of Western standards (76 mg/capita/year in the US; world average 5.6 mg/capita/year) [22].

In the past few years, Lebanon witnessed a major improvement in the availability and accessibility of opioid drugs. In 2006, MPH decree no 1/484 improved availability by extending the duration of treatment per single prescription from 15 days to one month. In addition, it improved accessibility by introducing drug certificates that transferred drug delivery rights from the Ministry of Public Health to pharmacists. Prior to the decree, patients were required to obtain approval from the Narcotics Department of the MPH for every prescription refill. In 2009, additional amendments to prescription laws further facilitated the process of pain management and drug delivery. Prior to 2009, only cancer patients were entitled to opioid products and only oncologists were extended the right to prescribe them. With the new law, every patient has the right to be free of pain. Opioids could now be prescribed to non-cancer patients by all qualified physicians specialized in pain management.

More importantly, the law facilitated the prescription process by limiting the requirement to a simple medical report describing the disease and cause of pain for non-cancer patients, although two doctors must sign the medical report, one of whom should be an oncologist or pain specialist.

These major changes in the Lebanese law were driven by the Limoges recommendations concerning the use of opioid products in chronic non-cancer pain [23].

As the prescribing process stands today under the wider accessibility policy, a patient can obtain opioid treatment by presenting to the Narcotic Department a copy of his/her identity card, the medical prescription, and a medical certificate describing the diagnosis.

The medical prescription is a customized form "carnet à souches" made available by the MPH to oncologists and pain management doctors only (intended to better track and control the use of opioids) and specifies the patient's name, age and address. Upon presenting these documents, the patient is issued an official card signed by the Narcotic Department of the MPH, with which a one month supply of the medication can be obtained from predetermined pharmacies for the duration of almost one year.

Prior to 2012, long-acting morphine sulfate (MST) was the only oral opiate available in Lebanese. MST tablets are known as prolonged release tablets. Fentanyl was only available in parenteral (transdermal) form (Table 2). The year 2012 was a pivotal one for increasing narcotic availability in Lebanon. In a major step forward, the MPH introduced new opioid products, allowing clinicians more flexibility and control in pain management (Table 3).

The MPH is currently considering the approval of other products. Oxycodone, hydromorphone, and immediate release morphine sulfate (MSIR e.g., Sevredol) are currently under consideration, and will be welcome additions to the armamentarium of drugs utilized in improving the quality of life of terminal patients.

Future Perspectives and Conclusion

Palliative care in Lebanon is still in its infancy though this discipline is now officially recognized by the MPH and is being integrated in the education and training of future healthcare providers. It is essential to involve policy-makers at this early stage of development in order to establish the framework and tools needed for future growth. It is also necessary to promote public awareness to the benefits of palliative care through community outreach and the media.

Table 2. Registered narcotic drugs in Lebanon prior to 2012

Narcotic	Brand	Composition	Dose	Delivery
Morphine	MST continus	Morphine Sulfate	10 mg	60 sustained release tablets
			30 mg	
			60 mg	
			100 mg	
	Morphine sulfate	Morphine Sulfate	1.5% (15 mg/ml)	10 ampoules
	Chlorhydrate de morphine (Renaudin)	Morphine Chlorhydrate	0.10 % (1 mg/ml)	100 ampoules
Fentanyl	Fentanyl (Hameln)	Fentanyl Citrate	50 µg/ml	10 x 10 ml ampoules
	Fentanyl (Panpharma)	Fentanyl Citrate	0.5 mg/10 ml	10 x 10 ml ampoules
			0.1 mg/2 ml	10 x 2 ml ampoules
	Fentanyl (Renaudin)	Fentanyl Citrate	0.05 mg/ml	10 x 10 ml ampoules
	Fentanyl	Fentanyl Citrate	0.05 mg/ml	50 x 10 ml ampoules
	Duragesic	Fentanyl	25 µg/h (4.2 mg/patch)	5 transdermal patches
			50 µg/h (8.4 mg/patch)	
			75 µg/h (12.6 mg/patch)	
			100 µg/h (16.8 mg/patch)	
Alfentanil	Rapifen	Alfentanil HCL	0.5 mg/ml	5 x 2 ml or 5 x 10 ml ampoules
Sufentanil	Sufenta	Sufentanil citrate	0.005 mg/ml	5 x 2 ml or 5 x 10 ml ampoules
	Sufenta forte	Sufentanil citrate	0.05 mg/ml	5 x 5 ml ampoules
	Sufentanil (Renaudin)	Sufentanil citrate	50 µg/ml	10 x 5 ml
			5 µg/ml	10 x 2 ml ampoules
				10 x 10 ml
Remifentanil	Ultiva	Remifentanil HCL	1 mg	5 vials – powder for injection
			2 mg	
			5 mg	
Buprenorphine	Buprenophine (Arrow)	Buprenophine chlorhydrate	0.4 mg	7 tablet
			2 mg	
			8 mg	
Pethidine	Pethidine (Renaudin)	Pethidine hydrochloride	100 mg/2 ml	10x 2 ml ampoules

Table 3. Registered narcotic drugs in Lebanon added to national formulary in 2012

Narcotic	Brand	Composition	Dosage	Delivery
Methadone	Methadone AP-HP	Methadone HCL	1 mg	7 capsule
			5 mg	
			10 mg	
			20 mg	
			40 mg	
	Chlorhydrate de Methadone	Methadone HCL	5 mg/3.75 ml	Single dose syrup
			10 mg/7.5 ml	
			20 mg/15 ml	
			40 mg/15 ml	
			60 mg/15 ml	
	Methadone Cloridrato Molteni	Methadone HCL	5 mg/ml	1000 ml oral solution
Fentanyl	Abstral (R)	Fentanyl Citrate	100 μg	10 sublingual tablet
			200 μg	
			400 μg	

Perhaps the biggest challenge facing us is winning the hearts and minds of patients and providers. In a culture where futile interventions are often requested and routinely granted, there is little appreciation for end-of-life discussions, which is viewed as "giving up". Recommending only comfort care in a nation where family ties are tight and tertiary care abundant is often met with suspicion or mistrust. Such misinformation is partly based on poor communications skills, conflicting accounts given to patients by various providers, and not taking sufficient time to establish trust and rapport. An underappreciated natural ally in the growth and acceptance of palliative care medicine in any community is the word-of-mouth of family members who have experienced the process.

Palliative care, done properly, provides better outcomes than curative care alone, is cost effective, and alleviates pain and suffering for patients and caregivers alike [24].

The interdisciplinary approach and continuity of care makes this possible. With a committed and talented group of clinicians working towards this goal, the future of palliative care in Lebanon is encouraging.

References

[1] Center for Disease Control and Prevention; National Vital Statistic System. http://www.cdc.gov/nchs/nvss.htm. Accessed November 26, 2013.

[2] *The World Factbook*, Central Intelligence Agency. http://www.cia.gov/library/publications/the-world-fact-book. Accessed November 26, 2013.

[3] United Nations, Department of Economic and Social Affairs, Population Division (2011). *World Population Prospects: The 2010 Revision*. New York.

[4] Hajjar, R. R., Sabra, M., Touriguian, S. Why Geriatrics? The Rational Behind the Science. *Lebanese Medical Journal*, 2012; 60(4):188-191.

[5] Lebanese Ministry of Public Health, National Cancer Registry (NCR). Beirut, Lebanon: Cancer in Lebanon 2004 with an update of 2003: http://cms1.omsar.gov.lb/en/Health Prevention/EpidemiologicalSurveillanceUnit/Cancer (accessed September 20, 2013).

[6] Hajjar, R. R. *Unpublished data; presented at the annual meeting of the American Geriatric Society – Special interest Group on Ethno-geriatrics*, 2013; Grapevine, TX.

[7] Daher, M., Tabari, H., Stjernsward, J., et al. Lebanon: Pain relief and palliative care. *Journal of Pain and Symptom Management* 2002; 24: 200-4.

[8] Huijer, H., Dimassi, H. Palliative care in Lebanon: Knowledge, attitudes and practices of physicians and nurses. *Lebanese Medical Journal* 2007; 55: 121-8.

[9] Lebanese Ministry of Public Health, National Palliative Care Committee. *Ministerial Decree no. 486,* May 4, 2011.

[10] Lebanese Ministry of Public Health, Patients Rights and Informed Consent. *Ministerial Decree no. 574,* Feb. 11, 2004.

[11] Daher, M., Estephan, E., Abu-Saad Huijer, H., Naja, Z. Implementation of palliative care in Lebanon; past, present, and future. *J. Med. Liban.* 2008; 56: 70-6.

[12] White paper on standards and norms for hospice and palliative care in Europe: Part 2. Recommendation from the European Association on Palliative Care (EAPC). *European Journal of Palliative Care* 2010; 17: 22-33.

[13] *The National Consensus Project for Quality Palliative Care (NCP).* (Second edition). Available at: http://www.nationalconsensusproject.org (accessed December 17, 2013).

[14] Crosswalk of JCAHO standards and palliative care with Palliative care policies, procedures and assessment tools. http://www.capc.org/capc-resources/capc_publica-tions/

[15] Palliative Care Nurse Practitioner Candidate Clinical Competencies. Available at: http://www.capc.org/capc-resources/capc_publications/

[16] The Canadian hospice and palliative care nursing competencies. Available at: http://palliative.info/mpcna/CHPCN_CaseExamples-RevisedFeb2010.pdf.

[17] Meier, D. E.: *Guide to Building a Hospital-Based Palliative Care Program: Center to Advance Palliative Care*, New York: CAPC, 2004.

[18] National Association for Social Workers (NASW), Standards of Social Work Practice in Palliative and End of Life Care. Available at: http://www.socialworkers.org/practice/bereavement/standards/

[19] Osman, H., Abboud, M., El Zein, L., Ghusn, H., Hanna, J., Kanazi, G. Setting practice standards for palliative care in Lebanon; Recommendations of the subcommittee of practice – National Committee for pain Control and Palliative Care. *Lebanese Medical Journal*, 2013; 61:199-203.

[20] Abu-Saad Huijer, H., Dimassi, H. Palliative care in Lebanon; knowledge, attitudes, and practices of physicians and nurses. *J. Med. Liban.* 2007; 55: 121-8.

[21] Antoun, J., Saab, B. R. A culturally sensitive audiovisual package to teach breaking bad news in a Lebanese setting. *Med. Teach.*, 2010; 32 (10): 868-9.

[22] Silbermann, M., Arnaout, M., Daher, M., et al. Palliative cancer care in Middle Eastern countries: accomplishments and challenges. *Ann. Oncol.* 2012; 23(Suppl. 3): 15–28.

[23] Perrot, S., Bannwarth, B., Bertin, Ph., et al. Utilisation de la morphine dans les douleurs rhumatologiques non cancereuses: les recommandations de Limoges. *Rev. Rhum. Mal. Osteoartic.* (Ed. Fr.) 1999; 6:651-7.

[24] Daher M, Doumit M, Hajjar R, Hamra R, Naifeh Khoury M, Tohme A. Integrating palliative care into health education in Lebanon. J Med Liban 2013; 61 (4): 191-198. http://www.lebanesemedicaljournal.org/articles/61-4/review1.pdf

In: Palliative Care to the Cancer Patient
Editor: Michael Silbermann
ISBN: 978-1-63117-709-5

Chapter 11

MOROCCAN EXPERIENCE

Mati Nejmi*[1,*], *M.D. and Leyla Hessissen*[2], *M.D.
[1]National Center of Pain and Palliative Care, INO, Rabat, Morocco
[2]Hospital of Pediatric Oncology and Hematology, Rabat, Morocco

"Fighting cancer is a lifelong mission. It implies a long struggle which enhances our humanity and teaches us humility, solidarity and hope."

HRH Princess Lalla Salma of Morocco

MOROCCO TODAY: THE PARAMETERS OF THE PROBLEM

Morocco (population 32.52 million people) is a country in Northern Africa that covers an area of 700.000 square kilometers. Its boundaries border the North Atlantic Ocean and the Mediterranean Sea, between Algeria and Mauritania. The capital of Morocco is Rabat. (Figure 1)

According to the United Nations human development index (HDI), Morocco is ranked 125/177 countries worldwide (value 0.620) and 6/45 African countries for which an index is available. [1]

This places Morocco in the group of countries with medium human development.

The age distribution of the Moroccan population is as follows: 0-15 years, 27.85%; 16-59 years, 64,54% ; and 60 years and above, 7,61%.

Population living in urban areas 57% and 43% lives in rural Morocco. The estimated life expectancy at birth is 72 years (for males, 70 years and for females, 74 years). Literacy rate among adults aged 15 years or more is 56,10%. GDP per capita is $3082,4. [2]

Morocco is currently in an epidemiological transition marked by a double burden due to the coexistence of infection and chronic diseases. While the prevalence of infectious diseases and the malnutrition is progressively declining, there is an increase in the prevalence of non communicable diseases, such as cardiovascular diseases, chronic diseases and cancers,

* Address for correspondence: mati.nejmi@gmail.com.

accountable for 56% of total morbidity. In particular, cancer burden is getting more and more overwhelming for the health system.

The main factors contributing to these changes are:

- The increasing live expectancy which rose from 47 years in 1962 to 72 years in 2008;
- The rapid socioeconomic development;
- The environmental change;
- The lifestyle changes: sedentary lifestyle, greater and quicker adoption of western diet, and high prevalence of smoking.

The only source of epidemiological information currently deemed valid on the epidemiology of cancer in Morocco is the Grand-Casablanca-Region Cancer Register (CCRCR). This register is based on a population sample accounting for 10% of the Moroccan population. [3]

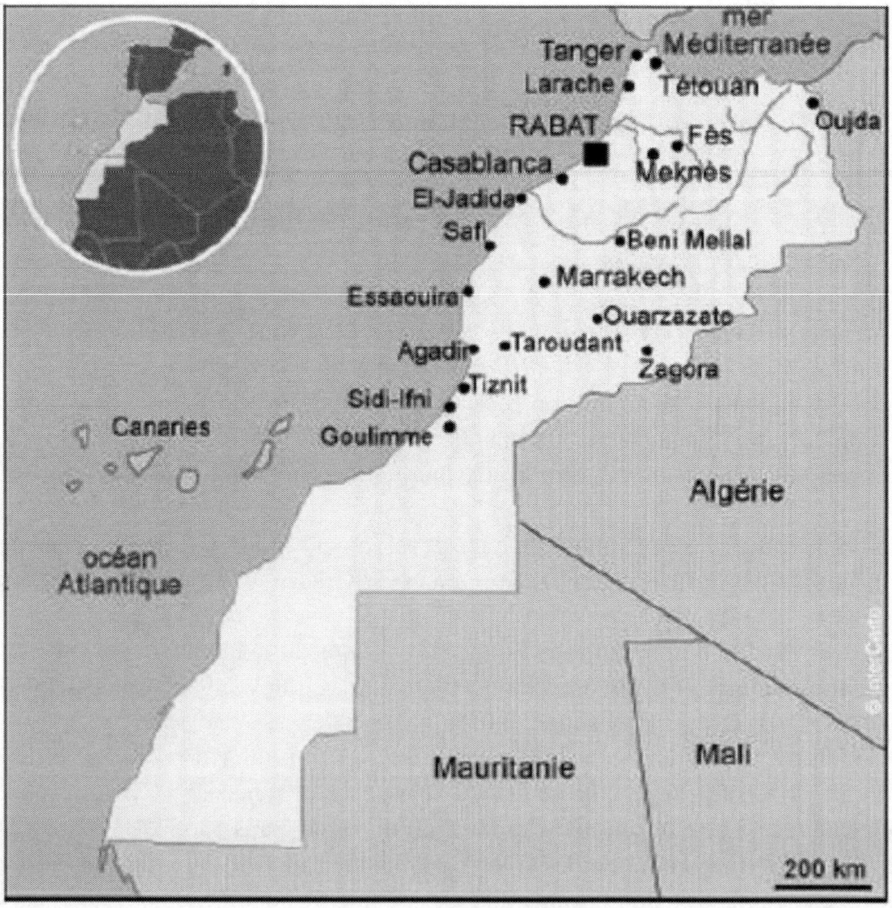

Figure 1. Map of Morocco.

In 2007, the extrapolation of the results to the total Moroccan population leads to a global 35.000 new cases of cancer registered each year. Unfortunately, treatment reaches only near

25.000 of those, leaving many with no treatment and significant pain. Moreover, 60% to 70% of all patients are metastatic and incurable at the time of diagnosis. Cancer is responsible for 8% of death each year.

The most common cancers are breast (36.1%), lung (31.5%), cervix (13.3%), colorectal (12.2%) and prostate (3.7%).

Regarding cancer in children, estimated crude incidence according to the CCRCR is 11.34 for 100.000 children. In children, each year, approximately 1.000 new cases of cancer are registered. This figure accounts for 3.2% of all cancer cases collated. Girls are greater in numbers with a proportion of about 53.8% versus 46.2% for boys. The most frequent cancers in children are malignant hemopathies (19.8%), followed by tumors of the brain and meninges (17.1%), then cancers of bones (12.33%), adrenal glands (11.3%) and eye (10.4%).

Current Moroccan National Plan of Prevention and Care of Cancer

Cancer has only recently emerged as a public health problem in Morocco. The cost of the management of cancer is high and the situation is all more worrying that more than two thirds of the population has no medical coverage. The results of impact studies on the costs related to cancer care are sufficient proof of the heavy burden incurred by households as well as the severe social and economic repercussions of cancer disease; up to 90% of the cost of certain cancers are incurred by patients [3]. As a result, cancer contributes inevitably to making families poorer.

Hence, under the guidance of HRH Princess Lalla Salma, President of the Lalla Salma Foundation for Prevention and Care of Cancer (FLSPCC) [3], and WHO Goodwill Ambassador for Promotion of Cancer Prevention and Care, Morocco has adopted the "International Strategic Approach" and has rallied efforts by the Minister of Health (MoH), civil organizations and other stakeholders, to design of the National Plan of Cancer Prevention and Control (NPCPC).

The NPCPC development project was prepared by the Lalla Salma Foundation for Prevention and Care of Cancer (FLSPCC) in 2005, validated by a steering committee and a joint panel made up of FLSPCC and MoH (joint committee). An ad hoc commission was created for follow-up and monitoring the project.

Situation Analysis

The NPCPC development project began with a situation analysis, carrying out 15 studies and collecting of data in all fields associated with incidence data, behavioral and professional factors, demographics, health care, information on prevention and early detection activities, diagnosis and therapeutic practices, management of pain and palliative care, information on applicable legislation and regulation of substances under the International Board Control, information on the needs of patients and their families, the needs of healthcare practitioners and individuals exposed to risk, population perceptions, knowledge, attitudes and practices toward cancer.

The NPCPC development project, launched in 2010 by the HRH Lalla Salma Foundation began the situation analysis making palliative care as part of the project. It revealed a series of major problems: the lack of a prevention policy and screening program; the absence of a health map; inadequate coverage and a high cost for management, causing treatment to become unaffordable for many patients; inadequate core training of healthcare practitioners in palliative care and a comprehensive patient approach; inadequate linkage between the psychological and ethical fields, a marked separation between health system and social organizations; understaffing of physicians, nurses, attendants, health care aides; and a lack of relief care hospitals adapted to general palliative care and lack of supportive care and cultural good assistance regarding end of life and death.

With regard of leadership of HRH Princess Lalla Salma, the existence of a political will, the recognition of cancer as a priority public health issue, the existence of a dynamic civil society, the availability of human skill potential, this situation requires specific objectives: The development of pain management and the organization of palliative care networks (in hospital, ambulatory care and at home); define family, close social support activities, and research axes.

A number of important measures in the field of palliative care were defined specifically in the situation analysis in order to make this humane project available and realizable:

A beginning must be made to institutionalize pain management at all health system levels, develop palliative care access legislation, and provide pain management training. "Morphinophobia" must be fought through protocolization and the decentralization of pain management activity, as well as by ensuring close familial and social support during cancer illness and the agonizing death phase. Palliative care must be developed and extended into a nationwide network with management structures and defined standards and norms. An information system and the development of research in the field of palliative care must be created.

To make this project a reality, the Minister of Health (MoH) must assume leadership, necessitating social mobilization and partnership at all levels.

Given the incidence and magnitude of its associated suffering, cancer is the logical entry point to begin implementing pain relief and palliative care in Morocco

Palliative Care Service Provision

Current Service

An initial sensitization to the magnitude of cancer pain occurred in 1990 when the first author of this report became head of the department of anesthesiology and intensive care at the National Institute of Oncology in Rabat. He was deeply affected by the severe pain that the majority of patients endured, not only in the post-operative period but also in large numbers of cancer patients coming for out-patient consultation. At that time, only injectable morphine was available and was used to treat emergencies and actually suffering inpatients. The problem was that after this relief, only Buprénorphine was prescribed after patient discharge because of the unavailability of morphine tablets in external pharmacies. We realized that patients soon returned to the department because the Buprénorphine relief was insufficient.

Facing this dilemma, we invited a friend from France, Dr Philippe Poulain, who was at the Institute Gustave Roussy - a famous hospital in Paris dedicated to cancer and palliative care, to come in Rabat to head a conference about how to manage cancer pain with morphine tablets correctly. Thereafter, we urged the hospital administration to buy slow- and immediate-release morphine tablets, and within a few weeks we were able to manage the most of the cancer out-patients correctly. In mars 1995, slow- and immediate- release morphine tablets became available in Morocco and it was easier for us to manage pain in the department and for out-patients.

The first data on the prevalence and management of pain in Morocco became available in late 1994 and revealed a high prevalence of pain (64%) in general practice. Surprisingly, not a single doctor prescribed morphine. More importantly, 2/3 of the Moroccan oncologists were unaware of the 3 steps in the WHO Recommendations for treating cancer pain. This data was presented in Paris in a conference organized by the French Society of Pain (September 1994). In a meeting with Professor Alain Serrie, the founding president of the NGO "Douleurs Sans Frontiers" (DSF) "Pain without Frontiers" based in Paris, he proposed to the first author of this report that he would help us train and support the implementation of pain management and palliative care in Morocco.

The Moroccan Society of Pain and Palliative Care was created (July 1996), located in Rabat.

With the goal of disseminating more information about the burden of pain, the necessity for treatment, and the promotion of palliative care, we organized the 1st Moroccan conference on Pain and Palliative Care (December 1996) in the presence of the past Minister of Health, the Dean of the Medical University in Rabat, and eminent international personalities : Professor Jean-Marie Besson (past président of IASP) ; Professor Charles S. Cleeland (past-president of the American Pain Society), and the president and vice president of "Douleurs Sans Frontières" (Professor Alain Serrie and Doctor Philippe Poulain). The media (TV and journalists) were also invited. This conference constituted the first Moroccan advocacy of the need to manage pain generally, and the treatment of cancer pain and the implementation of palliative care specifically.

Initial pain and palliative care training and education in Morocco was undertaken by the Moroccan Society of Pain and Palliative Care. In 1999, the 3rd Euro-Maghrebin conference on Pain and Palliative Care was held in Marrakech, attended by 300-400 healthcare professionals, Moroccan doctors and nurses, and all the North African health care leaders involved in this field. A panel of international health care leaders from France, Belgium and Switzerland also attended. Significantly, nurse educator Françoise Porchet and other European colleagues were invited to provide two full days of training. They reported:

> "This opportunity allowed us to provide our nursing colleagues in the Maghreb with up-to-date knowledge on palliative care through a process of exchange and constructive learning. It is very gratifying to note that the spirit of palliative care can transcend borders, cultures and languages. It is also important to realize all the possibilities that can arise from a training initiative put together between colleagues from the European countries and the extent to which this is a unifying event." [4]

This initiative has been repeated every two years and conferences have also been organized with other Moroccan Societies (Oncology, Internal Medicines, Anesthesia, Neurology and Nurses). Our organization prepares trainers in the field of disseminating palliative skills around the country.

In 2002, our department, in collaboration with a team headed by Prof. C.S. Cleeland (of Houston Texas), translated the "MD Anderson Symptom Inventory" into Arabic, with the goal of demonstrating the validity and reliability of an Arabic version of the M.D. Anderson Symptom Inventory (MDASI-A) - a multi-symptom assessment tool for use with cancer patients - to describe symptoms related to cancer and its treatment in patients being evaluated at the major cancer center in Morocco. We enrolled a sample of 165 Arabic-speaking patients with different types of cancer who were undergoing various treatments and experiencing pain and other symptoms. The majority of the patients in the sample (68%) had advanced cancers. The average age was 49 (+/-) years of age, 56% were females. 95% were educated below a high school level, and only 4% were employed at the time of the survey. Breast, gastro-Intestinal, lung and gynecologic cancers affected about 68% of the patients. Sixty-two percent of sample had an ECOG performance at level 3 or 4. Cancer-specific treatments were being given to 24% of these patients, with 8%, and 14% of the sample undergoing chemo and radiation therapy, respectively, in the month preceding their enrollment in the study. The most severe symptoms were pain, fatigue, poor appetite, sadness, sleep disturbance, shortness of breath and distress. Patient-reported fatigue, sadness, numbness, and poor appetite were most predictive of average interference with patient's daily life.

Based on this study, we concluded that the Arabic version of the MDASI is a valid and reliable patient-reported outcome instrument which can be used to evaluate patient's multiple symptoms in clinical practice for symptom management or in clinical research among Arabic-speaking cancer patients in Morocco. Furthermore, this assessment tool could be used by all stakeholders who are involved in cancer pain and palliative care in the Arab countries. [5] The findings regarding the majority of patients in severe pain were so important and dramatic, and the utility of MDASI-A for research in palliative care so evident, that the publication of the study won the Moroccan Medical Research award in 2002.

Attending this ceremony, the Minister of Health was so moved, that he decided to build the first National Center of Pain and Palliative Care in the National Institute of Oncology in Rabat. HRH Princess Lalla Salma, who laid the cornerstone for the Center, thereby demonstrated her support for the implementation of palliative care and the management of relieving pain for cancer patients. (See photo)

Implementation

Opened in 2005, this first National Center of Pain and Palliative Care (NCPPC) in Morocco provides the only palliative care service in the country, with 10-beds hospital inpatient unit and an outpatient clinic. At the time, the staff consisted of a coordinator (first author), an assistant, three physicians, one psychologist and four nurses. A median of 800 patients were hospitalized each year for cancer pain and palliative care and 7.000 patients have been treated following pain consultations in 2008. (Figure 2)

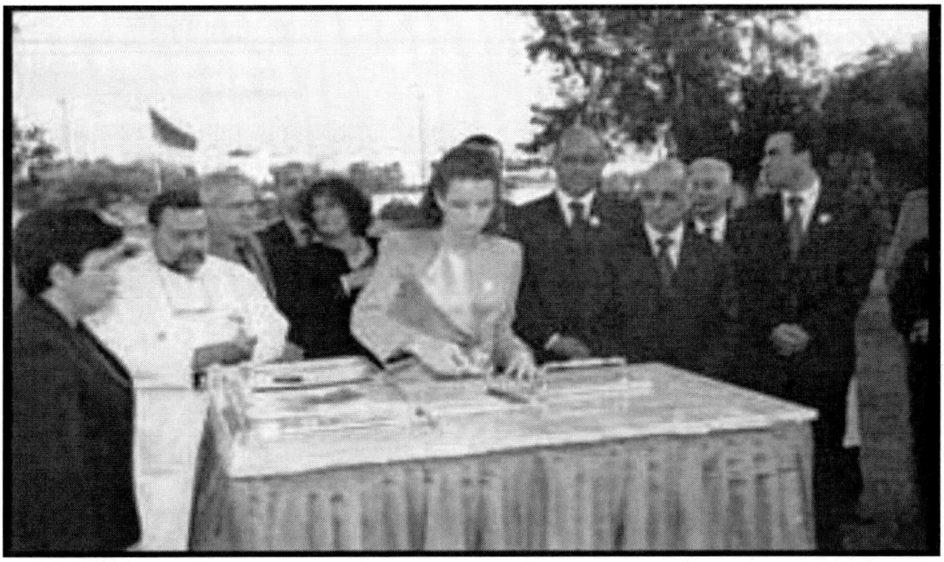

Figure 1. HRH Princess Lalla Salma laying the first cornerstone of the National Center of Pain and Palliative Care in Rabat.

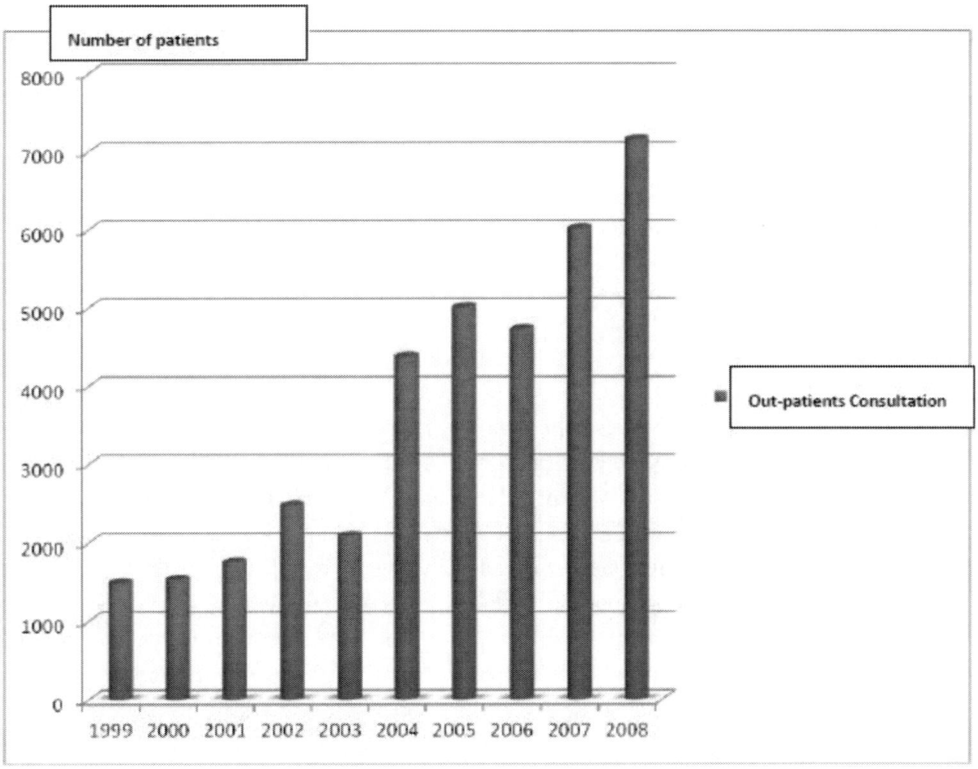

Figure 2. Number of patients in out-patients consultation.

The Main Objectives of the NCPPC Are: Care, Training and Research in Palliative Care

A pilot project was launched in 2012 in Rabat and the surrounding region, covering a population of 657.000 inhabitants. A Mobile team cares for cancer patient emergencies. A team of 4 doctors and 4 nurses trained in pain and palliative care respond to emergency calls from patient's homes. If necessary, they travel by medical ambulance to the home and evaluate the situation. If relieving the patient at home is possible, they provide all the necessary medications to continue treatment. If not, the patient is brought to the NCPPC and is hospitalized. A decision about the patient's condition is determined by the entire team by mobile consultation. This is the first project launched in Morocco to link the NCPPC with families and general practitioners in managing cancer or palliative care emergencies. It will be evaluated in terms of efficacy, and may be duplicated in other big cities in Morocco country as soon as possible.

Intermediate and Long-Term Outcomes

Drug Availability

Morocco suffered from outdated prescription rules and opioid regulation that did not allow for adequate pain control. The consequence was restricted availability and accessibility of opioids. While injectable morphine was used in a very few hospitals, only a seven-day supply of morphine tablets could be prescribed to out-patients.

Fortunately, this excessive regulation was changed by the Moroccan parliament in July 2013, amending the obsolete and restrictive law of 1922. Now, morphine could be prescribed for 28 days without maximal doses, and is available as necessary for patients. Nevertheless, in a country where only 35% of the population is insured, the cost of medications for a month of freedom from pain should be minimal. In practice and ideally, morphine must be given free of charge to the suffering in the same way that chemotherapy is delivered to cancer patients by the FLSPCC.

All physicians are allowed to prescribe opioids according to proper medical practice. The problem is that the prescription must be done on a "special book" for only opioids and all the physicians must ask and obtain it from the Health Ministry Division of Medicine and Pharmacy. The process is so problematic that many physicians are reluctant to ask for this "special book". This obstacle must be removed if we want to allow physicians to prescribe more morphine for pain medications. The "special book" must be replaced by immediate accessibility of the prescribed drug. Moreover, if a patient cannot come to the hospital in person, a reliable person should be entitled to receive the prescription and purchase the morphine on behalf of the patient. These simplifications will contribute to the elimination of the practitioners' opiophobia and encourage them, after proper training, to prescribe morphine as needed.

Prior to 1995, the International Narcotics Control Board (INCB) importation quota was extremely low. It began to progressing annually after 1996, but so slowly that the actual quota of 7.7 kg each year is totally insufficiency (Figure 3 and Figure 4).

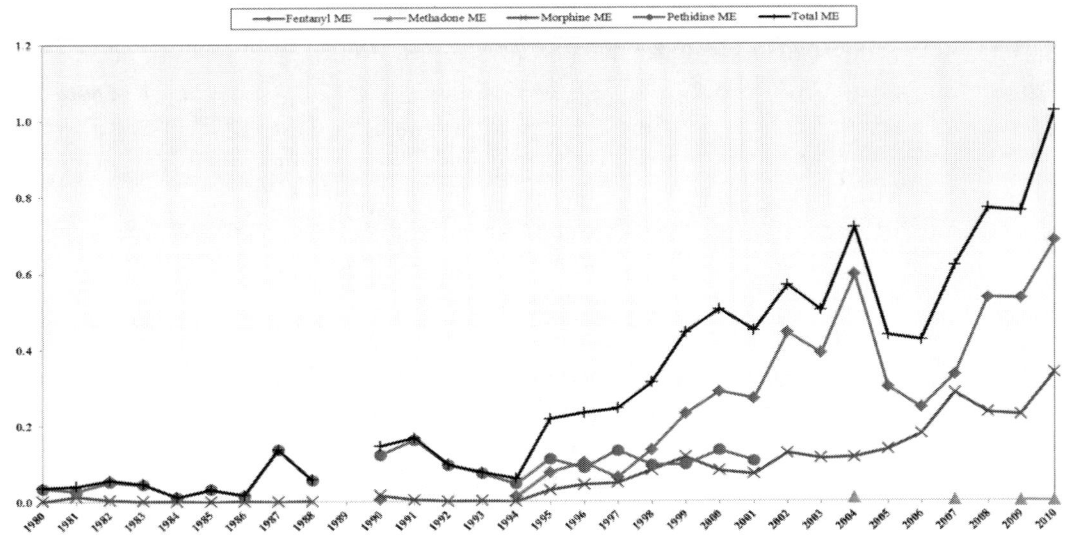

Sources:
Consumption – International Narcotics Control Board
Population – World Health Organization
ME Conversion factors – WHO CC Centre for Drug Statistics Methodolgy

Pain & Policy Studies Group
University of Wisconsin
Carbone Cancer Center
WHO Collaborating Center

Figure 3. Morocco. Opioid Consumption in Morphine Equivalence (ME), Mg/person.

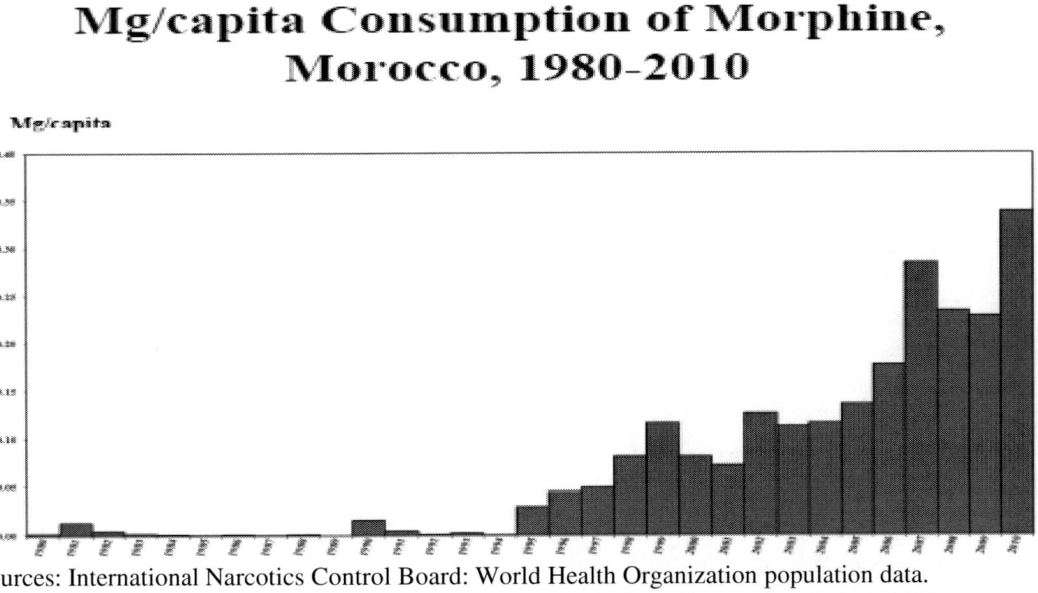

Sources: International Narcotics Control Board: World Health Organization population data.
By: Pain & Policy Studies Group, University of Wisconsin/WHO Collaborating Center, 2012.

Figure 4. Mg/capita consumption of morphine, Morocco, 1980-2010.

In December 2010, the Moroccan Society of Pain and Palliative Care organized a 2-days "Workshop on Availability and Accessibility of Opioids" in Marrakech with the support Dr. Willem Scholten representant of WHO; Dr. Martha Maurer of Pain and Policy Study

Group; Prof. Alain Serrie of DSF; Dr. Henry Dungu of African Palliative Care Association; representants of the Governmental Division of Control Substances and the Center of Pharmaco-Supervision in Morocco. During the sessions, size of the situation of cancer and HIV were discussed. Then the Barriers to Opioid Availability Test (BOAT) and the Self Assessment Checklist (SAT) in Morocco were evaluated, demonstrating the high burden of cancer in Morocco and the need for an action plan on an emergency basis.

A recent 2012 report from the Pain and Policy Studies Group at the University of Wisconsin, and Human Rights Watch pointed this failure. In 2009, a total of 14.278 cancer and 708 HIV patients were died. The opioids quota was at this time only sufficient to relieve pain from 31.6% of these patients. The result was that 11.777 patients died in unnecessary moderate-to-severe pain. The morphine necessary to meet the minimum demand of deaths due to HIV and cancer is 73 kg annually [6], which means that Morocco's 7.7 kg quota provides for only a tenth of those in need. Clearly, this is an insufficient amount. The main barriers to necessary availability and accessibility are the fear of addiction and the high cost of opioids.

This dramatic situation must be evaluated by the Governmental Division of Medicine and Pharmacy as soon as possible. WHO guidelines could help formulate a national drug control policy, estimate annual requirements, report consumption statistics to be submitted to the International Narcotics Control Board (INCB), and administer an effective distribution system to patients.

Another major problem is the unavailability of morphine both in the majority of the big Moroccan cities and in the rural area. Even in the big cities like Rabat and Casblanca, morphine is available only in the few pharmacies located near an oncology hospital or clinic. The major reasons for the paucity of pharmacies are the restrictive law, alongside the fear of robbery and misuse. We have begun sensitizing pharmacists regarding the need to make morphine accessible for patients, emphasizing their moral obligation to play a role in the humanitarian effort to improve the management of cancer pain in our country.

Education and Training

It is important that the goals of the National Plan of Cancer Prevention and Control (NPCPC) foundation are addressed in a coordinated way. Educational lectures on pain and palliative care during the conferences and seminars in the National Center of Pain and Palliative Care (NCPPC) have a sensitizing effect on health care professionals.

Since 1996, all doctors studying for an Anesthesiologist diploma in the Medical University of Rabat must spend six months in a training period in our department of Anesthesiology and Intensive care, and since we opened the NCPPC in 2005, they receive all the necessary education on the evaluation and management of acute and chronic pain. They have responsibility both in the intensive care and out-patient consultations about pain. Palliative care is also one of the curriculum.

Together with the Moroccan Society of Hemato-oncology and the Moroccan Society of Pediatrics and Hematology we participated in organizing training about pain management and palliative care in pediatrics in the major towns in Morocco in 2010, attended by 200 pediatrics.

Caravane douleur 2006/2007

	Date	Ville	Présence MG
2006	17-avr-06	Casa I	130
	25-avr-06	Rabat I	160
	18-mai-06	Marrakech	140
	01-juin-06	Tanger	190
	07-juin-06	Fès	200
	22-juin-06	Rabat II	130
	06-juil-06	Agadir	160
	13-juil-06	Meknès	200
	20-juil-06	Casa II	220
			1530
2007	26-avr-07	Guelmim	70
	11-mai-07	Oujda	200
	08-juin-07	Béni Mellal	80
	14-juin-07	Kénitra	167
	15-juin-07	El Jadida	125
	21-juin-07	Khémisset	60
			702
			2232

Figure 5. Attendance at "Caravan of Pain" conferences in 2006-2007.

In 2006-2007, we organized two "Caravan of Pain" conferences in all the main cities in Morocco aimed at sensitizing general practitioners about problematic pain management in our country. The conferences focused on the physiopathology, evaluation, opioid pharmacology and treatment of acute and chronic pain. Palliative care was also taught. Over 2.200 general practitioners attended. (Figure 5) They were also urged coming to Rabat for training and improving them practice in the management of the unnecessary pain of our thousands citizens.

Intensive follow-up bedside training is critical in order to provide hands-on experience in prescribing opioids. This is the fundamental rule that we apply when we introduced a University certificate "Management of pain and palliative care" in the Faculty of medicine in Rabat. Teaching was carried out with the support of doctors from "Douleurs Sans Frontières" (DSF) who came from France and gave 3-to-5 day theoretical seminars. Candidates worked 2 days weekly in the department of Anesthesiology and Intensive care and also in the National Cancer of Pain and Palliative Care (NCPPC), gaining hands-on experience in understanding how to evaluate the intensity of pain, start a titration of morphine, and prescribe a correct dosage to patients when they leave the hospital and continue their treatment at home.

During 2005-2010, each year 40 doctors took part in this training curriculum annually.

Once generic morphine became available in Morocco in 1996 and bedside training was introduced, greater confidence was built up in the use of opioids. Seeing positive effects in patients created enthusiasm for opioid use and helped the physicians overcome their opiophobia. Experience in India has demonstrated that if bedside training is not giving, clinicians will not use the available analgesics effectively or alter their clinical practice.

Moreover, introducing bedside training before drugs are available will also have little impact. Thus, it is imperative that training and availability of opioid analgesics be coordinated.

Nurses from DSF were also for great help. Two nurses were present at the NCPPC every month, taking part in the training our nurses in pain management, the philosophy of palliative care, and the encounter with physical, emotional and existential problems.

At the same time, training is offered to intern nurses in our hospital and in the Institute of Formation of Nurses in Rabat. Several nursing students have written papers about cancer pain and palliative care.

THE WAY FORWARD

Over the past 18 years, remarkable progress has been made in Morocco in overcoming the barriers to the integration of palliative care in cancer care, increasing knowledge and skills, and improving the experience of patients and families.

Significant accomplishments by the Moroccan Society of Pain and Palliative Care (MSPPC), its members, and other stakeholders since the establishment of the NPPCC project at the initiative of HRH Princess Lalla Salma in 2005 are as follows.

Clinical Accomplishments

From its beginnings, the MSPPC understood that the supply of optimal pain and palliative care requires access to and availability of care rendered by skilled clinicians, buttressed when necessary by palliative care experts. Moreover, the integration of pain and palliative in the curricula of all future doctors is necessary and should be introduced in all the Moroccan Medical Universities and the Nursing Schools.

Advocacy and Policy Statements

Internationally, the WHO, the International Narcotics Control Board (INCB) and other agencies advocate for palliative care as an integral part of cancer care. The insufficient quota of morphine and other essential drugs by our regulatory system must be amended, as recommended in “Achieving Balance to Availability and Accessibility of Opioids” edited by the Pain and Policy Study Group and the organization of Human Rights Watch. Opioids are absolutely necessary for medical and scientific research needs. Estimated annual requirements, the report of consumption statistics, and the submission of statistical reports to the INCB are fundamental. Our authorities should permit and encourage the distribution of opioid medications throughout the country, maximizing access while maintaining adequate controls.

In 2005, the 58th World Health Assembly fully integrated palliative care into its resolution WHA58.22 to improve cancer prevention and control. The resolution recognizes palliative care as an essential component of comprehensive cancer care, equal to medical, surgical, and radiation oncology. It urges member nations to fully integrate palliative care into their national cancer control programs.

Integration of Palliative Care

Several innovative models integrating palliative care in cancer care have been developed in the last decade. Adopting the model at the University of Texas M.D. Anderson Cancer Center (Houston, Texas) since 2005, Morocco has been integrating palliative care into its outpatient and inpatient services.

Educational Accomplishments

Moroccan physicians have demonstrated tremendous interest in learning about the evaluation and management of pain, along with the philosophy of palliative care. Moroccan Society members are proud to be part of this noble and humane mission.

Recognition of Palliative Medicine as a Specialty

With palliative care formally recognized as a medical specialty in several countries (Australia, Ireland, the United Kingdom, the United States and France), we hope that in the next few years, it will attain this recognition in Morocco as well.

References

[1] Report of the United Nations Development program 2004 (HDI 2002). See: http://hdr.undp.org/statistics/data/indic_8_1_1.html
[2] WHO. See: http://www.who.int/chp/chronic_disease_report
[3] Fondation Lalla Salma de Prévention et Contrôle du Cancer. www.contrelecancer.ma
[4] Porchet F, Schaerer G, Larkin P, Leruth S. Intercultural experiences of training in the Maghreb. *Eur. J. Palliative Care* 2005;12(1):35-37.
[5] Mati Nejmi, Xin Shelley Wang, Tito Mendoza, Ibrahima Gning and Charles S Cleeland. Validation and application of the Arabic Version of the M.D. Anderson Symptom Inventory in Moroccan Patients with cancer. *JPSM Vol. 40* n°1 July 2010. Pp 75-86.
[6] Pain and Policy Studies Group. University of Wisconsin. Carbone Cancer Center (USA) WHO Collaboration Center.

In: Palliative Care to the Cancer Patient
Editor: Michael Silbermann
ISBN: 978-1-63117-709-5

Chapter 12

PALLIATIVE CARE IN OMAN

Zakiya Al-Lamki, M.B., Ch.B, DCH, MRCP, FRCP (UK), FRCPCH, FRCP[1]*
and Shah Mohammed Wasifuddin, M.D., DCH, FRCPCH[2]
[1] College of Medicine & Health Sciences, Sultan Qaboos University, Muscat, Sultanate of Oman, Ireland
[2] The National Oncology Center, Royal Hospital, Muscat, Sultanate of Oman, UK

ABSTRACT

Background

The Oman Ministry of Health was able to establish a modern national health system that offers all its citizens accessible services free of charge. The rapid developments brought a significant decline in communicable diseases thus earning a global recognition. With the ageing population and changes of lifestyle, there is a rising trend of non-communicable diseases including cancer. The climbing rates further complicated by the advanced stage presentation of the disease and patients' late reporting of pain thus drew attention to the need for palliative care services. These efforts have been complimented by National Association for Cancer Awareness (NACA). Prior to that, there were patchy distribution of services mainly localized at the two tertiary institutions. Treatment of pain was mainly by traditional methods until the introduction of morphine after the early 1980s. The ministry of health has legislative control and restrictive regulations on use of narcotics.

Framework Development

There was a paradigm shift from only curative to palliative services. In year 2008 a workshop was held during a pediatric conference. In 2012, NACA jointly with the Middle

* Address for correspondence: zakiya.allamki@gmail.com

East Cancer Consortium (MECC), launched an introductory course in palliative care for nurses followed by a symposium in 2013. As part of capacity building two nurses from national oncology center were sent to North America for training.

Pain Management

Small teams of palliative care are established at the tertiary hospitals .The WHO Ladder for pain management is used as a guide. Pain management is family-centered, non-pharmacological measures, pharmacological and adjuvant therapy are used. Spiritual healing is widely applied by patients and education is important part of the management. Most analgesics drugs are available in Oman. Morphine consumption is 0.66mg/capita. (Figure 1)

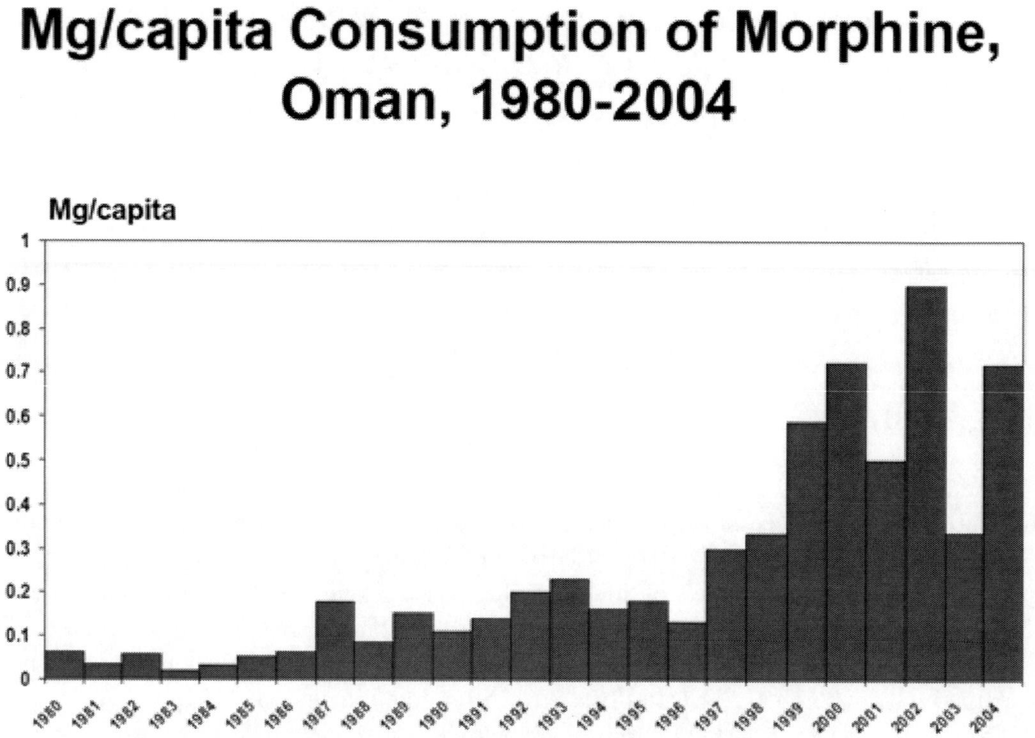

Source: International Narcotics Control Board, United Nations Demographic Yearbook.
By: Pain & Policy Studies Group, University of Wisconsin WHO Collaborating Center, 2006.

Figure 1. Mmg/Capita Morphine consumption.

Barriers and Future Reforms

Cost in Oman is not considered as a barrier to palliative care. Tradition, beliefs and culture are main barriers. Pain management is considered a luxury with worries about addiction and lack of awareness. There is late reporting of pain and highly restrictive policies for prescriptions. Analgesics are not readily available, palliative care training programs are limited and there is very little of support services. However, Oman is taking major steps to improve cancer care, addressing the need of palliative care and developing framework to integrate into a wider health service within the reach of the community. There is an urgent need of capacity building, educating and training both the professionals and the public.

INTRODUCTION

The Sultanate of Oman is the second largest country on the southeastern corner of the Arabian Peninsula. It covers a total area of approximately 309,500 square kilometers and a mid-year population (by the National Center for Statistics and Information) in 2012 of 3,623,001. More than 80% of the government revenues come from oil and gas with a GDP of about 78 billion United States dollars (USD).

To emphasize the importance of health and social development, the ministry of health was established soon after the renaissance in 1970. It was able to build from scratch through proper health planning, a modern national health system that offers all its citizens universally accessible health services free of charge. Directing the expansion of its services to primary health care and public health, brought a decline in preventable diseases and dramatic drop in infant and child morbidity and mortality rates. The improvements occurred at a high speed and much less time than in many other countries to the extent that the World Health Organization (WHO), in its analysis of health system documented in its Year 2000 Report, ranked Oman first among all 191 WHO member states on health level and 8th as regards health system performance. In 2010, the United Nations Development Program listed Oman as one among the world's ten leading countries for putting up the best performance in public health. [1,2]

CURRENT STATE OF AFFAIRS

Health statistics revealed that communicable diseases accounted for 43.2% of the total outpatient visits in 1996 compared to 31.5% in 2011 and non-communicable diseases was 42.5% in 1996 compared to 49.9% in 2011. During 1990, inpatient morbidity of communicable diseases had constituted 21.4% of the total discharges and this was reduced to 17.9% in 2011. Cancer ranges between the first to the third cause of mortality in the inpatients depending on the age group. [3]

The 2011 figures from the Oman Population Based Cancer Registry which was established in 1996 showed that the crude incidence rates for all cancer among Omanis were 55.2 per 100,000 for males and 56 per 100,000 for females. The age standardized rate, adjusted to the world standard population was 123.2 per 100,000 for males and 103.7 per 100,000 for females. Cancer among children aged 14 years and below, constituted 7.3% of the total cancers reported. Although the age adjusted incidence rates appear lowest in comparison to industrialized countries, it has been shown from the ageing population and increasing cancer risks due to lifestyle changes as observed elsewhere, that Oman is facing an upward trend in cancer incidence.[4] It is therefore witnessing a growing shift of its health problems, from communicable to non-communicable diseases. This led to the need of strengthening its secondary and tertiary care activities directed towards control of non-communicable diseases including cancer. This was complimented by the work of a Non-Governmental Organization (NGO), National Association for Cancer Awareness (NACA), founded in 2004, by a cancer survivor whose aim was to educate, train the public and support cancer patients and research. The climb in cancer rates further complicated by the advanced stage presentation of the disease and patients' late reporting of pain has restored attention of the health caregivers. For those patients the only realistic treatment option is pain relief and thus the need for palliative care services have emerged. Prior to that, attention to palliative care has been minimal with patchy distribution of services mainly localized at the two tertiary institutions namely the Royal Hospital in the Ministry of Health and the Sultan Qaboos University Hospital (SQUH) each with a total bed capacity of about 700 and a 550 respectively.

Historical Perspectives

Prior to 1970 cautery by the colloquial Arabic name of "wassam" was used as a form of traditional medicine to treat pain. This was similar to the Chinese old therapy of "moxibustion" but instead of using a fire heated dried herb, it uses metal sticks or iron nails that are heated red hot and applied at the site of the pain. Dry and wet Cupping was also used successfully as a form of local pain relief. Severe cases of pain were treated in hospitals with intramuscular pethidine (meperidine hydrochloride) whenever necessary. SQUH approved the use of both parenteral and oral narcotics in 1989 and started pain management after receiving its first consignment in the same year. The Ministry of Health has a legislative control of narcotic drugs thus preventing their misuse and illegal acquirement. Slow release oral morphine was only obtainable from the Royal Hospital Oncology department with special prescription signed by a senior consultant oncologist. In 1996, the central drug committee on the recommendation of the national cancer committee took the decision to allow oral morphine usage in some regional hospitals with oncology units.[5] Until 2006, SQUH was the only hospital, besides the Royal Hospital, allowed to procure, stock, and dispense oral narcotics. Health institutions are required to submit their annual opioid consumption to the regulatory authority, the Directorate General of Pharmaceutical Affairs and Drug Control in Ministry of Health who process the import authorization by providing country's detailed annual estimates and reports on the requirements to the International Narcotic Control Board. WHO assist access for permission to the country's requirements of narcotics and psychotropic drugs. Illegal possession or non- medical consumption of these controlled drugs is closely monitored by the local police. The country's total consumption of morphine is 0.66mg./capita (the global mean is at 5.57mg/capita). [6,7]]Fully licensed Doctors (and not nurses) are allowed to prescribe for inpatients as well as for ambulatory cases. Special prescription forms are in use, signed and stamped along with an electronic request (figs. 1,11).

EDUCATION AND TRAINING

It was not until the year 2008 when the first initiative was undertaken by a palliative care workshop held during the pediatric cancer conference (5th SIOP-Asia) under the umbrella of International Network for Cancer Treatment and Research (INCTR). In January 2012, ministers of the six Gulf Cooperation Countries (GCC) met in Muscat to respond to the call from United Nations General Assembly on political declaration and control of non-communicable diseases. One month later, the Middle East Cancer Consortium (MECC), American National Cancer Institute (NCI) and Oncology Nursing Society (ONS) in collaboration with the Oman National Association for Cancer Awareness (NACA) organized the first palliative care course for Omani nurses. As a direct follow up of that course, in February 2013 MECC jointly with NACA, ONC and the American Society of Oncology (ASCO) organized a training course which was followed by a research day in palliative care in the community as well as two international workshops in the geriatrics and pediatrics oncology respectively. Besides local health care professionals, a number of participants from regional countries as well as North America and Europe participated in those events.[8,9]

While palliative care is often associated with cancer, a much wider circle of patients with health conditions that limit their ability to live a normal life can benefit from it. It gradually became recognized by health care providers that palliative care is an integral part of health care system for cancer and therefore there is a paradigm shift from curative services to palliative care. Both medical and nursing staff is eager to make changes. As part of capacity building, two nurses from the national oncology center were sent to Calvary in United States of America for few weeks training in palliative care where they learnt on how to address the medical, psychological and mental needs of advanced cancer care patients and their families. They sat in on bereavement groups with social workers, and visited the hospice.

EXISTING SERVICES

There are pain management teams in both tertiary care centers namely the SQUH and the Royal Hospital. These were built gradually through the past few years and consist of a small multidisciplinary group of motivated nurses and physicians, mainly from the oncology and hematology units led by a senior anesthetist. The teams conduct independent joint clinics for the follow up of adult patients with chronic pain as well as newly referred cases internal and outside the hospitals. These are held twice and thrice weekly for cancer patients and all other types of pain. At SQUH, in addition, there is an interventional pain management clinic once a week. The team is responsible for answering inpatient calls on patients with intractable pain not responding to conventional treatment. It is also responsible for initiating patient control analgesia (PCA) give epidural, peripheral nerve blocks, articular joint blocks with steroids and occasionally permanent blocks with radiofrequency ablation. The Royal Hospital team provides training in pain management and conduct end of life courses for nurses quarterly around the year. Staff from other hospitals around the country also attends these courses thus extending training to the regions. Irregular meetings of the team members are being held. There is a continuous effort to develop national educational guidelines for cancer treatment, pain management, and palliative care. Pain control guidelines and standard protocols are in place at SQUH which are regularly updated. Clinical audits and peer reviews are conducted. [10] There are also minimal services rendered by a small team of two nurses and anesthetists established at the main trauma center, Khoula hospital. It mainly provides support for acute pain in cases that need postoperative analgesia and occasionally answers inpatient calls for interventional analgesia such as epidural blocks or PCA. They do not follow up patients with chronic pain and do not hold formal meetings or educational activities.

All treatment modalities of cancer are available at the two treating centers, the National Oncology Centre (NOC) at the Royal Hospital and the Oncology Units at the Sultan Qaboos University Hospital (SQUH). These facilities offer state of the art Medical Oncology practice, Radiation Oncology, Bone Marrow Transplantation and modern diagnostic facilities. Besides provision of tertiary medical care both institutions offer teaching and training to undergraduate and postgraduate medical students and nurses. There are no hospices yet but home visits activities not specific for palliative purposes, are being initiated by community nurses.

Pain Management

The WHO Ladder for pain management is used in oman as a guide. Linear analogue pain scales are used for assessing pain intensity and in children, the 'faces' scale is usually used. Pain management is Family-Centered and therefore family is an integral part of the palliative care team. Non-Pharmacological measures, pharmacological and adjuvant therapy are used. Patient education is an important part of the management mainly carried out by nurses who explain on the cause of pain and symptoms. They emphasize on the importance of reporting pain early and address patients' concerns. Most analgesics drugs are available in Oman, non-opioids as well as opioids such as acetaminophen, non- steroidal anti-inflammatory drugs, codeine, tramadol, morphine, pethidine and fentanyl. Slow release morphine as well as the oral suspension form and fentanyl patches are generally prescribed for chronic pain. Anticonvulsants are sometimes used for neurogenic types of pain. Patient Control Analgesia (PCA) and epidural blocks are also used in acute and postoperative pain. Non-pharmacological measures used are mainly distraction therapy, physical exercise and positive reinforcement in children. Transcutaneous Electrical Nerve Stimulation (TENS) is sometimes applied. Although modern medicine is recommended, but traditional practices and spiritual healing are equally important forms of treatment. Reciting verses from the holy Qur'an is found very comforting and help patients cope with pain. Drinking the holy "zamzam" water also provides a soothing effect.

Barriers to Palliative Care

Oman has put in place a functioning drug supply system. Cost and availability of the palliative care drugs is not considered a barrier to palliative care. However treatment is not evenly distributed amongst the tertiary and the secondary hospitals in the various regions. Pain management teams are not yet established in many of the hospitals and in those few where they do exist, their operational functions are still limited. Pain management is considered a luxury with fear of addiction equally among the health care professionals as well as the patients and that is why they are reluctant to take opioids. The lack of knowledge and awareness in both parties coupled by the unnecessarily restrictive drug control regulations and practices worsen the legitimate prescribing of narcotics. Tradition, public beliefs and culture are main barriers. As in the rest of the muslim community, when a bad event happens the Omanis believe that it is a divine fate. Because of their strong faith, they accept it better and they put all their trust in Allah. Pain is considered a test from God or spiritual trial which teaches understanding and better use of life. They tend to under report pain because they think it is part of the disease and believe that pain and suffering wipe away one's sins. They delay in seeking treatment and usually wait until pain and symptoms are severe before reporting. Care of the dying is considered an important responsibility of the family and friends. Death is preferred at home, surrounded by loved ones and prayers. Physicians avoid honest end of life conversations. Religious teachings say "Seek God's help with prayer and patience". The caring physician is therefore expected to strike a balance between alleviating the suffering while maintaining a level of consciousness that enables a patient to worship God till death. Another encountered barrier is the hectic schedules of the health care providers that rarely leave them time to focus on patients' and their families' well-being and there is very little in the way of support services. Palliative care in Paediatric Oncology is still in its infancy due to the highly specialized nature of the disease in this age group and also owing to bureaucratic restrictions. Most of the care is provided by the medical and nursing teams of the parent paediatric oncology teams. [11]

Opportunities and Future Developments

Combination of these barriers coupled by regulatory hurdles and the effect of the global war on drugs are largely to blame for the suboptimal palliative care offered to patients with cancer and other serious illnesses resulting in severe suffering and agonizing death. As part of best practices, there is need to address the existing barriers through comprehensive reform. Oman is taking major steps to improve cancer care and addresses the need of palliative care. In the anticipation of the rising numbers of patients with cancer, Oman requested the International Atomic Energy Agency (IAEA) imPACT review which was conducted under the WHO–IAEA joint program in collaboration with International Agency for Research on Cancer (IARC) and other partner agencies. In January 2013 a team of international experts in the areas of cancer control planning, carried out visits to various sites where cancer-related services are offered to get a fuller understanding of the organizational capacities, challenges and the quality of the services provided for the cancer patients and their families in order to assess the national cancer burden including palliative care. The imPACT Review Mission will submit a report to the Ministry of Health and provide recommendations to the Omani health authorities to better address the cancer burden and in the long term, give the Omani people increased chances of survival and a better quality of life. [12] The aim is to launch a national policy that integrates a palliative care program in the health care system and work on the need of developing policies and procedures for pain assessment and management. Development of palliative care curricula in nursing and medical schools is an essential requirement in addition to education and awareness of the public and professional community at large. The return from abroad of well trained Omani specialized doctors will have positive effect on scaling up the provision of such care, Hospices movement should be expanded and introduction of mind-body exercises to distress nurses and physicians in the care of the suffering is an essential tool for the success of this new modality of care.

Oman's developments so far and the ongoing efforts by the government, earned recognition by the European Society of Medical Oncology (ESMO). It designated centres including Oman of integrated oncology and palliative care program in their 10th anniversary this year. This highlights the growing importance of palliative care in cancer treatment worldwide. The accreditation is valid for three years and centres can reapply. We will need to maintain the ESMO designation.

Conclusion

Palliative Care in Oman received late attention but in the short time since the awareness and capacity building phase began, a lot has been achieved. Health authorities have shown their resolve by supporting and facilitating efforts to plan an organized and structured service in the country based on future requirements. International organizations and local NGOs such as NACA are also playing an important role in these efforts.

Conflict of Interest

We declare: No Conflict of Interest.

Acknowledgement

We wish to acknowledge the Pain Management Teams at SQUH, Royal & Khoula Hospitals

All reasonable precautions have been taken to verify the validity of information contained herein.

References

[1] The Public Versus The World Health Organization On Health System Performance, Health Affairs; Robert J. Blendon, Minah Kim and John M. Benson 2001.

[2] Healthcare earns global recognition; *Ministry of health Bulletin* 2012-2013.

[3] Annual Health Reports; Department of Health Information & Statistics; Director General of Planning, Ministry of Health; Chapter 9, *Morbidity & Mortality* 2011.

[4] Cancer Incidence in Oman, *Ministry of Health* 2011.

[5] Community Health & Diseases Surveillance Newsletter by MOH Vol. VII No.1 Jan-Mar 98.

[6] Oman Pharmaceutical Country Profile: Published by MOH in collaboration with WHO Sawsan Ahmed Jaffer.

[7] Opioids in middle eastern population Silbermann M. *Asian Pac. J Cancer Prev*. Apr 11 Suppl 1: 1-5.

[8] Impressions and Experiences of a Palliative Care Courses to Nurses in the Sultanate of Oman. Michael Silbermann *J Palliative Care & Medicine* 2012, 2-3.

[9] Nurses Paving the Way to Improving Palliative Care Services in the Middle East; Michael Silbermann and Manal Al-Zadjali; *J Palliative Care Med* 2013; 3-4.

[10] Historical perspectives and trends in the management of pain for cancer patients in Oman. Mahfudh SS *Asian Pac. J. Cancer Prev*. 2010 Apr, 11 Suppl 1: 93-6.

[11] Middle East experience in palliative care. Zeinah GF, Al-Kindi SG, Hassan AA. *Am J Hosp Palliat Care*, 2013 Feb; 30 (1): 94-9.

[12] Jennifer S. Temel, M.D., Joseph A. Greer, Ph.D., Alona Muzikansky, M.A., Emily R. Gallagher, R.N., Sonal Admane, M.B., B.S., M.P.H., Vicki A. Jackson, M.D., M.P.H., Constance M. Dahlin, A.P.N., Craig D. Blinderman, M.D., Juliet Jacobsen, M.D., William F. Pirl, M.D., M.P.H., J. Andrew Billings, M.D., and Thomas J. Lynch, M.D., Early Palliative Care for Patients with Metastatic Non–Small-Cell Lung Cancer *N Engl J Med* 2010; 363:733-742, August 19, 2010.

In: Palliative Care to the Cancer Patient
Editor: Michael Silbermann

ISBN: 978-1-63117-709-5

Chapter 13

PALLIATIVE CARE IN PAKISTAN

Rehana Punjwani**, R.N. and Muhammad Shamvil Ashraf, M.B.B.S. (DOW), DCH, MCPS, MRCP, FCPS
Children Cancer Hospital, Karachi, Pakistan

PALLIATIVE CARE IN PAKISTAN - CURRENT SITUATION

Palliative care in Pakistan, presently the sixth most populous country in the world [1], is still at its developmental stage. In 2002, the World Health Organization (WHO) National Cancer Plan was initiated in Pakistan [2] with the primary purpose of cancer control. The plan included up-gradation and consolidation of cancer registration, building capacity of health systems, prioritizing pain relief and palliative care alongside prevention and control efforts, and building a network of organizations at the national, provincial and local level.

The first Palliative Care Workshop was held in Karachi in February 2007 with the support of INCTR (International Network for Cancer Treatment and Research). Since then several workshops have been organized in Pakistan and in addition representatives from Pakistan have participated in international palliative care meetings and workshops organized by MECC (Middle East Cancer Consortium) and other organizations.

However despite a decade since implementation, services have slowly evolved and its implementation has been poor, particularly with regard to development of services for early detection, palliative care, and morphine availability. As a result, most patients still present with advanced disease in need of palliation from the start, face abandonment when terminally ill and usually die of poorly controlled pain [3].

HUMAN RESOURCES AVAILABILITY

By WHO classification, Pakistan falls into the lower middle income category with nearly 22.3% of the population living below the poverty line [4]. Health expenditure has always had

* Address for correspondence: rehana_punjwani@yahoo.com

a low priority with total per capita health expenditure being 1.8% of the GDP or approximately USD 21.8 per capita [5]. Health professionals are few with WHO 2010 health statistics estimating 8.1 physicians, and 5.6 nurses and midwives per 100,000 people [6].

As such, primary, secondary and tertiary governmental healthcare facilities do exist but due to political and economic instability, poor infrastructure and budget, the access and services are far from satisfactory particularly for life threatening illnesses like cancer. Private sector hospitals are too expensive and health insurance system is very limited. Treatment is therefore beyond the reach of majority. Fortunately there is tremendous philanthropic support in healthcare in Pakistan.

The precise annual incidence and mortality rates for cancer patients in Pakistan are not known. However, according to WHO estimates, as many as 61,624 incident cancer cases and 42,624 cancer deaths occur annually among men and 75,095 incident cancer cases and 43,188 cancer deaths among women [7].

Population-based national statistics for childhood cancer incidence do not exist in Pakistan. Pediatric cancer incidence, based on the calculated total pediatric population, and generalization of pediatric cancer occurrence from the Karachi Cancer Registry figures, gives an estimated ranging between 6000-8000 new cases per year [8].

Even though the need for palliative cancer care is recognized, in the current conditions, it is not a primary focus among many other competing needs for health care within the government sector.

Manpower is also lacking. With the exception of two foreign qualified palliative care physicians, there are no formally trained palliative care doctors in Pakistan. Furthermore, in a country with a large cancer burden, there is no formal academic training for palliative care at the undergraduate and postgraduate level. In most places, palliative care is led by oncologists working in the organizations.

Palliative care in nursing is also very undeveloped. Very few institutions have nurses specialized in palliative care on their oncology team. Most of the nurses are trained on the job by physicians and some may have attended short courses or workshops. Pakistan Nursing Council, the licensure body of nursing in Pakistan, does not offer any certification or diploma in palliative care nursing.

Palliative care services are offered only in few hospitals and hospices in Pakistan. There are no community-primary health centers services for palliation. At Aga Khan University Hospital in Karachi there is a home-based service but only for paying patients.

There are few hospices limited to three major cities with no systemic approach to palliative care. These centers are mainly used for terminal care. At some of these centers, chemotherapy is also provided and they function more like a cancer hospital. They are looked after by oncologists and nurses. Psycho-social support is non-existent or minimal. Most of them are run by NGO`s with philanthropic support. Many of them have morphine available but there is no multidisciplinary and pain management team.

Very few institutes have developed some form of palliative care team and services. They have physicians and nurses in the team whereas some have psychologists, spiritual counselors, and social workers as well. Most places are still following an old model where patients are referred to the palliative care team once curative options are exhausted. A full multidisciplinary palliative care team exists only in one or two institutions. The members of the team include nurses, anesthetists, oncologists and physicians. Nurses play a key role in collaboration and delivery of palliative care. The major focuses are symptom control, particularly pain management. Other aspects like psychological, social and spiritual support are mostly unmet.

At the moment, the following institutes have a palliative care team in Pakistan:

Shaukat Khanum Memorial Cancer Hospital, (SKMCH) Lahore has a well developed palliative care team including two physicians, nurses, social worker and a psychologist. They have regular palliative care clinics, four in-patient beds and 24 hours on call consultant and helpline line for patients. *ga Khan University Hospital* (AKUH)in Karachi has a palliative care team consisting of physicians and nurses. They have a pain management team lead by an anesthesiologist and pain management nurse. In patient and out-patient coverage is available and home care is well developed for those who can afford. Intravenous and oral morphine are available. PCA are available for inpatient whereas outpatients are prescribed with oral morphine.

Children Cancer Hospital (CCH) Karachi, has a pediatric palliative care program which has gradually developed since 2008. The team is now fully developed with physicians, nurses, a psychologist, social workers and a spiritual counselor. Intravenous and oral morphine is available. Pain management has become a fifth vital sign. Regular multidisciplinary meetings are held and education sessions to increase the awareness among parents has also increased. Palliative care unit at Children's Hospital Lahore was initiated with mentorship of Dr Aziza Shad as a project of My Child Matters Grant of Sanofi Aventis. The program is moving ahead with a dedicated psychosocial support team.

PAIN MEDICATION: AVAILABILITY AND ACCESSIBILITY

As far as drug availability is concerned, acetaminophen, ibuprofen, tramadol, nalbuphine and benzodiazepines are easily available and can be prescribed by any physician. Among opioids, only IV morphine sulfate (50mg/ml ampoule) and capsule morphine sulfate (medium release) 10 mg, 30mg are available after approval of relevant departments. Fentanyl patches are not easily available but can be procured through some medical stores.

Procurement of morphine by any institution is a difficult, complicated and drawn out task. It has to go through four authorities Federal and Provincial health ministries, narcotic board and Department of Excise. (Figure 1) The whole process takes six to eight months and by the time it is received, the drug expiry is limited to 1.5 years. The process of disposing off remaining/expired drugs is even more troublesome than acquiring it. In the past, morphine supply was sporadic but now with increase in demand and usage, it is available most of the time.

Only authorized physicians are allowed to write morphine prescription. Complete data of use has to be submitted to government. Intravenous morphine can only be given in the hospital and ampoules have to be saved and given back to authority. Oral morphine can be prescribed for out-patient but for limited period of 7-10 days.

Majority of the parents coming from distant areas prefer to take their child home to die. Very few of them can get morphine and most of them die in pain. Among the residents living closer to the healthcare facility, most parents prefer to take the child home to die with approximately 30% children actually die in the hospital. In institutions where palliative care services are developed (SKMCH and AKUH), residents and nurses take the emergency calls and place where it is in and in the developmental phase the duty doctor takes the emergency calls.

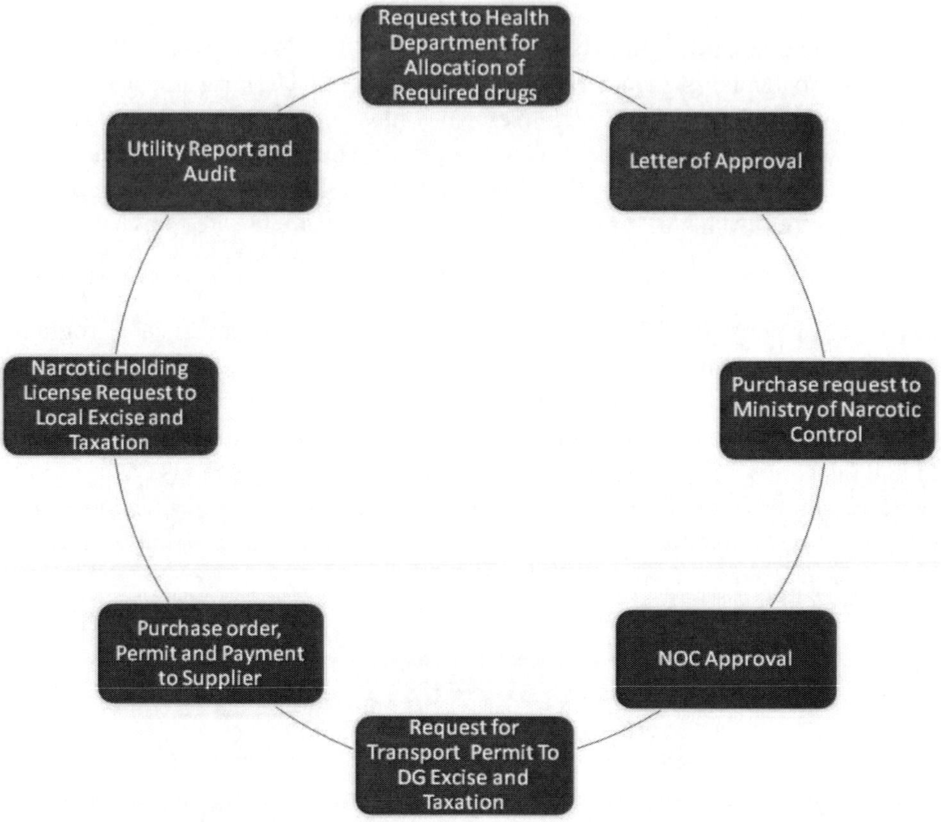

Figure 1. Processes in procurement of morphine.

PALLIATIVE CARE BARRIERS

At present in Pakistan, there are many barriers to palliative care. The major factors are:

Uncommitted government: Care for people with life limiting diseases is not seen as a priority. There is no national program for palliative care, although Pakistan has established National Cancer Control program in 2002 with objectives to improve palliative care and availability of morphine but the implementation has been very poor.

Drug availability: Although morphine is available but the procurement procedure is too complicated and exhaustive. Supply is often interrupted.

Unrecognized specialty: Due to absence of palliative care module in undergraduate and most postgraduate curriculums the specialty remains unrecognized and regarded as a less prestigious discipline among healthcare givers. This entrenched attitudes within the medical profession results in very few professionals entering in the field.

Low public awareness: There is a taboo around death and disclosure of diagnosis in culture and beliefs and care is often not demanded by the patients.

Lack of education and training: There is no formal training and accreditation of any palliative care program

Overburdened oncologists: In an oncology setting one of the important barriers is huge workload on oncologists dealing with new and actively treated patient. They have hardly any time to fulfill the demands of palliative care.

Palliative Care Training and Education

Palliative care remains unrecognized at all levels of medical education in Pakistan. There is no module of palliative care in any undergraduate and postgraduate medical curriculum except in oncology. There is no formal training, course or diploma offered by any medical and nursing institutions. Apart from two physicians trained abroad in palliative care, most of the care givers have no formal training.

Most of the nurses are trained on the job by physicians or through workshop and seminars. Post RN oncology diploma for nurses at Shaukat Khanum Memorial Cancer Hospital, Lahore and Oncology Nurse Technician course at Children Cancer Hospital, Karachi has a palliative care module. Private institutes like SKMCH and AKUH send their nurses to developed countries for couple of weeks or months for clinical exposure to palliative care.

Certified education and training in palliative care whether it is a diploma or masters developed locally is the need of the day. These can be done on -line with few weeks on hand training with certified physicians. Shaukat Khanum Cancer Hospital has a plan to start this once they get approval for certification from a university.

Future Needs

To establish and improve palliative care in Pakistan, two areas that need priority focus are the availability of opioids and education and training in palliative care. The procurement of morphine has to be simpler and restrictions on its use have to be minimized. Until and unless a palliative care module is incorporated in undergraduate and postgraduate curriculums in medical and nursing colleges the specialty will not be recognized and services will not grow.

References

[1] South Asia: Pakistan [Internet]. 2013 [cited 2013 Jul 10]. Available from: https://www.cia.gov/library/publications/the-world-factbook/geos/pk.html

[2] Nishtar S. The National Action Plan for the Prevention and Control of Non-communicable Diseases and Health Promotion in Pakistan--Prelude and finale. *J. Pak Med Assoc.* 2004 Dec;54 (12 Suppl 3):S1-8. PubMed PMID: 15745321.

[3] Shad A, Ashraf M, Hafeez H. Development of palliative-care services in a developing country: Pakistan. *J. Pediatr. Hematol. Oncol.* 2011 Apr;33 Suppl 1:S62-3. PubMed PMID: 21448040.

[4] Pakistan Economy [Internet]. 2013 [cited 2013 July 24]. Available from: http://www.theodora.com/wfbcurrent/pakistan/pakistan_economy.html

[5] Pakistan Health Profile [Internet]. WHO.,; 2013 [updated Jul 15, 2013; cited 2013 May]. Available from: http://www.who.int/gho/countries/pak.pdf.

[6] Pakistan Health Services [Internet]. 2013 [cited 2013 Jul 22]. Available from: http://www.tradingeconomics.com/pakistan/health-expenditure-total-percent-of-gdp-wb-data.html.

[7] Bhurgri Y, Bhurgri A, Nishter S, Ahmed A, Usman A, Pervez S, et al. Pakistan--country profile of cancer and cancer control 1995-2004. *J. Pak Med. Assoc.* 2006 03/;56(3):124-30.

[8] Ashraf M. Pediatric oncology in Pakistan. *J. Pediatr. Hematol. Oncol.* 2012 Mar;34 Suppl 1:S23-5. PubMed PMID: 22357147.

In: Palliative Care to the Cancer Patient
Editor: Michael Silbermann
ISBN: 978-1-63117-709-5

Chapter 14

PALLIATIVE CARE IN PALESTINE

***Mohamad Khlief, M.H.P.M.*[1,•] *and Amal Dweib, B.S.N.*[1]**
[1]Pall Nurse Specialist, Al-Sadeel Society for Palliative Care,
Bethlehem, Palestine

ABSTRACT

Cancer is a devastating condition that depletes resources on both the individual and community level. In Palestine it is the second leading cause of death (12.4%) (MOH, 2012), with most cases diagnosed at late stage (Husseini et al., 2009), and having very low levels of pain control and palliative care (AL-Sadeel Society, 2013). This chapter is exploring the situation of cancer patients in Palestine and the burden of this disease on them and their families, as well as on the healthcare providers and system. It is also looking through available services to cancer patients from a palliative care point of view.

This chapter provides overview of the current conditions in Palestine regarding palliative care service availability, some vital statistics for cancer mortality and morbidity, pain and symptom control, and quality of life (QoL) of cancer patients. It provides also data regarding current human resources in palliative care and need for such multidisciplinary team. Moreover, pain and other symptoms are discussed in this context, showing some results of current state of these symptoms and the available control modalities. Availability and accessibility of Opioids and some cultural issues are also discussed. Financial, administrative, political, societal, and cultural barriers are explored within the current situations in Palestine and in the view of available data and studies.

In addition to that, education and training needs are discussed in this chapter. This included current situation of education, training, and research for palliative care and what would be the best method of such education. Opportunities for palliative care in Palestine are discussed in the scope of available national and international strategies and resources. And finally, needs and recommendations for further development of palliative care service in Palestine are argued in the scope of evidence-based results from national and international research and data.

• E-mail: mkhleif@yahoo.com.

1. INTRODUCTION

Quality of life for the cancer patients is a vital issue in the presence of this devastating condition that depletes all resources on both the individual and community level. Palliative care for cancer patients is the advanced and most up to date choice that should be provided for them. Unfortunately, palliative care service is not yet integrated within the Palestinian healthcare system. There is no systematic designated palliative care service provided to patients. Control of some symptoms is arbitrary and done as response to nagging need in a non-constant manner.

However, there is a non-governmental organization in Bethlehem, AL-Sadeel Society for Palliative Care, who initiated in 2008 the first professional conference for palliative care in the country. This organization is the first and only one so far in this field. It tries to spread awareness and knowledge, among healthcare providers and clients, about the importance of having palliative care service to be integrated within the healthcare system. These efforts are still in the beginnings and need a lot of support both on the national and international aspects. Now, this NGO is providing consultations to patients and their families for issues in palliative care, and plays a role in supporting and participating in research in the field of palliative care and quality of life of cancer patients in Palestine. also, it is in direct communication and contact with the ministry of health and its higher education arm, Ibn Sina college for nursing and midwifery, to include palliative care education within the curriculum for the nursing students.

Statistical wise, Cancer is one of the first leading causes of death globally, approximately 70% of cancer deaths occur in low- and middle-income countries (WHO, 2013). Cancer is the second leading cause of death in Palestine, accounting for 12.4% of all deaths with the most common cancers to be breast cancer (11.8%), colon cancer (9.7%) and stomach cancer (9%) (MOH, 2012). According to the Palestinian health information center (PHIC) report, the reported new cases of cancer in West Bank of Palestine were 1,498, with an incidence rate of 64.2 per 100,000 populations with highest incidence in Bethlehem governorate (111.3/100,000), 38% of the cases were over 65 years of age, 54.3% of them were females, and mortality from cancer was 897 persons (MOH, 2012). This confirms that those newly diagnosed cases of cancer are at an advanced stage and terminally ill, and in need for palliative care service. Also, National statistics showed that most of the cancer cases are diagnosed at the end stage of the disease (Husseini, et al., 2009); this late diagnosis makes it difficult to treat and control symptoms and results in low survival rates and poor QoL of the cancer patients. This represents a significant need for Palliative Care service in the Middle East region, including Palestine (Bingley and Clark, 2009).

Moreover, very low level of pain control and palliative care, low level of staff training, and also low number and level of health facilities that care for cancer patients in Palestine (only three main centers in West Bank) are available. This is based on a need assessment survey in the West Bank of Palestine that was done by a local non-governmental organization for palliative care (AL-Sadeel Society, 2013).

According to WHO 30% of cancer deaths can be prevented by implementation of evidence-based strategies for cancer prevention, early detection and management (WHO, 2013). Furthermore, it has been stated in the literature that at least 100 million people would have improved quality of life (QoL) if today's knowledge of palliative care was accessible to everyone of the public (Stjernsward et al., 2007 a).

Moreover, QoL assessment is a vital instrumental tool to adopt, especially at the primary steps, in developing data bases for future use in formulation of country wide programs to support the efforts for better QoL. Guner et al. (2006) cited in their study that QoL assessment considered the most important indicators of the outcome of medical service; provides understanding of nature of disease and experiences of patient, and works as index of efficiency for treatment. Additionally, this will facilitate the implementation of palliative care programs in the community and aim for providing care for all people in need of that, and ensures equitable access to affordable medications and therapies (Stjernsward et al., 2007 b).

2. Current Human Resources

To recognize the value of palliative care, there is need for competent palliative medicine. This can be done through system redesign that has palliative care as essential part of its standard cancer care, protocols, and delivery models. This will need, off course, necessary investments in resources; both human and logistic (Meier and Brawley, 2011). Multi disciplinary teams play an important role in addressing patients' needs early and providing them with advice for better access to the best benefits and least costs (Rogers et al., 2012).

Unfortunately, there is no organized palliative care team working in Palestine yet. To our best knowledge, there is no hospital, community-primary health centers or home-based services available for cancer patients. As well, there are no hospices or hospice care available for such patients.

However, the AL-Sadeel society for palliative care is working on formulating a palliative care team through sending professionals from nurses and doctors for training in palliative care issues to USA and Israel. The author added that the society, which is the first palliative care facility in Palestine, succeeded to get scholarship from the American National Cancer Institute for one doctor to be specialized in palliative care for oncology patients in Israel. Also, it succeeded to recruit a psychologist, social worker, nutritionist, yoga specialist, and communication specialist to be part of the society team so far. As well, and from the experience in work with patients and families, there is need for using some different tools to ease the introduction of such new concepts of care, both to patients and professionals; we have to use puppets theatre players, doctor clown team, and story tellers as tools to attract the people to the new idea and ensure their understanding of the concepts and instructions we provide them with.

The society also works on integrating palliative care in the curriculum of nursing students through signing an agreement with the Ministry of Health's College of nursing to do so. Finally, the society activities have place in the local community and in the main governmental hospital that provide cancer care in Palestine in Bethlehem District. It provides its services free of charge to patients and families, and it depends mainly on funding from the local community and sometimes from other international donors, but this is so far still in the form of small funds that can only allow for very minimal services. These services include consultations in palliative care issues to patients and their families in the hospital, limited visits to homes of patients to provide assistance and care for them and their families, awareness campaigns in local community and through media toward the importance of palliative care for better quality of life for cancer patients, and scientific workshops and conferences for professionals who are working in the field of cancer care.

3. Relieving Pain and Other Symptoms

While pain is considered one of the most important symptoms when talking about cancer; it is also considered one of the main factors that have an apparent effect on the QoL of patients with cancer. Quality of life for the cancer patients is a vital issue in the presence of this devastating condition that depletes all the resources on both the individual and community level. Thienthong et al. (2006) found a high correlation between the average change of pain intensity and QoL scores; a change of scores of pain of at least 3 points out of 10 had a significant statistical and clinical effect on the QoL of 520 cancer patients. The conclusion of this study suggests the high importance of pain management for better QoL of cancer patients. This unnecessary burden, which can be prevented, has a negative impact on QoL, especially on physical health (Bostrom et al., 2003).

The most distressing symptoms and difficulties among cancer patients in Palestine were fatigue (66.6%), financial difficulties (64.6%), and pain (63%). Most of the QoL functions were below the half of the full function. The means were between 46% and 60.5% (Khleif and Imam, 2013). Pain and fatigue were found to be significantly and strongly correlated in a negative relationship with QoL, all the functions, and adverse outcomes (Khleif and Imam, 2013; Meier and Brawley, 2011; Alawadi and Ohaeri, 2009; Pud et al., 2008).

General look at the results of different studies presents variations in QoL functions that were lower for Palestinian cancer patients (Khleif and Imam, 2013; Thweib, 2011; Alawadi and Ohaeri, 2009; Samara and Saca, 2009; Scott et al., 2007). This is another indicator for the bad situation for Palestinian cancer patients. This emphasizes the need for in-depth studies to explore in more details all aspects of the cancer patient life and needs.

Availability and accessibility of Opioids in Palestine are limited. Only three out of the seven essential opioids (Codeine, Morphine oral Controlled release (MoCR), and Morphine injectable (MoINJ) are available occasionally in Palestine for free, Fentanyl transdermal patch (FentTD) is available occasionally and in full cost, while the other drugs (Morphine oral immediate release (MoIR), Oxycodone oral immediate release (OcIR), and Methadone oral (MoPO) are not available at all. Furthermore, not all essential drugs for palliative care are available in Palestine. Also, there is no official list of such drugs within the official documents of the ministry of health.

Currently, only oncologists can prescribe such drugs, and the process of doing so is bit complicated and has a lot of bureaucratic procedures. Also, there is limit of the amount that can be prescribed by each physician and for each patient. Moreover, these can be obtained from specific places only, which are the governmental pharmacies in hospitals or some main governmental primary healthcare centers. These drugs are not available in pharmacies in the community at all. In addition, the prescription is valid only once as it should be taken by the pharmacist upon dispensing to patient. So, if the patient in need for more medication he needs to go to his treating oncologist for another prescription or maybe admitted to hospital. The maximum number of days these opioids supplied is usually seven days. In the community, the only available drug is MoCR 30mg. There are no other available forms such as rectal or injectable forms.

Cancer patients in Palestine prefer to die mainly at home. This is as the familial and social relationships are strong among people in the Palestinian culture and of great importance for the patients and their families. Moreover, most of cancer patients, in the Middle East region, prefer to die at home due to presence of multiple traditional and social reasons. This stresses the need for home-based services as a high priority in the health care system for better QoL (Silbermann, 2012). But on the ground, patients are actually dying at the hospital. This is as a result to unavailability of home-based palliative care, the thing that force them go for hospitalization. This happens sometimes only for simple tasks like controlling their pain or constipation, the thing that can be done at home with better cost-effective interventions for both the patient and the health system.

4. Barriers to Palliative Care in Palestine

Palliative care is not present in Palestine yet, and so, not integrated within the health care system (Khleif and Imam, 2013; Khleif and Shawawreh, 2011; Khleif, 2010; Bingley and Clark, 2009). One study findings illustrated the main problems in the region in lack of fund or governmental support, and lack of awareness for need for such service among the public as well as the policy makers and professionals (Bingley and Clark, 2009).

There is high cost of care; indirect loss of production, and the societal stress as a result of the high morbidity and mortality of cardiovascular and cancer diseases as major killers in Palestine, and that a large proportion of the expenditure on health is on expensive curative care outside the area (Husseini et al., 2009). Also high concentration of cancer cases is in the districts that are considered metropolitan and where the referral hospitals are located (Bailony et al., 2010).

Meier and Brawley (2011) stressed the importance of promoting quality of care for cancer. They suggested new delivery and payment models aiming for promoting quality of care which may increase the incentives toward whole-person quality care.

The poorer QoL of Palestinian cancer patients, on comparison with other similar populations, might be due to the deteriorating socio-economic and political situation in the country, or lack of professional and specialized care to support cancer patients (Khleif and Imam, 2013). Also, the lack of secured funds for organizations working in the field, and no enough cancer care facilities are of the main factors in not having palliative care service in Palestine yet.

Cancer in Palestine is diagnosed at late stage, and the surveyed sample, in one study, had high spirituality beliefs (Samara and Saca, 2009). Silbermann (2012) discussed the culture of taboo and stigma of cancer and its pain. He said that people in this region consider pain as part of the disease and accept it, they use non-pharmacological modalities. The stress is on assessment of pain and distress to be routine practice. He concluded that of the barriers to palliative care are also the protective attitudes of the family of patient (Silbermann, 2012). Lamas and Rosenbaum (2012) explained that the root of the problem, in a way or another, lays in physician's perception about palliative care, as many physicians believe that discussing pain control is admitting defeat; they are afraid of treating pain as they are afraid of patients' addiction to morphine.

Moreover, the challenge of chronic diseases, including cancer, is not the only one. The national economy, strategic planning, health-care policy formulation, and national priority setting are affected by the prevailing geopolitical situation. The geographic and administrative fragmentations of Palestine, and the barriers to movement, are all having their damaging effects on the health care system abilities and deliverability. In addition to adding to the physical suffering of patients and the financial costs since they have to travel for treatment (Husseini et al., 2009; Physicians for Human Rights website, 2012).

5. Training and Education of Caregivers

It is recommended in the literature that to recognize the value of palliative care there is need for competent palliative medicine. This can be done through including palliative care requirements in the training programs of oncology trainees, and through system redesigns that has palliative care as essential part of its standard cancer care, protocols, and delivery models. This will need, off course, necessary investments in resources; both human and logistic (Meier and Brawley, 2011). The tragedy is the non-availability of palliative care for most of the world's population (Stjernsward et al., 2007a), as it is the case for Palestine now.

To the best of our knowledge, there is no any specialized educational or training program in palliative care in Palestine; neither in medical nor in nursing schools. Also, there is no specialty training in the field of palliative care; neither as residency in oncology, internal medicine, pediatrics, anesthesia, surgery, nor nursing specialties. Moreover, no formal educational courses are available in this field so far for professionals working with cancer patients. However, there is a collaborative effort to integrate palliative care education at the undergraduate level for nurses. This is still the beginnings for palliative care education in the country.

There is no official or evidence-based recommendations for what would be the best method or approach of training or education of palliative care in Palestine. But suggestions include integrating it in the curricula of undergraduates of medicine and nursing, special training courses for professionals working in the field, exchange programs with other countries that have palliative care service, and organizing scientific conferences and workshops for professionals on regular bases. This should be arranged and supported by the government and the ministries of health and education, the local partners who work in the field of cancer care and education, and the international donors and supporters. All of that would be doable only when the issue of palliative care got the attention of the policy makers and achieve the success to be put on the priority agenda on the national and international aspects.

In addition to that, health related QoL researches are necessity in these endeavors toward initiating palliative care in Palestine. Such researches have shown the human side of cancer care and played a strong role as a predictor for survival. As well as, they helped in the decision making process for both the physician and the patient, throughout weighing costs and benefits of the deferent care modalities (Schwartz and Sprangers, 2002). So, encouraging research in this field has its implications in supporting such endeavors.

6. Opportunities for Palliative Care in Palestine

Of the opportunities for palliative care in Palestine are some of the national and international strategies and policies. The Palestinian national health strategy vision is to have "Better quality of life for the Palestinian people through controlling cancer prevalence in Palestine" (National Strategy for Cancer Prevention and control, 2009). This is also in harmony with international standards and rights. Palliative care is considered as human right in many universal declarations. Of these declarations are the Universal Declaration of Human Rights for the right to standard living and healthy well-being, equal access to preventive, curative and palliative health services, avoidable pain management, and essential drugs. The goal is to have palliative care and pain treatment on the agenda of the policy makers in each country health system (Breitbart, 2011). It is a public health strategy adapted by the WHO since 1990, who produced the WHO public health model for palliative care; also it is a public health issue to deal with people with cancer in the proper way (Sepulveda et al., 2002; Stjernsward et al., 2007a).

Other opportunities include international attention to such issues and putting up the evidence to solve the problem and bridging the gaps. For example, the WHO defined gaps to bridge in the way to implement palliative care programs. Of these; are considering palliative care as a priority public health problem, by countries, and integrating it into the national health policies. As well, it advocated for key components of comprehensive palliative care programs such as policy development, education and training, drug availability, and providing good quality care (including home-based care) (Sepulveda et al., 2002; and Stjernsward et al., 2007a).

Moreover, the availability of good education system through many universities in Palestine is an opportunity. These universities, which already provide education in many health fields; such as medicine, nursing, and other health professions, and in collaboration with other available resources; such as hospitals, NGOs, and international supporters, are good candidates for hosting and initiating educational programs in palliative care at the undergraduate and post graduate levels.

Within this scope, there is a process in progress now in Palestine, in collaboration between the only governmental nursing college (Ibn Sina College for Nursing and Midwifery) and the only palliative care organization (AL-Sadeel Society for Palliative Care), to integrate a palliative care education and competencies in the curriculum of the undergraduate nursing students. This, maybe, will be the start of a systematic approach toward building up the bases for palliative care education and service in the country.

7. Ongoing Needs for Further Development

Palliative care medicine and practitioners work with other specialists on providing care to patients with curative and life-prolonging therapies (Theofilou, 2012; Meier and Brawley, 2011). The need for earlier and greater involvement of palliative care in the treatment of cancer was argued, as a result of the accumulated evidence of benefits of palliative care in alleviating symptoms distress in those patients and improving outcomes of care and provides them with better QoL (Meier and Brawley, 2011; Temel et al., 2010; Stjernsward et al., 2007a; Uzun et al., 2004).

The main areas for attention in the scope of ongoing needs for development and initiation of palliative care services in Palestine, as well as it is same with other places, are professional training, public awareness, health policies regarding opioids use and dispensing, accessibility to essential palliative care drugs, and integrating palliative care into the health system, service provision and health education (Khleif and Shawawreh, 2011; Khleif, 2010; Bingley and Clark, 2009).

Good policies to avoid unnecessary suffering and costs for patients, families, and society in general are needed. Stjernsward et al. (2007b) suggested development of national cancer control policy in order to integrate palliative care into the health care system and as a priority aspect in the national health plan. But unfortunately, Silbermann (2012) explained that the Middle East countries still lack governmental policies that recognize palliative care. Also, patients, mostly, prefer to die at home due to presence of multiple traditional and social reasons in the Middle East region. This stresses the need for home-based services as a high priority in the health care system planning (Silbermann, 2012).

On the other hand, outcome measurement, which are based on measured reported outcome by patients, has major role in improving, not only the quality of palliative care, but also its efficiency and availability. It is considered an effective tool to assess and monitor care and QoL in palliative care services for cancer patients. Furthermore, this can help focusing on improving quality of services (Theofilou, 2012).

Following that and to show the massive need, it was found that QoL of the cancer patients in Palestine were very poor scoring 41.8% (Khleif and Imam, 2013). This result was worse than national and international results for QoL (Thweib, 2011; Samara and Saca, 2009; Alawadi and Ohaeri, 2009; Dehkordi et al., 2009; Scott et al., 2007; Pinar et al., 2003).

Furthermore, there was significant relationship between QoL of Palestinian cancer patients and educational level, income, department of care, stage of cancer, duration of treatment, and region. As well as, there were significant effects on QoL from fatigue, nausea and vomiting, pain, dyspnea, insomnia, appetite loss, constipation, diarrhea, and financial difficulties. While, predictors of QoL were stage of cancer (β= -0.3, $p<0.001$), monthly income (β= 0.19, $p=0.001$), educational level of patient (β= 0.12, $p=0.04$), and duration of treatment (β= -0.12, $p=0.04$) respectively. While, there was no significant relationship between QoL and center of treatment, marital status, age, or gender. Patients' expressed their needs for better perception and understanding of their disease and its treatment, better QoL, less administrative, financial, political and societal barriers to service delivery, and better community perceptions for their disease (Khleif and Imam, 2013).

This poor QoL results stress the need for intervention to preserve the QoL of Palestinian cancer patients by better care, early detection, holistic multiple team approach, and better pain and symptoms control. This is of high value in determining the most vulnerable patients within the general population of cancer patients. Also, it would be of great value for policy makers and health care planners, for health care providers and professionals, and for fund raising and allocation. As well, it would help in determining the priorities, especially under the current scarce resources and weak economy in Palestine. This should be done on all levels including policy maker, health professionals, organizations in the field of cancer care, patient support groups, and patients and their caregivers.

Further recommendations, in order to narrow the gap of needs, for policy makers include considering palliative care as a priority public health problem, integrating it into the national strategy for cancer, integrating it into the health care system within the efforts toward quality improvement, and as a quality measure that is economically efficient and cost-effective, providing good quality care including home-based care, especially as most patients prefer to die at home, valuing competent palliative medicine through education and training, and including its requirements in the training programs of health care professionals, promoting quality of care toward whole-person quality care; through system redesign and family social and institutional support, having effective comprehensive prevention programs for cancer, to be implemented through health care system redesign, improving quality health information systems, especially the cancer registry program, in order to improve data availability, consistency and accuracy; this will facilitate further researches and will provide better quality data for decision makers and stakeholders. Moreover, financial support for cancer patients, through effective role of the government ministries, especially the Ministry of Social Affairs, having palliative care and symptoms management facilities in all areas around country, ensuring drug availability, especially those for control and management of cancer symptoms, and adopting essential drug list based on the international essential drug list for palliative care, promoting health policies toward better advocacy and increasing awareness about cancer screening and early detection and treatment, also, address stigmatization of patients, and finally, monitoring system for proper practice and provision of oncology health services.

The healthcare organizations in the field of cancer care should promote education on pain management and ensure correction of wrong beliefs and myths, such as those related to pain management and addiction, should educate and train staff on issues related to palliative care, pain and symptom management, and communication skills, and should work on formation of multidisciplinary teams to care for cancer patients.

Conclusion

There is need for early detection and awareness among cancer patients and their families in Palestine, as well as awareness and education of health care providers for better care and symptoms management to achieve better QoL for patients. More important is the desperate need for integrating palliative care into the health care system and to gain high priority on the health policy planning agenda in Palestine.

The main problem lies within two main streams; the socio-economic factors of the patient, and the ability of the health care system to early detect, diagnose, treat, and provide professional support for cancer patients in Palestine, such as qualified and trained healthcare providers in palliative care and symptom management. Stjernsward et al. (2007a) found that 35 million people around the world are in need and can benefit from palliative care service.

The integration of cost-effective palliative care services in Palestine is seen as solution to the burden on the healthcare system and patients. This can be done through education, training, and awareness to both professionals and patients. This is of high importance for health system policy makers and professionals. Additionally, as cancer is the second leading cause of death in Palestine (MOH, 2012), and there is extremely poor QoL of the cancer patients in Palestine, severe symptoms, and extra financial burden (Khleif and Imam, 2013), there is need for palliative care service integration into the health system to improve quality of care and as an economically efficient and cost-effective measure.

Uzun et al. (2004) suggested incorporating palliative care and pain management in service delivery for improving QoL of cancer patients. Also, Sepulveda et al. (2002) suggested that it is a public health issue to deal with people with cancer in the proper way. Moreover, palliative care and pain control is a human right (Breitbart, 2011). This emphasizes the importance of such public health need, especially in this region of the world.

Within these endeavors, many gaps defined internationally to bridge in the way to implement palliative care programs. Of these; are considering palliative care as a priority public health problem, integrating it into the national health plans and develop national cancer control policy, effective cancer registry, education and training, drug availability, providing good quality care including home-based care especially as most patients prefer to die at home and not able sometimes to afford coming to the hospital, valuing competent palliative medicine, including palliative care requirements in the training programs of professionals, promoting whole-person quality care, and family social and institutional support (Sepulveda et al., 2002; and Stjernsward et al., 2007a; Alawadi and Ohaeri, 2009; Meier and Brawley, 2011; Silbermann, 2012; Khleif and Imam, 2013).

References

Alawadi, S., and Ohaeri, J. (2009). Health-related quality of life of Kuwaiti women with breast cancer: a comparative study using the EORTC Quality of Life Questionnaire. *BMC Cancer*, 9: 222.

AL-Sadeel Society website: http://www.sadeel.org [access date 2013-9-04].

Bailony, R., Hararah, M., Salhab, A., et al. (2010). Cancer registration and healthcare access in West Bank, Palestine: a GIS analysis of childhood cancer, 1998-2007. *International Journal of Cancer*, UICC, DOI: 10.1002/ijc.25732.

Bingley, A., and Clark, D. (2009). A Comparative review of palliative care development in six countries represented by the Middle East Cancer Consortium (MECC). *Journal of Pain and Symptom Management,* 37(3): 287-296.

Bostrom, B., Sandh, M., Lundberg, D., Fridlund, B. (2003). A comparison of pain and health-related quality of life between two groups of cancer patients with differing average levels of pain. *Journal of Clinical Nursing*, 12: 726–735.

Breitbart, W., (2011). Palliative care as a human right: update. *Palliative and Supportive Care*, 9: 345-349.

Dehkordi, A., Heydarnejad, S., Fatehi, D., (2009). Quality of life in Cance patients undergoing Chemotherapy. *Oman Medical Journal*, 24(3): 204-207.

Guner, P., Isikhan, V., Komurcu, S., et al. (2006). Quality of Life and sociodemographic characteristics of patients with cancer in Turkey. *Oncology Nursing Forum*, 33(6): 1171-1176.

Husseini, A., Abu-Rmeileh N., Mikki N., et al. (2009). Cardiovascular diseases, diabetes mellitus, and cancer in the occupied Palestinian territory. *Lancet*, 373: 1041-1049.

Khleif, A., Shawawreh, M. (2011). Palliative Care Situation in Palestinian Authority. *Journal of Pediatric Hematology Oncology*, 33(1): S64-S67.

Khleif, A. (2010). Workshop on Psycho-Oncology: Alleviation of Fear, Frustration and Sense of Loss through Non-Pharmacological Treatment Modalities, (Abstracts); Palliative Care Situation in Palestinian Authority. *Journal of Pediatric Hematology Oncology*, 32(1): 18-20.

Khleif, M., Imam, A. (2013). Quality of Life of Palestinian Cancer Patients in the Absence of Palliative Care Service. Unpublished study, AL-Quds University, Jerusalem, Palestine.

Lamas, D., Rosenbaum, L. (2012). Painful Inequities; Palliative Care in Developing Countries. *The New England Journal of Medicine,* 366(3): 199-201.

Meier, D. and Brawley, O. (2011). Palliative Care and the Quality of Life. *American Society of Clinical Oncology, Journal of Clinical Oncology*. 29(20): 2750-2752.

Ministry of health (MOH), (2012). Palestinian health information center (PHIC), Health Status in Palestine 2011, Palestine.

National Strategy for Cancer prevention and control (2009). National committee for cancer control, Ministry of Health, Palestinian National Authority. http://www.moh.ps

Physicians for Human Rights-Israel website; http://www.phr.org.il/phr

Pinar, R., Salepci, T., and Afsar, F. (2003). Assessment of quality of life in Turkish patients with cancer. *Turkish Journal of Cancer*, 33(2): 96-101.

Pud, D., et al. (2008). The symptom experience of oncology outpatients has a different impact on quality of life outcomes. *Journal of Pain and Symptom Management*, 35(2): 162-170.

Rogers S., Harvey-Woodworth C., Hare J., Leong P., Lowe D. (2012). Patients' perception of the financial impact of head and neck cancer and the relationship to health related quality of life. *The British Association of Oral and Maxillofacial Surgeons*. Published by Elsevier Ltd. 50(5):410-6.

Samara-Awad, M., Saca-Hazbon, H. (2009). Factors influencing quality of life for women with breast cancer in Palestine. *Online presentation*, http://www.google.ps/url?sa=tandrct=jandq=mariam%20breast%20cancer%20palestineandsource=webandcd=2andcad=rjaandved=0CCIQFjABandurl=http%3A%2F%2Fwww.jnc.gov.jo%2Fjncconfweb%25202%2Fthe%2520third%2520JNC%2520international%2520conference%2Fsession%2Fday2%2FSession%2520B%2FSession%25205%2F11-12%2FMariam%2520Samara.pptandei=Dn9xULX7F6X80QWejoBAandusg=AFQjCNEJhAM3CY6X5ZXTmyfnft8ZTLUPCQ, [accessed 7/10/2012].

Schwartz, C., Sprangers, M., (2002). An Introduction to Quality of Life Assessment in Oncology: The Value of Measuring Patient-Reported Outcomes. *The American Journal of Manged Care*, 8:S550-S559.

Scott, N., Fayers, P., Aaronson, N. et al. (2007). The relationship between overall quality of life and its subdimensions was influenced by culture: analysis of an international database. *Journal of Clinical Epidemiology*, 61: 788-795.

Sepulveda, C., Marlin, A., Yoshida, T., Ullrich, A. (2002). Palliative Care: the world health organization's global perspective. *Journal of Pain and Symptom Management*, 24(2): 91-95.

Silbermann, M. (2012). Availability of Pain Medication for Patients in the Middle East: Status of the Problem and the Role of the Middle East Cancer Consortium (MECC): Implications for Other Regions. *Journal Palliative Care and Medicine,* 2(6):e118. doi:10.4172/2165-7386.1000e118.

Stjernsward, J., Foley, K., and Ferris, F. (2007 a). The Public Health Strategy for Palliative Care. *Journal of Pain and Symptom Management*, 33 (5): 486-493.

Stjernsward, J., Foley, K., and Ferris, F. (2007 b). Integrating palliative care into national policies. *Journal of Pain and Symptom Management*, 33 (5): 514-520.

Temel J. S., Greer J. A., Muzikansky A., et al. (2010). Early palliative care for patients with metastatic non–small-cell lung cancer. *The New England journal o f medicine,* 363: 733–742.

Theofilou, P. (2012). Outcome measure in palliative care: quality of life. *J. AIDS Clinic Res.,* 3(5):159. doi:10.4172/2155-6113.1000159.

Thienthong S., Pratheepawanit N., Limwattananon C., Maoleekoonpairoj S., Lertsanguansinchai P., Chanvej L. (2006). Pain and quality of life of cancer patients: a multi-center study in Thailand. *Journal of Medical Association Thailand*, 89(8):1120-1126.

Thweib, N. (2011). Quality of life of Palestinian cancer patients. *Journal of Pediatric hematology oncology*, 33: S68–S69.

Uzun, O., Aslan, F., Selimen, D., and Koc, M. (2004). Quality of life in women with breast cancer in Turkey. *Journal of Nursing Scholarship*, 36(3): 207-213.

World Health Organization (WHO) website, >cancer. [Accessed 2013-9-08]. http://www.who.int/cancer/

In: Palliative Care to the Cancer Patient
Editor: Michael Silbermann

ISBN: 978-1-63117-709-5

Chapter 15

PALLIATIVE CARE IN SUDAN

Nahla Gafer, M.D.[1,*], Esther Walker, M.B.E., B.Sc.[2] and Mohja Khair Allah, M.B.B.S.[3]

[1]Radiation and Isotope Center, Khartoum, Sudan
[2]St. Catherine's Hospice. Crawley, Sussex, UK
[3]Soba University Hospital, Khartoum, Sudan

INTRODUCTION

In 2011 Sudan was geographically the largest country in Africa with a population of 42 million. After many years of civil war it peacefully divided into two independent countries: the Republic of Sudan (Sudan) and South Sudan. Khartoum remained Sudans' capital after the separation and is located at the confluence of the Nile. Sudan now has a population of just over 31 million it remains a country with heavily populated towns and vast sparsely populated deserts. The only oncology services are located in Sudan and prior to this separation, all patients affected by cancer needed to travel to the Radiation and Isotope Centre in Khartoum or a smaller oncology center – the National Cancer Institute of the University of Gezira in Wad Medani. The following paragraph predates the secession of South Sudan.

As in the rest of the developing world Sudan is experiencing an alarming increasing incidence of cancer, estimated to have an annual incidence of 21,900 cases [1a], with the most common cancer being non-Hodgkin lymphoma in men and breast cancer in women. Other common cancers include: nasopharynx, cervix uteri, oesophagus, oral cavity, Hodgkin's disease and Leukaemia [1]. In reality very little is actually known about the true incidence of cancer, as until very recently there was no national population based cancer registry [1]. Consequently statistics are based upon reported hospital case series [1].

Nearly 80% of the patients presenting at these two oncology centers have stage III or IV disease [2]. The reason for such late presentation is common to many developing countries: there is low public awareness, weak healthcare services, stigma and reliance on traditional

* Address for correspondence: nahla.gafer@yahoo.com.

medicines and a population living in mainly rural nomadic communities - many days' travel away from Khartoum.

CURRENT STATE OF AFFAIRS

Palliative care in Sudan developed from the enthusiasm and commitment of a few clinicians, who were themselves supported by the wider international palliative care community. Despite great achievements in advocacy, education, service development, improving access to opioids and improving standards of care, it remains an embryonic service, with very limited governmental funding.

Palliative care is yet to be recognised as a specialty or universally taught in pre or post graduate nursing or medical education. The services described continues to be provided to a large degree by enthusiastic doctors, nurses and other health care professionals, trained in basic palliative care, who seek to improve the care and lives of Sudanese affected by advanced cancers. The majority provide this care by working as volunteers.

The Radiation and Isotope Center, Khartoum (RICK)

RICK is the main oncology center in Sudan, 60% of patients arrive from outside the Khartoum state. It is a public hospital with about 100 beds for inpatients and about 100 beds for chemotherapy administration. The state covers 70% of the cost of treatment with some charitable monies to cover the remaining fees for those in need. It has two functioning Cobalt machines and one linear accelerator. RICK receives about 8,000 new patient referrals annually [3].

RICK was the site for Sudan's first palliative care service and from here palliative care developed and spread to the other two centers.

The service includes:

- An out-patient clinic that accepts patients daily five days a week, from other oncology units at the center or from outside the hospital. To date (October 2013) 1,200 patients have been referred and offered PC services. Through joint working between the palliative care unit and the pharmacy, oral morphine has been made available through RICK pharmacy and with education it's appropriate use has been spread throughout RICK.
- A 9 bedded in patient ward area opened in 2011, with 3 female, 3 male and 3 paediatric beds. It acts as a demonstration site for holistic nursing care, continuity of care, networking, and effective communication with patient and family members. Patients are usually admitted for symptom control or end of life care, the majority of admissions are for a duration of less than five days. To date 561 of patients have been admitted to this unit.
- In Sudan patients are admitted along with a family member who also provides care and psychological support and is known as the 'co-patient'. In the palliative care unit, the nurses and doctors train the co-patient in how to care for the patient,

including how to dress fungating wounds, exercise the limbs, prevent the development of pressure sores and foster good nutritional activities. Interestingly, the PC unit has the lowest mortality rate among the hospital units mainly due to staff being open with patients and families about their situation and possible prognosis, therefore patients have the opportunity to make the decision to leave RICK and return home to die, whereas in other departments this issue is rarely broached.

- Patients living close to RICK are able to be discharged home and supported by a limited home care service which started enthusiastically in May 2011 when the use of a vehicle on Saturdays was possible through an NGO. Currently the administration of RICK is unable to provide any transportation to support this service. Volunteering personnel (usually a doctor, a nurse and a psychologists) offer their time after official hours, but the service is not regular and unsustainable.

PC services at RICK introduced major changes in the hospital practices including: proper pain assessment and management; the concept that the patient comes first; continuity of care (including contacting patients by phone); use of metronidazole crushed tabs for fungating wounds (a practice exported from Hospice Africa Uganda); good communicating skills; addressing psychosocial issues. All these simple procedures lead to better outcomes. With the introduction of palliative care principles, patients and families receive improved care and a greater level of support when admitted to the palliative care unit.

The National Cancer Institute (NCI)

The NCI is part of Gezira University and is situated in Medani 180 km south of Khartoum. With RICK they form the major oncology centers in the country that provide chemotherapy and radiotherapy services. Other public and private centers are emerging. NCI was established in 1999 and currently more than 1700 new cases are treated at the center annually [4]. The patients are mainly from Gezira State usually in more advanced stages of the disease and a poorer financial condition than patients presenting to RICK.

The PC team at NCI (Medani) started with 2 nurses, a doctor, a psychologist and a pharmacist. Currently due to lack of commitment from a leading doctor, there is only the one well-trained nurse, who is actively engaged in demonstrating and teaching the other nurses how to deal with symptoms besides providing pain management and care of wounds.

Soba University Hospital (SUH)

SUH is a referral hospital, with more than 700 beds. Most of the patients come from all across the different states of Sudan. The patients are referred for advanced surgical, medical, paediatric, obstetrical and gynaecological services, e.g., paediatric surgery, mycetoma center … etc. It is affiliated to the University of Khartoum.

The PC services provided at SUH started as a weekly in-patient consultation for pain and symptoms management at the wards, including surgery, medicine, obstetrics and gynecology and pediatric wards. A PC outpatient clinic commenced in April 2013 for follow-ups of patients and morphine dispensing.

The team includes a doctor and a nurse both trained in palliative care. The head of the palliative care services at RICK, Dr. Nahla Gafer provides a weekly consultation service to support this team.

HIV/AIDS and Palliative Care

Sudan is estimated to have an HIV prevalence of 0.53% with just under 100,000 people living with HIV in Sudan in 2011 [5]. The annual AIDS related deaths are approximately 8,000 [5]. The Sudan National NIV/AIDS Control Program (SNAP) is leading Sudan's' response to the control of its spread, education, treatment and services offered to people living with HIV and AIDS. Despite some initial contact between SNAP and the palliative care service at RICK, no progress has been made towards offering palliative care services to PLWHA. Only those patients who develop HIV related cancers and are consequently referred to either of the oncology centers, currently receive palliative care.

There is likely to be a huge unmet need for palliative care amongst the 8,000 people dying each year from an AIDS related illness. However, without adequate funding of the palliative care team and training of more personnel in palliative care, this need is likely to remain unmet [6].

National and Governmental Levels

The overall quality of the national response to cancer is determining for palliative care. Obviously, where there is no adequate health care, there is no regular morphine supply. Similarly, where effective cancer statistics are not available, as is still the case in many EMR countries, evidence to support new care-giving policies and practices will not be readily available. There is a need to develop adequate structures for assistance and morphine supply to all patients who need help, independent from their social levels.

Itinerary of Training and Service Development

Over a three-year period, to initiate and develop palliative services the following training activities have been conducted:

June 2009 Esther Walker a British palliative care nurse living in Khartoum, volunteered to conduct a series of weekly lectures in Palliative Care to interested nurses both at RICK and SUH. Dr. Nahla Gafer a clinical oncologist was translating for Esther from English to Arabic, soon enough she herself became greatly interested in PC.

Oct 2009 Hospice Africa Uganda initiators course had it's first two candidates from Sudan Dr. Nahla Gafer (funded by IAHPC) and nurse Elfaki Adam both encouraged by Esther Walker to attend this comprehensive 5 weeks training of trainers course in PC.

Jan 2010 Dr Anne Merriman founder of HAU together with Dr. Jack Jagwe made a 1-week advocacy visit to Khartoum; meeting personnel from the Ministry of Health and different NGOs.

Mar 2010 Introductory Palliative Care Course: 24 medical officers and nurses were trained at RICK for 1 month. Esther Walker joined forces with nurse trainer Catherine Nwangi (from HAU and Dr. Nahla Gafer). The candidates came from different hospitals in Khartoum, from the Ministry of Health and from NCI (Medani). A one week training course was also held for 32 volunteers who were also trained in supportive palliative care. Candidates included pharmacists, psychologists, medical students and members from different NGOs working with cancer patients.

May 2010 Two doctors and one psychologist from Khartoum were invited by Dr Omer Shamieh – a PC specialist working at the National Guards Hospital, KSA to attend a 3 day intensive education course in Palliative and End-of-Life Care (EPEC-O)..

December 2010 A workshop “Palliative Care in Practice” was conducted at SUH. Esther and Dr. Nahla were joined by visiting PC Professor and Head of the PC Unit at MD Anderson, Texas, USA Associate Professor Ahmed Elsayem. 32 health professionals attended the 3-days workshop which included patient clerking, management, reassessment and communication skills training.

January 2011 The palliative care ward was opened with special funding from Africa Palliative Care Association and the generosity of individuals at RICK. The hospital administration provided the rooms but were only able to provide limited nursing cover, eventually after eighteen months dedicated nursing staff were provided for this ward, prior to this the nurses duties included covering other ward areas. The ward consists of 3 rooms with 9 beds, a nursing and doctors’ station.

March 2011 Dr. Mhoira Leng Head of Palliative Care Department, Makerere University Kampala, visited Sudan for 1 week. During the week she met with the University of Khartoum, Soba University Hospital and the Sudanese Board of Medical Specializations … advocating for them to include Palliative Care in undergraduate and postgraduate educational programs.

October 2011 Nurse Osama Khider from RICK PC Unit attended the Initiators Course in PC at Hospice Africa Uganda. Osama returned with great knowledge and enthusiasm. He raised the standards of care at the PC ward and helped greatly in executing the home-care visits.

November 2011 Esther Walker from UK revisited the unit and together with Catherine Nwangi and Rachael Dipo from Hospice Africa Uganda conducted an Advanced Palliative Care Workshop for the 17 personnel already involved in the Unit. After that another 10 days were spent at NCI (Medani) were 25 medical personnel attended an Introductory Course in Palliative Care.

January 2012 A Palliative Care team was appointed at NCI (Medani) formed of 2 nurses, a doctor, a psychologist and a pharmacist. Their work consisted of identifying in-patients with PC needs and addressing these needs. They did a good job especially in availing oral morphine. Currently the nurses are able to provide pain management and conduct a wound clinic (addressing fungating offensive-smelling wounds) but the PC services have stagnated without a doctor to lead this service.

One of the PC nurses is currently doing an MSc in PC nursing. She was also involved in PC training at Kuwait, Oct 2012 – a WHO PC training workshop.

2012 Following joint working and lobbying by the PC team, pharmacy department with the Poisons and Medicines Board. Sudan increased its' estimated requirement of morphine with the International Narcotics Control Board from just 1.3 kg for a population of 42 million to 30 kg. This was achieved as a result of the increased use of morphine by the palliative care team at RICK, demonstrating a need for greater access to morphine.

Feb 2012 Dr. Nahla Gafer attended a one-week course in Research in Palliative Care "Making a Difference Internationally" at the University of Edinburgh. Contacts with Prof Scott Murray and Dr Liz Grant among others were established.

April 2012 The International Atomic Energy Agency sent a team of experts working with the Programme of Action for Cancer Therapy to Khartoum. They were invited by the FMoH and conducted a comprehensive assessment of the country's cancer control capacity and needs. Crucially palliative care is included as a key component of any cancer programme by the IAEA and the team visited the palliative care team at RICK and received a report from the team.

May 2013 Sudans first Pediatric Palliative Care Workshop was conducted in Khartoum. 36 personnel attended this intensive one-week training. It was organized by International Children's Palliative Care Network who sent Dr. Julia Ambler and Tracey Brand from South Africa. Candidates included pediatric specialists, medical officers, pharmacists and nurses from different hospitals.

October 2013 The Federal Ministry of Health Guidelines for Medications in the major 15 health problems is drafted. It includes a chapter about Chronic Pain Management. Thanks to clinical pharmacist Dr. Alyaa Faisal working with the PC at RICK. She is advocating for greater availability of oral morphine at primary health care centers throughout Sudan.

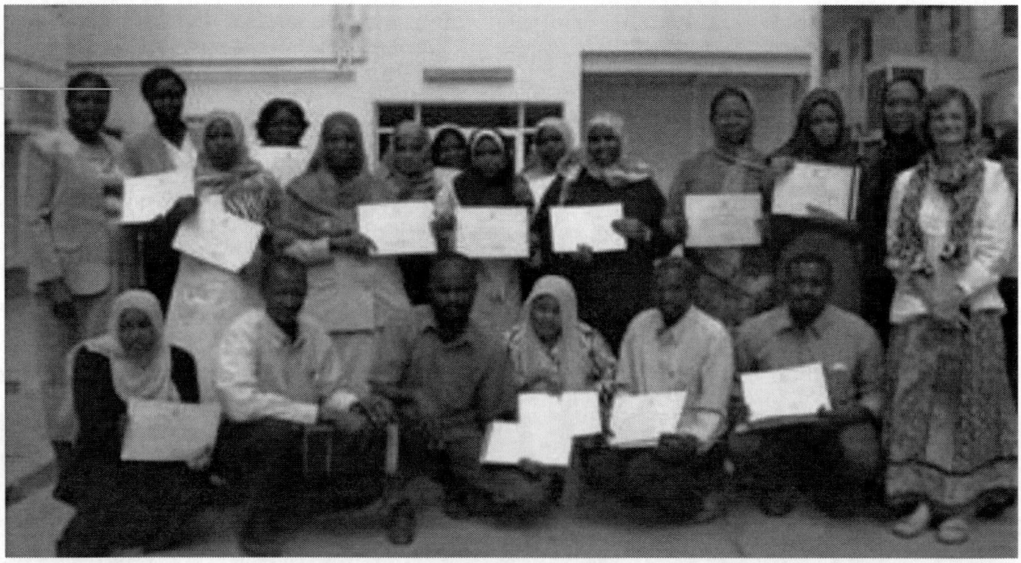

First Palliative Care Training Mar 2010. Organized at RICK, conducted by Esther Walker & Catherine Nwangi (HAU).

Current Clinical Challenges

- A lack of interest from the medical professioals in Sudan.
- Lack of knowledge and information about the palliative care and opioids.
- RICK and the FMoH continue to be unable to provide sustained funding for the appointment of adequate numbers of nurses and doctors for the PC unit.
- Underestimation of the importance of the palliative care and many medical personnel still view it as only applicable in the terminal stage of a patient's illness.
- The palliative services are not provided for all patient; unequal distribution due to lack of interested and well trained staffs.
- Reluctance amongst some doctors to refer their patients to the palliative care team for fear of their care being taken over by another team.
- Oral morphine is available only at RICK & SUH and only in the official hours and official days.
- The PCU at RICK and elsewhere face sudden shortages in morphine. For example one time only oral liquid form is available, and patients who use 30 mg 4 hourly have to take 60 cc of LOM every 4 hours. Sometimes stocks run out of all forms of morphine.
- Current team members need further development and training in palliative care. In particular; there is a need for them to develop skills in research so they can gather evidence in the effectiveness of their work and demonstrate the need for sustaining such services.
- Cancer patients self-reported greater burden from unmet existential and interpersonal problems [7].

Administrative Dilemmas

- Being honest and open and sensitive with the patient about the diagnosis and prognosis needs training of health professionals in communication skills. Discussing diagnosis and prognosis is also not viewed as conventional and culturally appropriate by many doctors. Despite anecdotal evidence in the palliative care clinic that many patients welcome the opportunity to know more and discuss their situation with honesty.
- A lot of health professionals believe there is no time to discuss such issues with the patients. Lack of time is the main reasons doctors do not probe into patient's symptoms and complaints.
- No budget specifically for the PC service at RICK
- Lack of Advocacy
- PC is not covered by health insurance.

Cultural Dilemmas

- The concept of palliative care is new. Some medical practitioners think of it as a luxury in these times of financial difficulties. The main reason is that they do not know what palliative care is.
- Families are always looking for cure and sometimes because of their good economic situation they cannot imagine that it is time to profit of the remaining time for the patient and not seek futile means to extend life. Some families will fly loved ones out of Sudan in the hope of finding a cure, only for the patient to find that no further treatments are available and they die in a foreign land away from family and friends.
- There is a strong propensity not to administer morphine usually because of misunderstandings. When the doctors are convinced how to provide pain management and the pharmacy convinced to provide it, we find sometimes the patient is not taking it regularly.
- Part of the Sudanese culture is the habit of visiting the sick almost every day. So patients who are very sick or terminally ill will be surrounded by large groups of people – visitors who are friends of friends, relatives and acquaintances. The family of the patient has to run into great expenses hosting these visitors while precious time for patient care or adjustment is lost.

Future Plans

In September 2013 the Sudanese MOH were invited to present their plans for the development of palliative care in Sudan at the African Palliative Care Association conference. The following commitments towards the development of palliative care in Sudan were made and are extracted from a paper presented by the Sudanese MoH representative Dr. Abdalla Awad Alkarem.

Training

- Approval of a post-graduate diploma for nurses in Oncology and Palliative Care
- Continuous courses for different health professionals in Khartoum
- Sequential training of health professionals from different states at Khartoum coming from different regional hospitals in Sudan in the hope of developing palliative care teams in these regional hospitals.
- Inclusion of PC training at undergraduate and post-graduate education of doctors and nurses.

Drug Provision

- Ensuring continuous uninterrupted supply of different forms of oral morphine at the main palliative care centers: RICK, NCI and SUH.

- Availing oral morphine and tramadol in at least one private pharmacy open 24/7.
- Availing these drugs also at the regional hospitals, were the staff are to be trained in palliative care.

Services

- Setting up satellite services at the regional hospitals.
- Supporting the palliative care teams at RICK, SUH and NCI through appointing needed staff, continuous training and provision of cars for home-care.

CONCLUSION

Palliative care is a core aspect of any integrated system for comprehensive caner control and a human right for all people affected by life limiting illness regardless their location in the world. Sudan faces an uncertain future with conflicts in Darfur and border disputes, the recent separation of the South, and economic difficulties.

Nevertheless the seed of palliative care has been planted and is growing. In 2011 the Worldwide Palliative Care Alliance published the latest report mapping palliative care development globally: Sudan is now recognized as having "isolated provision". With support from international groups and individuals, Sudanese health care provisional have used available resources and developed a service that demonstrates how the introduction of a holistic model of assessment combined with access to opioids reduces patients suffering.

The challenge will be to grow this service so that it can reach out the thousands of Sudanese currently suffering unrelieved pain and distress. There is need for a strategy; how to go forward with a realistic step-by-step programme in Sudan. In contrast to centralisation of cure for curable patients, in case of incurable patients de-centralisation of care is the way forward [8].

REFERENCES

[1a] World Health Organisation. GLOBOCAN.

[1] Awadelkarim KD, Mariani-CostantiniR and Elwali N E. Cancer in Sudan: an overview of the current status of knowledge on tumor patterns and risk factors. *Science of the Total Environment.* 2012. 423: 214-228.

[2] Hamad HM. Cancer initiatives in Sudan. *Ann. Oncol.* 2006;17(8): viii32-6.

[3] Radiation and Isotope Center Statistics for 2006 – 2012.

[4] Nationl Cancer Institute Statistics for 2000 – 2010.

[5] Sudan National AIDS Control Programme. Global AIDS Response Progress Reporting 2010-2011. Federal Ministry of Health. Mar. 2012.

[6] Concept Paper for Country Wide Initiation and Development of Palliative Care for Sudan, Anne Merriman, Jan 2010.

[7] Harding, Richard: Multidimensional Palliative Care problems among Cancer Inpatients in North Sudan, APCA Conference Abstract, September 2013.

[8] Tanneberger, Stephan, Cancer in Sudan: Palliative Care is the Most Rapid Way to Less Suffering, SMJ, August 2012.

In: Palliative Care to the Cancer Patient
Editor: Michael Silbermann

ISBN: 978-1-63117-709-5

Chapter 16

PALLIATIVE CARE TO THE CANCER PATIENT IN TURKEY

Rejin Kebudi, M.D.[1,*], Fatma Betul Cakir, M.D.[2] and Murat Gultekin, M.D.[3]

[1] Istanbul University Cerrahpasa Medical Faculty and the Oncology Institute, Istanbul, Turkey
[2]Bezmialem Vakif University Medical Faculty, Istanbul, Turkey
[3]Cancer Control Department, Ministry of Health, Ankara, Turkey

INTRODUCTION

This chapter focuses on the current status of palliative care (PC) in Turkey. The PC Project of the Ministry of Health, the current medical and nursing education in Turkey, pain management, ethical issues, barriers to PC are evaluated. The Pallia-Turk project is a national cancer control programme including palliation of the patients with chronic diseases including cancer implemented by the Turkish Ministry of Health since 2010.

Although, postgraduate education programs on pain and other symptom management and PC are held in meetings and courses, PC should be incorporated into the curriculum in medical and nursing schools. Pain and symptom management is satisfactorily done in most oncology centers, however formal PC unit/teams are available in few centers.

In recent years, most patients and families in urban cities prefer to stay in the hospital in terminal stage. Parallel to the development in diagnosis and specific treatment and supportive care in cancer, survival rates in both adults and children have increased significantly in Turkey, however PC still needs improvement.

The World Health Organization (WHO) defines palliative care (PC) as an approach that improves the quality of life of patients and their families facing the problem associated with

[*]Corresponding author: RejinKebudi. Istanbul University Cerrahpasa Medical Faculty and the Oncology Institute, , Istanbul, Turkey. E-mail: rejinkebudi@yahoo.com.

life-threatening illness, such as cancer, through the prevention and treatment of symptoms and side effects of the disease and its treatment, by means of early identification and impeccable assessment and treatment of pain and other problems, physical, psychosocial and spiritual [1].

In a patient diagnosed with cancer, PC should begin at diagnosis and continue through treatment, follow-up care, and the end of life.

In developed countries, both elderly and pediatric PC is well developed, but in the rest of the world, these kinds of services are still uncommon. An organized PC system was also lacking in Turkey before 2010. One of the pillars of Turkish Cancer Control Programme is PC [2,3]. The Pallia-Turk project in this respect has been implemented by the Ministry since 2010. The project is population based and organized at the primary level [2,3].

Turkey, according to the World Bank's classification for income is considered as an upper middle income country. The population in Turkey is about 73 million. The male-female ratio is about 1:1. One fourth of the population (18.9 million, 25.6 %) is 14 years of age and younger. Sixty-seven percent of the population is 15-64 years of age, 7.2 % are 65 years of age and older [2,4,5].So, there is a relatively a large young population. The gross national income was reported as 10830 US dollars per capita in 2012. The population annual growth rate is 11,2 ‰ for 2013. The average life expectancy is 75 years (F 77, M 72) [3-7].

Both adult and pediatric oncology national groups are established in Turkey. The Turkish Society of Medical Oncology (TSMO) was established in 1996. Palliative Care Society was established in 2006 and cooperates with European Society of Medical Oncology (ESMO) Palliative Group. The Turkish Radiation Oncology Group (TROG) was established in 1993. The Turkish Pediatric Oncology Group (TPOG) Society was established in 1997. The group has the main role of management of children with cancer (leukemias and solid tumors) and improvement of pediatric oncology in Turkey via meetings and courses.

The Turkish Pediatric Hematology Society (TPHD) is the other pediatric group which is established in 1999. This group chiefly focuses on non-malignant hematology, also leukemias and transplantation. The aforementioned three oncology groups (TSMO, TROG, TPOG) together organize the national cancer meetings with parallel sessions for medical doctors and nurses. There are also other multidisciplinary national oncology groups that participate in the education and improvement of oncology and related issues in Turkey. ESMO (European Society Medical Oncology), ESTRO (European Society for Radiotherapy and Oncology), MECC (Middle East Cancer Consortium) and SIOP (Society of Pediatric Oncology) post-graduate courses have been organized in Turkey. Pain and symptom management, palliative care including end of life issues are the topics included in most of these meetings and courses.

Furthermore, these societies and other non governmental organizations (NGOs) come together at the National Cancer Week Symposium held by Ministry of Health, annually.

Turkey is a member of the MECC, initially set up for the population-based cancer registries of the members of Middle East countries. MECC aims to promote preventive health care and training in cancer registry, to monitor cancer epidemiology and mortality and encourages cancer education and research. MECC has been supporting the improvement of Palliative Care in Cancer in the region by conducting various education and training programs in Palliative Care in Cancer since 2004. MECC meetings are held in various Middle East countries, including Turkey. Many medical oncologists, pediatric oncologists and nurses from Turkey have attended these courses and meetings [8-11].

Cancer is the second cause of death with a rate of 20% after cardiovascular diseases (39.9%) in Turkey [12].

The incidence of cancer is 227 per 100.000 which means about 175.000 new patients each year [13]. The most frequent cancers in adult females are breast (28%), thyroid (10.3%) and colorectal (8.5%); and in adult males are lung (31.2%), prostate (13.7%) and bladder (8.9%) [14]. The cancer stage at diagnosis is high (stage III or IV) in 52% [7,14].

In 2009, the infant mortality rate was reported as 19 % (in 1990 it was 69 %), the neonatal mortality rate as 12 %. According to childhood mortality, cancer is the fourth cause of death (7.2 %) after infections, cardiac deaths and accidents [7,10].

Each year in Turkey, 2500-3000 new childhood cancer cases are expected [15,16]. According to the TPOG and TPHD Registry, that was initiated in 2002, about 2000 new pediatric cancer cases are reported each year [15]. The distribution of major cancers in children are leukemia (32 %), lymphoma (17 %), central nervous system neoplasms (13 %), neuroblastomas (7,5 %), soft tissue sarcomas (6,5 %),bone tumors (6 %), renal tumors (5,5 %). The 5 year survival rate in children with cancer in Turkey is reported as 65 % [15]. Among 2179 patients, mostly solid tumors, diagnosed and treated between 1990-2012 in the Istanbul University, Institute of Oncology, Division of Pediatric Hematology Oncology, the 5 year survival rate is reported as 74 % [17]. Due to delay in diagnosis and late referral to oncology centers, the majority of patients in Turkey were diagnosed with quite advanced stages in the previous decade; in the current decade there is a trend for earlier diagnosis of cancer. In the current decade, the supportive care in cancer have improved a lot. We think that this is partly due to the result of the collaborative education program on “recognizing the signs and symptoms for early diagnosis of pediatric cancer and symptom management” organized by the TPOG and the Turkish Ministy of Health for primary physicians and nurses given in many different cities and the emphasis on pediatric and medical oncology topics in the medical school curriculum [16].

CURRENT STATUS OF PALLIATIVE CARE IN TURKEY

The Turkish Ministry of Health has launched a national cancer control programme in 2009 [2,3]. The programme includes five main headings: Registry, Prevention, Screening and Early Diagnosis, Treatment and Palliative Care. The Pallia-Turk project in this respect has been implemented by the Ministry since 2010. Among these, PC is the weakest part of current cancer control activities in Turkey [2,3]. The main reason for this might be the traditional Turkish family style. Relationships between the generations are still very intimate and when a family member becomes ill, all others support this person both physically and psychologically [18]. Turkish family is usually suitable for caring patients at home. In rural areas, home is still the most common place for death. Between 1980 and 2000, there has been a radical shift for the place of death in Turkish people toward hospitals, particularly those who have migrated to urban areas [19]. With this change in socioeconomic patterns, fewer women are available to care for relatives at home as they are working out of home.

The Pallia-Turk project focuses on two main topics: First; implementation of a PC model with family physicians, nurses and home care teams so that every citizen including cancer patients and others with chronic diseases will have the chance to receive basic PC services and integration of NGOs and local governors (municipals) to cover the psychosocial, economic and religious needs of patients and secondly; opioids availability [2,3].

The Pallia-Turk Project has three levels of organization: Primary, Secondary and Tertiary Palliative Care Centres. Primary Level Organization includes family physicians and home care teams. Patients who cannot be managed at this level are referred to secondary and tertiary level centres. Each ministerial hospital in Turkey will have a home care team [2,3,20]. Each team is composed of one general practitioner and three nurses. Home care teams will be responsible for simple acute measures such as pain relief, constipation, wound dressing and parenteral drug administration. Currently, Turkey has 20,700 family physicians. Each Turkish citizen has one family physician who will take care of him or her.

The patients who could not be managed by family physicians will be admitted to a hospital to get necessary consultations. Two beds will be reallocated for PC patients in each hospital. Secondary and tertiary level centres are responsible to take care for patients with severe symptoms and for patients who are in need of acute–subacute and chronic palliation that cannot be managed by family physicians [2,3,21].

Secondary teams will include at least one physician as the head of the team educated and experienced in PC and co-physicians, nurses, physiotherapist, nutrition expert, psychologist and social workers. Tertiary centers take care of complex patients who cannot be managed at the primary or secondary levels. These centers will work in a multidisciplinary approach and include all the physicians (internal medicine, surgery, medical oncology- usually the head of the team-, radiation oncology, cardiology, thoracic diseases, psychiatry, physical treatment and rehabilitation, anesthesiology or algology, general practitioners), experienced oncology nurses (one for two patients), social workers, physiotherapists, nutrition experts, psychologists and religious people. These centres will also plan and take role in research and training activities and certification facilities of doctors, nurses and social workers and interact with NGOs and local governors within time [2,3,20,21]. Recently, 290 home-care units related to the ministerial hospitals have been planned in 71 cities (Table 1). Several private home-care programs are present [14].

After the first International Home Care Congress held in October 2010, approximately 38,358 people have been visited at home in the first 8 months of 2011 [2,3,22]. This number has increased significantly in 2013 (Figure). However, the majority of the patients who received home care had neurological disease (45%), cardiovascular disease (21%) and other chronic diseases, only 4 % had cancer. Thus, most patients with cancer have not received home care. Lack of funds, the high number of cancer patients, the limited number of healthcare staff in the home care system are some barriers to the widespread use of this service. In addition, most cancer patients, even in the terminal phase, where most of the time they are not told of the eminent death, because of their family members wish, will like to see his/her oncologist and nurse that they know and not another doctor/nurse in the home care system.

Training and Education Facilities and Opportunities in Turkey

Turkey has a large population and a big surface area. Accordingly, health care services are difficult to implement and are expensive for investments. All medication and hospital costs for adults and children with cancer are provided by the government in university or government training hospitals.

Table 1. Development of Turkish home care services

Home Care Services	2010	2011	2012	2013 (first half)
Patients	16.651	124.085	244.961	316.603
Teams	407	642	715	762
Employees	478	3512	4143	4163

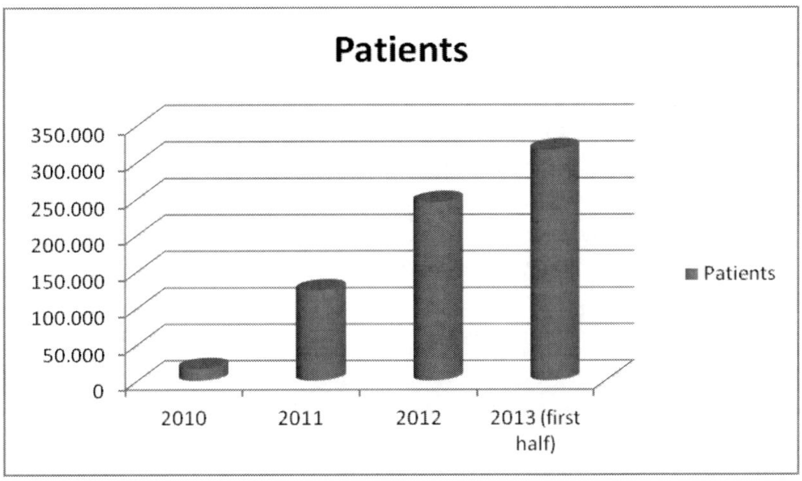

Figure 1. Number of patients who received home care service since 2010, Turkey.

Taking into account the large number of patients, especially in big cities where the majority of patients are located or travel to get medical treatment, the hospital beds are always full; the number of patients per doctor is high; and the number of nurses experienced in medical or pediatric oncology is low. Currently, Turkey has 10 structured PC units, 5 in governmental hospitals and 5 in university hospitals. Additionally; there is a private unit for pediatric cases and many pain units across the country [19, 23]. In 2010, the first pediatric PC unit was established at the Cancer Institute, Dokuz Eylul University Hospital in Izmir [24,25]. This team is continuing the PC both for children and adults very successfully and has been an important model for many centers. The Algology Division of the Anesthesiology and Reanimation Department in the Istanbul University, Istanbul Medical School, was initially established in 1986 as an outpatient one-room unit; improved to a 14 bed inpatient clinic in 1990, the first algology inpatient service in Turkey. Patients suffering from pain due to any form of chronic disease including cancer, can be hospitalized and have nutritional support, hemodynamic or wound care other than pain if required in this unit. Ankara Oncology Hospital is another important PC unit and has 18 beds for hospitalization of adult patients. Ege University, Tulay Aktas Oncology Hospital PC Unit was activated in 2005 for adults in Turkey. In a study performed in this unit, it was reported that the inpatient palliative oncology clinic has an enormous effect for improvement in symptom control and satisfaction with care [26]. Patient and family satisfaction levels were higher in the PC based case management intervention group with no extra direct health costs [26]. Although formal PC units or team are not available in many oncology centers in Turkey, most medical oncologists, pediatric oncologists, internists, anesthetiologists and family physicians provide some form of PC in their inpatient or outpatient clinic by way of consultations with the related disciplines.

Although there are some education programs on pain and other symptom control, formal comprehensive PC curriculum is not yet present [7,19]. PC continuing education for residents and doctors are more satisfactory. According to our regulations, after completing 6 years of education in the medical faculty, the title of "medical doctor" (MD) is obtained [16].An MD has to complete a 4-year training resident program in internal medicine or pediatrics to be a "specialist in internal medicine or pediatrics". Afterwards, a further 3-year fellowship program in medical oncology/pediatric hematology- oncology has to be completed to become a specialist in medical oncology (medical oncologist) or pediatric hematology and oncology (pediatric hemato-oncologist). The specialty and subspecialty training is given in university hospitals or government training and research hospitals authorized to provide training by the High Education Council and the Ministry of Health. The specialty and subspecialty certificates are awarded by the Ministry of Health. During the fellowship program, there is no formal PC lectures in the curriculum, however, since most PC is done in the inpatient clinics, due to lack of hospice and few home care programs, residents and fellows mostly learn PC while caring for these patients. There is no certified PC specialization or resident program in Turkey [7,16].

The nurses in Turkey are either graduated from high school for nursing or from universities for nursing. Clinical nursing education is carried out by faculty members of nursing schools after completion of or in conjunction with theoretical courses. Since April 2007, men have been accepted into nursing programs in Turkey [27]. Most nurses in medical/pediatric oncology get the experience while working in the oncology ward, from more experienced nurses and the pediatric oncologist/hematologist and some of them get a certificate by attending postgraduate courses for nurses in oncology. In general, there are no certified PC/hospice care specialist nurses. PC in general has not been incorporated yet into the curriculum of nursing at both undergraduate and postgraduate level. Hence, most nurses lack the professional background needed for PC [27,28]. However, PC training is increasing via interdisciplinary care program in the inpatient clinics and via lectures and courses in national meetings. There are perminent psychologists and psychiatrists only in a few oncology centers, in most others a psychology/psychiatry consultation is requested from the related department as needed. There are almost no social workers nor art therapists employed in the pediatric oncology centers. An art therapist had worked voluntarily for over a year in two pediatric oncology centers, and her positive contribution to the children was immense [29].

There are no specifically trained spiritual counselors. The doctors and nurses try to cover the role of the psychologist, social care worker in many centers, which sometimes leads to a burn-out syndrome [30]. Recently, a Ministry and Ankara University collaborative training program has been started for spiritual counselors. Also, e-learning for family physicians has been launched. Furthermore a special training program at Hacettepe University for doctors and nurses is being conducted. Regular trainings for all nurses and MDs are currently being considered at the High Education Council [31].

A study examining the oncology healthcare professional's views on PC found that 53.7 % of nurses never received any education or training on PC, neither at school nor thereafter [28]. Although the physician remains the central figure in the treatment of cancer patients, oncology nurses also play an important role in monitoring the cancer patients' physical symptoms and their levels of physical and psychosocial functioning [32-34]. Nurses are in contact with patients at all stages of cancer, during treatment, and care settings, and they have more in-depth, day-to-day contact with the patient than the medical oncologist, and can be more proactive and innovative in the care efforts intended to maximize the health-related quality of life of patients with cancer [32-34]. A study performed in Istanbul University Oncology Institute to address the quality of life of Turkish cancer patients by using a validated Nightingale Symptom Assessment Scale clearly showed that patient satisfaction is superior with trained high-quality nurses who have a good interpersonal relationship, who know the medication and recognize and control the side-effects of chemotherapy and therefore can educate the patient about his/her disease [32].Effective patient education might help in earlier recovery, decreases anxiety and might improve the compliance to the chemotherapy regimen. Another factor having an effect on satisfaction is the awareness of the nurses of the technical aspect of care (transportation or the other instruments required in the clinic) [35,36]. In this study, patients were most pleased with the respect shown by the nurses, getting answers to their questions, being sincerely interested in them, and nurses having knowledge about their condition [35]. Oncology patients have been reported to be the most satisfied when they are kept informed, when time is set aside for them, when respect is shown to them and in keeping confidentiality when giving explanations to them [35-37]. It was also reported that the presence of nursing students, who were in training, in the ward, meaning more nurses caring for them, improve the satisfaction of the patients [35].In this study, a positive correlation was suggested between length of hospitalization and level of satisfaction. Education programs on PC, including theoretical and clinical aspects, that are carefully designed to train health care professionals is essential.

Table 2. Palliative care in multiple adult and pediatric oncology centers in Turkey based on two surveys (First survey by Nurdan Tacyildiz, MD, reference 7, adapted to this table by her permission and a second survey by MECC 2013, data evaluated by Rejin Kebudi, MD)

City, Center	PC Unit or PC Team[1]/ Pain management consultation or Team[2]	Algology Unit	PC Education in medical curriculum	PC Continuing Education for MDs and RNs	Social, physiotherapy and bereavement services for patients and families
Adana Çukurova University Hospital/ Medical Oncology		Yes	No	Yes	Limited
Çukurova University Hospital / Pediatric Oncology	+[2]	Yes	No	Yes	No
Başkent Private University /Pediatric Oncology	+[2]	Yes	No	Yes	Limited
Adana Public Hospital/ Pediatric Oncology	+[2]	-	-	No	No
Ankara Ankara Oncology Hospital/ Medical Oncology	-	Yes	-	Yes	Yes
Ankara Oncology Hospital/ Pediatric Oncology	+[1]	Yes	-	Yes	Yes

Table 2. (Continued)

City, Center	PC Unit or PC Team[1]/ Pain management consultation or Team[2]	Algology Unit	PC Education in medical curriculum	PC Continuing Education for MDs and RNs	Social, physiotherapy and bereavement services for patients and families
Ankara University Hospital/Medical Oncology	+[2]	Yes	Yes	Yes	Limited
Ankara University Hospital /Pediatric Oncology	+[2]	Yes	Yes+practical training	Yes+practical training	Limited
GATA / Pediatric Oncology	+[2]	Yes	-	-	Limited
Gazi University Hospital/ Medical Oncology	+[2]	Yes	Yes	Yes	Yes
Gazi University Hospital/ Pediatric Oncology	+[2]	Yes	No	Yes	No
Hacettepe University/ Pediatric Oncology	+[2]	Yes	No	Yes	No
Children's Hematology Oncology Education and Research Hospital	+[2]	-	-	No	No
Dr. Sami Ulus Pediatric Hospital/ Pediatric Oncology	-	Yes	-	Limited	Yes
Antalya Akdeniz University Hospital/Pediatric Oncology	+[2]	Yes	No	Limited	No
Aydın Adnan Menderes University Hospital/ Pediatric Oncology	+[2]	Yes	No	Limited	Limited
Bursa Uludağ University Hospital/Pediatric Oncology	+[2]	Yes	No	Limited	Yes
Diyarbakır Public Hospital/ Pediatric Oncology	+[2]	No	-	No	No
Erzurum Ataturk University / Pediatric Oncology	-	Yes	No	Limited	Limited
Istanbul IU Anesthesiology and Reanimation Department	+[2]	Yes^	Yes	Yes	Yes
IU Oncology Institute/ Medical Oncology	+[2]	Yes	Yes	Yes	Yes
IU Oncology Institute/Pediatric Oncology	+[2]	Yes	Yes+practical training	Yes+practical	Limited
IU Cerrahpasa Medical School/Medical Oncology	+[2]	Yes	Yes	Yes	Yes
IU Cerrahpasa Medical School/ Pediatric Oncology	+[2]	Yes	Yes + practical training	Yes	Limited
IU Oncology Institute - Nurse	+[2]	Yes	Limited	Yes	Yes
Bezmialem Vakıf University Hospital/ Medical Oncology	+[2]	Yes	Limited	Yes	Limited
Bezmialem Vakıf University Hospital/ Pediatric Oncology	+[2]	Yes	Limited	Yes	Limited

City, Center	PC Unit or PC Team[1]/ Pain management consultation or Team[2]	Algology Unit	PC Education in medical curriculum	PC Continuing Education for MDs and RNs	Social, physiotherapy and bereavement services for patients and families
Marmara University Hospital/Medical Oncology	+[2]	Yes	No	Yes	Yes
Marmara University Hospital/Pediatric Oncology	+[2]	Yes	No	Yes	No
Göztepe Education and Research Public Hospital	+[2]	Yes	-	-	Yes
KartalLütfiKırdar Public Hospital	-	No	-	-	Yes
Izmir Dokuz Eylül University Hospital/Medical Oncology	-+[1]	Yes[^]	Limited	Yes	Yes
Dokuz Eylül University/Pediatric Oncology	+[1]	Yes	Limited	Yes	Yes
Ege University Hospital-Medical Oncology	+[1]	Yes[^]	No	Yes	Yes
Ege University Hospital-Pediatric Oncology	+[1]	Yes	No	Yes	Yes
Tepecik Children Public Hospital	+[2]	-	-	-	-
Kayseri Erciyes University/ Medical Oncology	-	Yes	No	Limited	Yes
Erciyes University /Pediatric Oncology	+[2]	Yes	No	Limited	Yes
Konya University Hospital-Medical Oncology	+[2]	Yes	No	Limited	No
Konya University Hospital-Pediatric Oncology	+[2]	Yes	No	No	No
ManisaCelal Bayar University/Pediatric Oncology	+[2]	Yes	No	Yes	No
Samsun Ondokuz Mayıs University Hospital/Medical Oncology	+[2]	Yes	Yes	Yes	Yes
Ondokuz Mayıs University Hospital/Pediatric Oncology	+[2]	Yes	Yes+practical training	Yes	Yes
Van YüzüncüYıl University/Pediatric Oncology	+[2]	Yes	No	Yes	No
Zonguldak Bulent Ecevit University Hospital/Pediatric Oncology	+[2]	Yes	No	Limited	No
	+[2]				

[1]Palliative Care Unit or Palliative Care Team, [2]Pain Management Consultation or Team, [^]Inpatient clinics, MD: Medical doctor, RN: Registered nurse.

Based on two surveys conducted by NurdanTacyildiz, MD (Ref.[7], by her permission) and recent MECC survey 2013 (available data evaluated by RejinKebudi, MD).

More participation and benefit could be obtained through courses in the national language (most do not understand or speak a foreign language in a good level) or with simultaneous translation for nurses. In a previous survey and a similar recent survey, conducted within oncology centers in Turkey, medical/pediatric/radiation oncologists and nurses from different cities in the country, responded to the questionnaire that referred to the current situation with regard to PC services within their centers [7,38].A summary of the results of the previous and the recent surveys are shown in Table 2.

Both surveys show that the doctors and the nurses are familiar with the concept of PC. Despite very few formal PC units or teams in most centers in Turkey, most physician and nurses state that they try to do pain and other symptom management and get consultations from related disciplines such as anesthesiology, psychiatry or gastroenterology. They are aware of the burden of "cancer pain" to the patients and their families, they state that pain and other symptom management is satisfactorily done in most cancer centers. Most medical and radiation oncologists' state that they explain to some extent the diagnosis (most families will not wish the doctor to tell the patient that they have cancer),details of the treatment and the prognosis to the patients. The families are informed of all the truth also.

In pediatric oncology, in Turkey, all parents are told of the diagnosis of cancer and the prognosis in detail. Most families do not want the doctors to use the word "cancer" to their children, at diagnosis. The child is told that he/she has a tumor or according to age groups, in small children using phrases such as "naughty" cells have caused a lump in the child. Mostly during the course of the disease, by the family's permission, some children are told that they have cancer.

In this survey, it is well established that the high number of patients, the limited number of staff in the healthcare team, the limited time that may be allocated to each patient, and the cultural and/or educational background of the patient are important barriers. Due to the limited number of beds and the lack of rooms with one bed, the terminal stage patient may not be hospitalized or sometimes are sent to an intensive care unit (ICU) for pain or symptom relief just because the lack of PC beds. The ICU beds are also very scarce and the oncologist is confronted with the hard decision of whether to use the oncology bed or an ICU bed for a patient who has a high chance of cure or a dying patient. The centers state that conditions about end of life care should be improved immediately. PC continuing education programs for nurses, medical and pediatric oncology fellows are present in some centers and almost every doctor and the nurses wish to learn more about PC through workshops, meetings or courses. These meetings should be easy to attend and in native language (Turkish) particularly for nurses. Written policies or guidelines about PC should be established in each center. Both surveys show that there is limited number of nurses and other staff in almost every center and nurses having education on PC have to do chemotherapy and other nursing work and not only PC. There is a lack of community awareness about PC in Turkey, but surveys show that volunteers for psychosocial support, mostly in pediatric oncology are somewhat more active in big cities like Istanbul, Ankara and Izmir. Psychosocial support is very important but limited in many centers. Some NGO voluntary groups try to give psychosocial support especially to children by organizing parties, picnics, and celebrations which are very much appreciated by the patients and the parents. They also sometimes make home visits to the patients.

PAIN

Health Ministry of Turkey has actually a good regulatory system for prescribing opioids. Legal trade (i.e., import, export, production, consumption, stock status control) of psychotropic substances used in cancer therapy is under the responsibility of the Ministry of Health.

Table 3. Available and non-available of opioids in Turkey

Morphine sulfate 10 mg/amp/1 ml	A	Red prescription
Morphine sulfate 30 mg/amp/1 ml	NA	
Morphine sulfate 10 mg tabs 20 mg tabs 30 mg tabs 60 mg tabs	A: M-Eslon 10 mg-20mg-30mg-60mg micropellet capsules	Red prescription
Morphine oral suspension 10 mg/5ml	NA	
Morphine sulphate suppository 10 mg	NA	
Pethidine 50 mg/amp	NA	
Pethidine 100 mg/amp	A: Aldolan 100 mg /2 ml amp	Red prescription
Oxycodone 10mg, 20 mg, 40 mg tabs	NA	
Codeine 30 mg	A: Codeincashe (majistral) 10,20,30 mg is made according to prescription	Red prescription
Dihydrocodeine 60 mg	NA	
Tramadol 50 mg tabs	Contramal capsule 50 mg	Green prescription
Tramadol 100 mg tabs	Contramal Retard 100 mg capsule	Green prescription
Tramadol 100 mg drops	Contramal 100 mg/ml	Green prescription
Tramadol 100 mg ampul	Contramalampul 100 mg/2ml	Green prescription
Methadone 5 mg tabs	NA	
Fentanyl 0.785 mg/ml, 1 amp/2ml	Fentanyl 0,5 mg / 10 ml amp	Red prescription
Fentanyl TDS 2.5 mg patches	NA	
Fentanyl TDS 12,5 µg/h (16.8 mg) patches 25 mcg/h (16.8 mg) patches 50 mcg/h (8.4 mg) patches 75 mcg/h (16.8 mg) patches 100 mcg/h (16.8 mg) patches	Durogesic 12,5 mcg transdermal 25 mcg transdermal 50 mcg transdermal 75 mcg transdermal 100 mcg transdermal	Red prescription
Hidromorfon Hidroklorür	Jurnista 8 mg capsule 16 mg capsule 32 mg capsule	Red prescription

A: available, NA: not available.

Each prescription is closely followed by the local health governours and also narcotic divisions of the police departments [19,23]. There is still "opiophobia" in many physicians, and they may avoid opioid prescription, especially morphine. According to the WHO and International Narcotics Control Board, Turkey was categorized along with countries that are not able to provide sufficient amounts of opioid products [3,23,39]. While many countries have shown an increase in consumption since 2000, Turkey still has 'inadequate' consumption as defined with a defined daily dose for statistical purposes per day per million people (S-DDD) of <200 mg oral morphine equivalents [39]. This is a dose <10% of the anticipated Adequacy of Consumption Measure (ACM) for opioids [40]. According to data in 2011, among cancer patients in Middle East Countries, morphine consumption is still limited in Turkey, although opioid consumption including fentanyl, hydromorphone, morphine, pethidine is close to that of Israel in Turkey [39,41]. Pallia-Turk Project aims at first new legislations for morphine prescription, to increase morphine availability in the markets, and train the medical staff against "opiophobia" [3,23].

Cancer Control Department is now in close collaboration with some professional national (Turkish Society of Palliative Care, TSMO, and Turkish Society of Oncology Nursing) and international societies (MECC, WHO, The Catalan Institute of Oncology Center) to implement nationwide training modules to all family physicians and their nurses [42]. Each family physician needs to be trained for pain management algorithms, use of morphines, and management for morphine-related side effects. Despite major improvements in pain management in most oncology centers, many children and adult patients are still under medicated for pain [43]. Turkey has a color-coded prescription system; red prescription sheets for strong opioids and green ones for sedatives and weak opioids (Table 3). White prescription sheets are used for all other drugs. There is a dosage limit for morphine and other opioids. Supply is limited to no more than 300 mg of morphine-HCl ampoules, 2700 mg morphine sulfate tablets, 1 g of codeine, and 1500 mcg transdermal fentanyl per prescription [7,19,23,39].

Patient controlled analgesia morphine pumps (intra-venous, intrathecal, epidural) and all types of nerve blocks are performed in algology departments in university hospitals. Opioids can be prescribed by family physicians and any specialist doctors. Ministry of Health has also planned to censor red prescriptions by 2015, to decrease the unnecessary bureaucracy, and e-prescriptions, as are currently being used for most medication in Turkey, are planned to be used for opioids. Existing opioid prescription legislations is also planned to be updated in accordance with European Union guidelines by Ministry of Health. In Turkey, in both university and in most educational government hospitals, anesthesiology departments have outpatient algology clinics for pain relief for all the patients having chronic diseases. PC begins at diagnosis. In all patients, "no pain" in invasive procedures is important. In children especially, all invasive procedures such as bone marrow aspiration/biopsy and/or lumbar puncture should be done under sedation or anesthesia. In some centers this is accomplished [44]. However, in many centers, this is not yet accomplished. Codeine, tramadol, slow-releasing morphine, hydro-morphone, and fentanyl are the available opioids in Turkish markets. Transdermal fentanyl usage has increased a lot for the last 3 years, as morphine was not generally available in the Turkish market (Table 3) [19,23,39]. Local production of opioids has been promoted to overcome opioid accessibility.

The Ministry of Health has agreed with Hacettepe University and local opioids will be ready by March 2014 for immediate and slow release oral forms (Table 3).

Ethical Issues

Medical oncologists and other professionals believe that each person diagnosed with cancer, should be informed of his or her diagnosis; but in Turkey, despite the significant improvement in survival, cancer diagnosis may be regarded as death in the community, family members often want to withhold the diagnosis from the patient.

While this is dishonesty, it is also an expression of the individual's desire to protect a loved one from bad news. However, while protecting the person from the hard truth, the family members also deprive the patient of the right to make decisions about his or her end of life [26]. This paternalistic attitude is the characteristics of the Turkish society.

Approximately 50% can talk about cancer, but some do not want to talk about it at all. Hence, most doctors act according to the patients' and families' desire and readiness to determine how much to talk [7,19,26].

Similarly, some health professionals, especially if new in their career, may face difficulties in talking to patients and their families about death and the dying period [16,19,45-47]. Family members often request to withhold "bad news" from the patient and thus prevent the dying patient the opportunity to make choices related to PC. The right of dying patients has not yet been established by law in Turkey, and do-not-resuscitate (DNR) order or practice of euthanasia for patients suffering from refractory symptoms is not yet legal [46,47]. A legal basis should be established to allow dying patients to give advanced directives related to their treatment.

End-of-life care is given mostly in the inpatient setting. Although most of the patients or family members in rural areas prefer to stay at home at their end-of-life period, most patients in urban areas and most families of children with cancer prefer to stay in the hospital in the terminal stage, in contrary to many countries in the Middle East, where the patient or families prefer the patient to die at home where they are cared for by their family [7,16]. In children, sending the child home to die is frequently considered by the families as "giving up on us" and the hospital sometimes becomes more "home" for the sick child than his/her own home [7,16]. However if hospice or home care were available, they could prefer it. As a result, the pediatric patient and the family should be offered an integrated model of PC that continues throughout the course of the illness, regardless of the outcome [16,48].

Sometimes, families resist PC consultations because this may symbolize evidence of the patient's deterioration, which may be difficult to face. All cancer care must be provided respecting families' spiritual, cultural background. It is obliged to promote a sense of well-being and to ease suffering in the patients. So health care professionals should be sensitive and tolerable of various traditions or religious beliefs in order to meet the unique spiritual needs of patients and families and ensure a "good death" and healthy bereavement [7,16, 26,48].

Barriers and Recommendations

There are a number of barriers providing optimal PC to patients in Turkey. Health care professionals other than oncologists and nurses working in the other services are not fully aware about PC. Thus, a core education from the onset of medical or nursing schools should be established. Physicians and nurses should have a certification for PC postgraduate. There are very few formal PC units/teams. There are some home-care units for chronic diseases, although according to data to date, few cancer patients are using it. There is no hospice in Turkey [7,16,19,23,26].

Physicians and nurses carry the major load of cancer palliation both for adults and children.

In a recent survey among Turkish oncology nurses, 114 nurses (working in medical oncology and surgical oncology services) indicated that the most commonly perceived barriers in the management of pain were system-related; the most frequent obstacles were patient-to-nurse ratio and lack of psychological support services [26].Patient to physician and nurse ratio is very high; so health care professionals are devoted and working more than their capacity. Many patients also come from other cities to the big crowded cities like Istanbul for the diagnosis and the treatment. The hospital beds are all full and not enough even to hospitalize patients with a new diagnosis of cancer needing an urgent intervention. These patients sometimes have to be transferred to other hospitals even in other cities after the patient is medically stable with the necessary interventions, for further oncologic treatment.

Problems of delays in chemotherapies sometimes may occur. Shortages of nurses are a serious barrier in Turkey. Most of the time, nurses having experience or education on PC have to work in regular patient treatment care in services.

There is a serious lack of psychological (psychologist and psychiatrist) support services specific for cancer patients; no social worker, no art therapist in most centers. Pediatric psychiatrists are able to consultate mostly the very problematic cases and usually prescribe medication. A liason psychological support is very helpful in the centers that have the team to perform it. When there is not a constant psychological support team, frequently, the doctors/psychologists change in every consultation, and the patient whether it is a child or adult, want to see the same person to feel confident. At pediatric setting, sometimes families do not control their feelings and may have unrealistic expectations or they may deny their children' diagnosis and/or the news of end of life. The families also need psychological support. Thus every center should have a permanent psychological support team. The same nurse group also stated that there is lack of guidelines for pain management [26]. Recently the use of opioids, mostly other than morphine has increased significantly, which means the awareness that cancer pain should be relieved, is increasing in the medical community.

There is always a need of funding for the organizations necessary in the PC setting. This funding issue should be supported by the government, also the support of NGOs may be incorporated. To increase the awareness of the importance of PC in the public, thus facilitate the support of the public and NGO's the media including TV, internet (facebook, twitter) newspapers may be used.

Conclusion

It is essential that improved PC program should be integrated into national health-care systems to control the suffering of all adult and pediatric cancer patients. This national policy enables to develop quality standards, funding, and accessibility of adequate care for most patients and families and serves a major role in facilitating to establish the PC units/teams and education like PC curriculum and availability of essential drugs for health-care professionals. PC units/teams, hospices and home care services should be established both for adults and children. Health-care professionals should have postgraduate PC education. Governmental attempts are needed to increase the number of nurses, psychologists, psychiatrists, social workers and art therapists and in the centers. Evidence-based pain and symptom management and PC written guidelines should be available for the clinical use of doctors and nurses in all oncology centers. Non-governmental organizations may be incorporated in the PC efforts. The media may be used to improve the awareness of PC in the public. Government, non-governmental organizations and health care professionals should collaborate to improve PC in Turkey.

ACKNOWLEDGMENTS

We thank Prof. Gul Koknel Talu, MD, from Istanbul University, Department of Anesthesiology and Reanimation, Division of Algology; Prof. Adnan Aydiner, MD, from Istanbul University Oncology Institute, and Istanbul Medical Faculty, Division of Medical Oncology; and Gulbeyaz Can, PhD, RN, Istanbul University Florence Nightingale School of Nursing for their valuable contribution.

REFERENCES

[1] WHO. http://www.who.int/cancer/palliative/definition/en/

[2] Tuncer, M., editor. *National cancer program, 2009-2015,* Ankara: Ministry of Health (Turkey), Department of Cancer Control; 2009. Ministry of Health publication no.760.[Turkish].

[3] Ozgul, N.,Gultekin, M., Koc, O., Goksel, F., Bayraktar, G., Ekinci, H., et al. Turkish community-based palliative care model: aunique design. *Ann. Oncol.* 2012;23 Suppl. 3: 76-8.

[4] Kutluk, T. The epidemiology of childhood cancer. In: Tuncer, M.,ed. *Cancer Control in Turkey.* Ankara: the Turkish Republic Ministry of Health, Department of Cancer Control; 2008:159–167.

[5] url: data.worldbank.org/country/tr.

[6] url: sbu.saglik.gov.tr (2011).

[7] Silbermann, M., Arnaout, M., Abdel Rahman Sayed, H., Sedky, M., El-Shami, M., Ben-Arush, M., et al. *Pediatric Palliative Care in the Middle East.* In: Knapp, C. Madden, V., Fowler-Kerry, S., eds. *Pediatric Palliative Care: Global Perspectives.* Springer Science+Business Media B.V.: Amterdam, The Netherlands; 2012:127–159.

[8] Middle East Cancer Consortium. Available at http://mecc.cancer.gov.Accessed August 15, 2008.

[9] Freedman, L., Al-Kayed, S., Bassam Qasem, M., et al. Cancer registration in the Middle East. *Epidemiology* 2001;12:131e133.

[10] Bingley, A. F., Clark, D. Palliative care in the region represented by the Middle East Cancer Consortium: a review and comparative analysis. National Cancer Institute. *NIH Pub. No. 07-6230 Bethesda*, MD, 2008.

[11] *The International Observatory on end of life care MECC country reports*. Available at http://www.eolcobservatory. net/global_analysis/mecc.htm. Accessed August 17, 2008.

[12] TurkishNationalStatisticsInstitude, 2012. Url: http://tuikapp.tuik.gov.tr/demografiapp/olum.zul.

[13] TurkishMinistry of Health, *CancerStatistics, 2008*. Url: http://www.kanser.gov.tr/daire-faaliyetleri/kanser-istatistikleri.html.

[14] Silbermann, M., Al-Hadad, S., Ashraf, S., Hessissen, L., Madani, A., Noun, P., et al. MECC regional initiative in pediatric palliative care: Middle Eastern course on pain management. *J. Pediatr. Hematol. Oncol.* 2012;34 Suppl. 1:S1-11.

[15] Kutluk, T., Yeşilipek, A. Turkish National Pediatric Cancer Registry 2002-2008 (TurkishPediatric Oncology Group and Turkish Pediatric Hematology Society).*J.Clin.Oncol.*31, 2013 (suppl.; abstr. 10067).

[16] Kebudi, R.; Turkish Pediatric Oncology Group. Pediatric Oncology in Turkey. *J. Pediatr. Hematol. Oncol.* 2012;34 Suppl. 1:S12-4.

[17] Kebudi, R., Uludag, D. Demographic characteristics and treatment results of children with cancer 1990-2012. *Thesis in pediatrics, 2013*, Cerrahpasa Medical Faculty, Istanbul, Turkey.

[18] Ddungu, H. Palliative care: what approaches are suitable in developing countries? *Brit. J. Hematol.* 2011;154:728–735.

[19] Komurcu, S. Current status of palliative care in Turkey. *J. Pediatr. Hematol. Oncol.* 2011;33 Suppl. 1:S78-80.

[20] http://saglik.gov.tr/TR/belge/1-570/evde-bakim-hizmetleri-sunumu-hakkindayonetme-lik.(legislation for home care programs) html (December 2013, date last accessed).

[21] Türkiye'deÖzellikliPlanlamaGerektirenSaglıkHizmetleri (*Healthcare Services that need a special program in Turkey*) 2011–2023 (Turkish). Turkish Ministry of Health, General Directorate of Curative Services Publications, Ankara, 2011.Available at http://www.tedavi.saglik.gov.tr/kutuphane/oplgsh.pdf. (December 2013, date last accessed).

[22] Evdesaglikilhizmetverileritablosu (*Table of home care programs in various cities*). Available at http://www.tedavi.saglik.gov.tr/ (December 2013, date last accessed).

[23] Ozgul, N., Koc, O., Gultekin, M., Goksel, F., Kerman, S., Tanyeri, P., et al. Opioids for cancer pain: availability, accessibility, and regulatory barriers in Turkey and Pallia-Turk Project. *J. Pediatr. Hematol. Oncol.* 2011;33 Suppl. 1:S29-32.

[24] Mutafoglu, K. Current Palliative Care Practice in a University Hospital. *J. Pediatr. Hematol. Oncol.* 2010;32(suppl. 1):S36–S38.

[25] Mutafoglu, K.; DEU Palliative Care Strategy Group. A palliative care initiative in Dokuz Eylul University Hospital. *J. Pediatr. Hematol. Oncol.* 2011;33 Suppl. 1:S73-6.

[26] Ozcelik, H., Fadiloglu, C., Karabulut, B., Uyar, M. Palliative care activity in the field of oncology in Turkey. *J. Palliat. Care.* 2010;26(4):305-10.

[27] Can, G. Nursing education in Turkey. *Nurse Educ.*2010;35(4):146-7.

[28] Elcigil, A., Maltepe, H., Esrefgil, G., Mutafoglu, K. Nurses' perceived barriers to assessment and management of pain in a University Hospital. *J. Pediatr. Hematol. Oncol.* 2011;33:S33-8.

[29] Kebudi, R., Ozcan, A. Understanding psychological states of children with cancer: Art therapy as a communication tool. *Psycho-Oncology* volume 20:supp. 2, October 2011, (abstract AA-3) p.83.

[30] Alacacioglu, A., Yavuzsen, T., Dirioz, M., Oztop, I., Yilmaz, U. Burnout in nurses and physicians working at an oncology department. *Psychooncology* 2009;18:543–548.

[31] http://www.kanser.gov.tr/daire-faaliyetleri/egitimler-farkindalik-calismalari/176-egitim-ve-farkindalik-calismalari.html. AccessedDec. 2013.

[32] Can, G., Aydiner, A. Development and validation of the Nightingale Symptom Assessment Scale (N-SAS) and predictors of the quality of life of the cancer patients in Turkey. *Eur. J. Oncol. Nursing*. 2011;15:153-11.

[33] Hilarius, D. L., Kloeg, P. H., Gundy, C. M., Aaronson, N. K. Use of health-related quality-of-life assessments in daily clinical oncology nursing practice – a community hospital-based intervention study. *Cancer* 2008;113, 628–637.

[34] Turgay, A. S., Khorshid, L., Eser, I. Effect of the first chemotherapy course on the quality of life of cancer patients in Turkey. *Cancer Nursing* 2008;31(6), E19–E23.

[35] Can, G., Akin, S., Aydiner, A., Ozdilli, K., Durna, Z. Evaluation of the effect of care given by nursing students on oncology patients' satisfaction. *Eur. J. Oncol. Nurs.* 2008;12(4):387-92.

[36] Radwin, L., Alster, K., Rubin, K. M. Development and testing of the oncology patients' perceptions of the quality of nursing care scale. *Oncology Nursing Forum* 2003;30(2):283-90.

[37] Thomas, T. *Patient satisfaction survey July–October 2004*. Cheltenham general hospital. Patient and Public Involvement Department. Gloucestershire Hospitals NHS Foundation Trust 2004.

[38] Tacyildiz, N. (2011) *Personal communication*. Ankara University: School of Medicine. Ankara, Turkey. Accessed March 2011.

[39] Cleary, J.,Silbermann, M., Scholten, W., Radbruch, L., Torode, J., Cherny, N. I. Formularyavailabilityandregulatorybarrierstoaccessibilityofopioidsforcancerpainin the Middle East: are port from the Global Opioid Policy Initiative (GOPI). *Ann. Oncol.* 2013;24 Suppl. 11:xi51-xi59.

[40] International Narcotics Control Board. *Report of the International Narcotics Control Board on the Availability of Internationally Controlled Drugs*: Ensuring Adequate Access for Medical and Scientific Purposes New York: United Nations. 2011;pp. 88.

[41] Silbermann, M., Hassan, E. A. Cultural perspectives in cancer care: impact of Islamic traditions and practices in Middle Eastern countries. *J. Pediatr. Hematol. Oncol.* 2011; 33(S2): S81–S86.

[42] Silbermann, M., Kutluk, T., Tuncer, M. Middle East Cancer Consortium (MECC) International pediatric oncology meeting abstracts. *J. Pediatr. Hematol. Oncol.* 2007; 29:S1–22.

[43] Mutafoglu, K. Challenges and obstacles facing the oncologist in pain management. *J.Pediatr.Hematol.Oncol.*2010; 32:424–425.

[44] Cakir, F. B., Umutoglu, T., Bakan, M., Topuz, U., Kebudi, R., Zulfikar, B. Experience on deep sedation anesthesia given to children with malignancy for invasive procedures at the pediatric ward. *45th SIOP Congress, Pediatr. Blood and Cancer*, 60;S3,173, Hong Kong, China, 25-28 September, 2013.

[45] Shad, A. T., McGee, M. E., Biel, M. B., et al. Collaborations in psychosocial care in pediatric oncology: The Middle East as a case example. In: Kreitler, S., Ben Arush, M., Martin, A., eds. *Pediatric Oncology: Psychosocial aspects and clinical intervention.* 2nd Ed. London, UK: Wiley, Blackwell. 2010.

[46] Aksoy, S. Ethical consideration on end of life issues in Turkey. In: Song, K. Y., Koo, Y. M., Macer, D. R. J., editors. *Bioethics in Asia in the 21st century.* Bangkok; Eubios Ethics Institute;2003.

[47] Oguz, N. Y., Miles, S. H., Buken, N., et al. End of life care in Turkey. *Comb. Q Health Ethics* 2003;12(3):279-284.

[48] Wolff, J., Wolff, B. Quality of death in children: where is it higher-at home or in the hospital. *Pediatr. Blood Cancer* 2008;50:945–946.

In: Palliative Care to the Cancer Patient
Editor: Michael Silbermann
ISBN: 978-1-63117-709-5

Chapter 17

ESTABLISHING A NEW PALLIATIVE CARE PROGRAM IN A UNIVERSITY HOSPITAL: CURRENT ACHIEVEMENTS AND CHALLENGES

Kamer Mutafoğlu, M.D.*
Centre for Palliative Care Implementation and Research,
Dokuz Eylul University, Izmir, Turkey

The road to establishing a new palliative care program in a place where palliative care has not existed before is full of challenges [1]. According to the International Observatory on End of Life Care's mapping levels of palliative care development, Turkey was among the countries where capacity building activity was taking place until recently [2]. Although awareness on palliative care has been developing among some health professionals in Turkey, great majority of physicians and nurses receive minimal or no education on the concept of modern palliative care during their undergraduate and postgraduate education [3]. This leads to confusion even around the definition of "palliative care". For instance, some of the oncologists define their supportive care efforts, which are mainly composed of *some* symptom control and transfusions, as "palliative care". Oncology and algology (pain) departments at some major hospitals provide pain control and some symptom management. Some hospitals use some of the beds for symptom control in deteriorating cancer patients. At some of the previous reports, these services have been called a "palliative care unit" as a misnomer [2]. Health care services which are established according to the modern palliative care concept have not been developed and integrated into the standard patient care yet. The Turkish MoH (Ministry of Health) has been working on a national palliative care project [4]. In parallel with the increasing state of awareness, some developments have been occurring for the last couple of years. This chapter is about the development of a palliative care program in a teaching hospital in Turkey.

Dokuz Eylul University (DEU) Hospital is a university hospital in Izmir, Turkey. The focus of patient care in this 1000-bed hospital is on investigation, diagnosis, and curative /disease modifying treatment. The hospital receives around 2000 new cancer patients / year,

* Address for correspondence: kamer.mutafoglu@deu.edu.tr

and almost 60% of these cases present with advanced stage disease. This big teaching hospital has been equipped with modern diagnostic and therapeutic facilities for cancer treatment, and has been serving for both adult and pediatric cancer patients through multidisciplinary teams that includes experts on medical and surgical oncology, radiation oncology, tumor imaging and pathology, and other diagnostic and therapeutic disciplines. However, there had been challenges and obstacles to provide holistic cancer care due to the lack of a palliative care (PC) program. The term "palliative" was only referring to palliative chemo or radiotherapy, and palliative surgery, as it has been the case in most of the hospitals in the country. Symptom management used to remain a fragmented approach to cancer care. Some detail on the situation with regard to PC was previously presented [5]. The lack of a PC program was leading to a variety of patient and family sufferings [6,7] and staff exhaustion and burnout syndrome [8].

The First Step

Being one of the physicians who had been experiencing challenges and obstacles to holistic patient care in pediatric oncology, the author had started working on developing a PC program for both adult and pediatric oncology teams in June 2008. During her pediatric oncology fellowship education and training, the author had the privilege of working with Prof. Faik Sarialioğlu, a master who had been emphasizing the importance of interdisciplinary teamwork, family-centered care, realistic goal-setting, non-abandonment, and continuing support, starting from the cancer diagnosis to the end of life (EoL). The motivation to initiate a palliative care program took its origin from two Middle East Cancer Consortium (MECC) meetings, which the author participated. (The "Workshop on the Stresses and Burnout of Working with Cancer Patients" in 2007, and the "Workshop on Psycho-Oncology: The role and involvement of the patient's family" in 2008). Being inspired by the presentations of the participating interdisciplinary palliative care team members, the author made a call to a small group of colleagues (Rüksan Çehreli; nutritionist ,Rıza Çetingöz; radiation oncologist, Tuğba Yavuzşen medical oncologist, , Ayfer Elçigil; oncology nurse, Can Cimilli; psychiatrist, Leyla İyilikçi; anesthesiologist) who were all very receptive to the patients' and families' needs. This small group of volunteers from the Medical and Nursing Faculty started an initiative at the end of 2008 with an aim to raise awareness and to develop an education program for health professionals, and to implement palliative care principles to the standard medical and pediatric oncology clinical practice.

Institutional Attempt

The group decided to establish this program through the Oncology Institute since four members of the core group were faculty at this Institute. Although the institution has no direct patient services, the clinical academic staff of the Oncology Institute has been working in affiliation with the university hospital. Therefore, an application was sent to the Council of Higher Education for establishing a Palliative Care and a Psychooncology Department within the structure of the Oncology Institute to promote education and research, and to provide clinical services in the DEU hospital on January 29, 2010. Unfortunately, this application was not approved. This was the first major barrier to development, but the group did not give up. They decided to develop an interdisciplinary palliative care working group at the hospital.

Table 1. DEU Palliative Care Working Group 2013

Health Care Professionals	Affiliation in Dokuz Eylul Hospital	Number of Participants
Nurses (n:12)	School of Nursing	**2**
	Dep. Nursing Administration	**2**
	Oncology Hospital	**3**
	Day Chemotherapy Unit	**4**
	Pediatric Oncology	**1**
Physicians (n:13)	Medical Oncology	**1**
	Pediatric Oncology	**1**
	Radiation Oncology	**2**
	Anesthesiology	**2**
	Psychiatry	**1**
	Child &Adolescent Psychiatry	**1**
	Physical Medicine & Rehabilitation	**2**
	Neurology	**1**
	Internal Medicine	**1**
	Cancer Surgery	**1**
Psychologist (n:3)	Mental Health Liaison Unit	**2**
	Child &Adolescent Psychiatry	**1**
Nutritionist n: 2)	Inst. of Oncology	**1**
	Dept. of Nutrition	**1**
Physiotherapist (n: 2)	Sch. of Physical Therapy & Rehabilitation	**2**
Total		**32**

*The names of the professionals taking part in the DEU Palliative Care Working Group by 2013 *(Names in alphabetical order)*

Nurses: Aslı Akdeniz, Deniz Arslan, Şule Baysak, Selda Kalem, Hatice Küçükkurt, Saliha Özdöker, Goncay Öztürk, Selda Paçal, Özlem Uğur, Mahdume Ulusoy, Tuğba Ülgen, Solmaz Zeybekci,

Physicians: Aynur Akay, Can Cimilli, Rıza Cetingoz, Ayşe Demiral, Özlem El, Yüksel Erkin, Leyla Iyilikçi Karaoğlan, Kamer Mutafoglu, Vesile Öztürk, Özlem Senocak , Selman Sökmen, Mehmet Tunca, Tuğba Yavuzsen

Psychologists: Ceyhan Çelikoglu , Figen Erkan, Esmahan Orçin,

Nutritionists :, Ferya Bertan, Rüksan Çehreli

Physiotherapist : Didem Karadibak, Özge Çeliker Tosun

An invitation from the Oncology Institute was sent out to the directors of related departments and hospital administrators on March 23, 2010, with whom earlier interviews were conducted by the author. The written invitation for this meeting included an attachment, highlighting the sufferings experienced by the cancer patients, briefly describing how PC has been improving the QoL (quality of life) of patients, families, and oncology staff in developed countries, and finally explaining the aim to set up a PC program in the hospital. This meeting took place on March 31, 2010, with participants from 13 different disciplines (School of Nursing, Nursing Administration, Departments of Radiation Oncology, Medical Oncology, Hematology, Pediatric Oncology, Pediatric Hematology, Chest, Algology, Psychiatry, Child and Adolescent Psychiatry, Physical Medicine and Rehabilitation, Nutrition Unit and the School of Physiotherapy). During this meeting, the author made a presentation about the current definition and scope of modern PC, emphasizing the need for a PC services for cancer patients.

Right after this meeting, "DEU Palliative Care Working Group" (PCWG), a multiprofessional voluntary working group was established at the hospital on May 2010. Thirteen volunteer professionals from different disciplines including the Nursing School, Nursing Administration, DEU School of Medicine Departments of Pediatric Oncology, Medical Oncology, Anesthesiology, Psychiatry, Child and Adolescent Psychiatry, Physical Medicine and Rehabilitation, and Nutrition Support Unit, Mental Health Support Unit, and School of Physical Therapy and Rehabilitation joined this working group.

The group had their first meeting on May 26, 2010 and defined the goal of the working group as increasing awareness and knowledge of palliative care among health care professionals, developing and implementing educational programs for multidisciplinary health care teams at the hospital who work with cancer patients, and eventually implementing the modern PC principles to the standard cancer care [9]. Since June 2010, this voluntary PCWG has been actively working and the number of participants has risen to more than 30 by 2013 (Table 1). The group has been led by the pediatric oncologist who has started the initiative. There have been regular weekly meetings for strategy planning, education, and for discussing palliative care needs of the cancer patients.

Achievements by the Palliative Care Working Group

1. **Group Education Program:** The PCWG first started a group education program. All the volunteer professionals in the group were receptive about the needs of the patients/families, and they had some education about some of the PC topics, and most of them had significant experience with cancer patients, however the level of knowledge and experience on PC was not uniform within the group. Three members of the PCWG had PC education at overseas. The medical oncologist had worked up to 2.5 years as a research fellow in Palliative Medicine in the Cleveland Clinic previously. She was trying to implement PC principles to her clinical practice, however the high number of the new adult cancer patients and lack of a PC program were major barriers. Except for her education, all the education and training support at overseas came from the Middle East Cancer Consortium (MECC) for some group members. The MECC provided valuable palliative care education and training support through inviting some members of this group to the scientific meetings on PC that were organized by MECC. The oncology nurse from the nursing received PC education and training at New York Calvary Hospital, and the author had been in New York Calvary Hospital and San Diego Hospice and the Institute for Palliative Medicine as a visiting fellow through MECC grants. With the aim of sharing knowledge and experience, developing a common language and to be able to work as a "team", the first step was a group education program. The weekly group education program on 2010-2012 focused on almost all the aspects of PC starting from the theoretical basic principles, continuing with clinical practice during patient rounds.

2. **Documentation of Unmet Needs:** An important approach to overcome denial is to document the level of unmet need in patients and families in the hospital. Surveys were conducted by the group members to document the uncontrolled symptoms or unmet needs experienced by cancer patients and care givers, as well as barriers to palliative care. Depending on these results, the group defined pain & distress management as a priority.
3. **Changes at Symptom Management Practice in the Hospital**
   Clinical practice on management of symptoms in cancer patients has been changing with the advocacy, education and application provided by the PCWG members. Several examples on the changing practice are given below.
   - **Pain as the 5th Vital Sign:** The first hospital-wide revolution achieved by the group on 2010 was the development of a new nursing chart for the whole hospital incorporating pain as the 5th vital sign. The first group education module was on pain control. One of the main goals of the module was overcoming opiophobia and disseminating knowledge on "total pain" and its management.
   - **Pain and Distress Scales:** The group provided all the nurses and residents a pocket scale for pain and distress. More nurses and physicians started using pain assessment scores. Oncology nurses and physicians started using these tools regularly.
   - **Pain Management with Morphine:** The pediatric PC program focused on pain management initially. Aggressive pain control was advocated for children with cancer. Since oral immediate release morphine is not available in the country, oral morphine solution is made out of ampoules, and is used for pain management in children and adolescents for the first time. Oral morphine solution prepared by the staff and transdermal fentanyl are drugs of choice for treatment of severe pain in children depending on the available drugs. The pediatric oncology team also started using morphine mouth wash for severe mucositis pain. Medical oncology team started using subcutaneous and intravenous morphine more often than before.
   - **Distress Management:** The oncology teams started using distress thermometer and "how do I feel meter" in order to briefly assess distress. Two psychologists and a child psychologist working with the group have began seeing patients in distress, and making connections with the busy Psychiatry Departments for a psychiatry consultation when needed.
   - **Terminal Dyspnea Management:** The pediatric oncology team started using opioids & benzodiazepines for management of dyspnea in cancer patients, a practice which was totally new to the whole hospital units. The group members have been advocating for the use of systemic opioids for the management of severe dyspnea in patients with advanced life threatening diseases during the patient rounds, and education hours.
   - **Delirium Management:** The awareness on the frequency of delirium in cancer patients & knowledge on its management have been increasing in oncology clinics.

- **Overcoming "Adverse/Side Effect Phobia"**: In pediatric oncology, the barriers to good symptom control were defined, and "adverse/side effect phobia" and lack of knowledge on opioid analgesics emerged as the major barriers. Some drugs, which are effective and can easily be provided was not being used for the fear of side effects. The clinical practice was largely changed with education, and being a role model for the residents and fellows.

4. **Changes at "Cancer Care Concept":** Before the initiative, cure from cancer was almost the only indicator of clinical success. As the group members' level of knowledge on palliative care topics such as communication skills , breaking bad news, goal setting, QoL issues , and end of life (EoL) care have increased, other indicators of success have been emerging within the group, such as the importance of good care, quality of care, patient/family centered care, continuity of care/ non-abandonment, and respectful death.
   The group members made interdisciplinary patient rounds for cancer patients with complex problems once a week both at the pediatric and medical oncology wards.
5. **Mental Health Support:** The needs assessment surveys at the early days of the initiative showed that only 4% of the pediatric cancer patients were receiving professional mental health support [7]. A self-report questionnaire given to adult cancer patients in the Day Chemotherapy Unit showed that 70% of the adult cancer patients had been experiencing distress to some extend (unpublished data). The psychiatrist member of the PCWG, Prof. Can Cimilli, who has been the Head of the **Liaison Psychiatry Unit,** provided connection with the Mental Health Support Unit of the Hospital. With this attempt, psychological evaluation and support has become possible for more cancer patients. A child psychologist from the group started seeing children and adolescents in distress, and making connections with the busy child psychiatrists. The Child and Adolescent Psychiatry Department has been trying to give priority to the kids with cancer when consultations are requested.
6. **Management of Interventional or Refractory Pain:** There are two anesthesiologists taking part in the group. One is from the Pain Unit of the Hospital; the other is the Head of the Non-Operating Room Anesthesiology Team. All the painful interventions in cancer patients like endoscopic procedures, biopsies, embolizations, percutaneous endoscopic gastrostomy, percutaneous biliary drainage, endoscopic retrograde cholangiopancreatography, insertion of double J stents, esophageal stents, and brachytherapy have been performed under sedoanalgesia. This team has been giving sedoanalgesia to pediatric cancer patients during bone marrow aspiration/biopsies, and intrathecal chemotherapies, and when needed, during radiotherapy and radiological interventions. The Pain Unit has been providing various invasive pain management techniques, including somatic and sympathetic nerve blocks and spinal analgesia (epidural, intrathecal) for refractory cancer pain.
7. **Nutrition:** Cancer patients have been regularly offered either enteral (oral, tube-feeding, gastrostomy) or parenteral nutrition (by central venous catheters/ports) throughout the whole disease trajectory in our center. The goals for medical nutrition therapy in cancer patients are to prevent or reverse nutrient deficiencies, preserve lean body mass, help patients better tolerate treatments, minimize side effects and complications. Discussing nutritional issues during rounds and tailoring nutritional support to the particular patient, goal setting with patients and families, and

withdrawing unnecessary aggressive nutritional support at the end of life are some examples of the changing practice.

8. **Physical Therapy and Rehabilitation:** Before the initiative, physical therapy and rehabilitation was provided to occasional cancer patients only on demand of the oncologists. With the major contribution of two therapists and two specialists taking part in the PCWG, the need for physical therapy has been evaluated for more cancer patients either during inpatient rounds or on demand of the oncologist at the outpatient clinics. The aim of the exercises and physical activities is to help condition muscles, restore strength / movement, and restore normal function. They also provide lymphedema treatment. Physical therapists are encouraging patients for strength training and exercise to counteract fatigue.
9. **Changes at the Curriculum and Training Programs**
   Keeping in mind that a major cultural change is needed at places where PC programs and services have not existed before, the group believes that providing education at all training levels and having formal curriculum space has a pivotal role in changing culture. The group members aimed to promote formal PC education and training at the health campus of the university. With the advocacy of PCWG, palliative care has got some formal curriculum space at the DEU School of Medicine, School of Nursing and School of Physiotherapy. The PCWG has been seeding the "palliative care" concept to every area possible within the Hospital and the Schools of the DEU.
   - **Formal Curriculum Space**
     - **The Nursing School Curriculum:** The Nursing Faculty added PC topics (pain and symptom management, palliative care, and integrative medicine) to the "Oncology Nursing" Module at the 3rd grade of the undergraduate curriculum. They also opened an elective course on "Palliative Care Nursing" at the Nursing Post-Graduate Program
     - **The Medical School Curriculum:** The Medical Faculty added a 2-hour panel on "Palliative Care in Cancer" to the curriculum for the 3. Grade medical students, starting from 2011.
     - **The Physiotherapy School Curriculum:** The School of Physiotherapy added PC topics to the "Oncologic Physiotherapy " (FTR 3035) block at the 3rd grade curriculum, including role of physiotherapy in palliative care for cancer, symptom control (pain, fatigue, others), and integrative methods for symptom control in cancer patients
   - **Nursing Education Program**
     - Nursing Orientation Program: The DEU Hospital Nursing Administrators added "Nursing approach to pain" as a new title to the nursing orientation program.
     - CME for Hospital Nurses: "Nurses' role in pain management" and "palliative care" sessions were added to the CME program.
   - **Resident and Fellow Education Program:**
     - The education for residents and fellows in pediatric and medical oncology have focused on good symptom control, communication skills , breaking bad news, goal setting, QoL issues , and EoL care.

- Education for Residents : Annual "Palliative Care" lectures for the residents have been given since 2010 at the Internal Medicine , Anesthesiology , and Child & Adolescent Psychiatry Departments

10. **Proactive Advocacy (lectures, conferences):** The group members have been investing time in proactive advocacy. The group members have been advocating for adding PC topics to scientific meetings' programs. They have been giving lectures and panel talks on PC at the local and national meetings.

ESTABLISHMENT OF THE PALLIATIVE CARE IMPLEMENTATION AND RESEARCH CENTER

A formal PC Program needs designation of an administrative structure like a department or a division [1]. The DEU PC initiative has been developed with volunteer professionals, all of whom have other primary responsibilities (patient care, education, research and administrative duties) within the hospital and the university. The first attempt for establishing a department within the Oncology Institute was not approved. The second attempt was applying for establishment of a "center" at the hospital. The intensive preparatory work included meetings with the Rector and the Vice- Chancellor of the University, Dean of the Medical School, The Medical Director of the Hospital, and the Senate Committee members of the DEU. During these meetings, representatives from the PCWG told these administrators about the modern PC concept, its importance for providing holistic and comprehensive cancer care, about the need for PC education and service development in a hospital receiving great number of cancer patients, and about the ongoing efforts of the voluntary PCWG. The University Senate approved the application, and sent it to the Council of Higher Education. This application was approved on Sept 2012, and a formal structure, namely DEU Palliative Care Implementation and Research Center was established by law.

After formal recognition of the palliative care center, the PCWG has been continuing their activities under the frame of this center. The first executive board was established on October 2012, composing of the seven professionals who initiated this program. Table shows the composition and names of the professionals currently taking part at the Center's activities.

Education Program for the Health Campus: The Center developed an education program as its first activity. The aim of this year-long, weekly education program was disseminating knowledge and skills required to provide proactive palliative care for all health professionals in the hospital. This weekly education program on palliative and end-of life care in oncology was based on EPEC-O series [10]. It was first translated to Turkish, and then the scientific context was updated with recent publications on the subject. These meetings are open and free to all health care providers and students, and are announced to all the health campus of the university with e-mail notifications. These meetings attracted new professionals' attention, like oncology surgeons, neurologists, new nurses, who developed an interest in palliative care.

The first year's education program focused on symptom management in cancer, the barriers to good symptom control, and the impact of quality PC on patients' and families' life.

Patient referral to the palliative care team is not possible yet due to the lack of regulations by the Social Security Administration. However, the team members are actively treating and caring for cancer patients, so they implement the palliative care principles to their standard patient care. Most of the members are faculty at the DEU Health Campus. Therefore, they use this opportunity to disseminate knowledge and skills during the education and training they have been giving both at the undergraduate and postgraduate level. On the other hand, the physician members of the team see patients on a consultation basis on the demand of the treating physicians. These consultations are significantly different than it used to be before. The team members are very sensitive about the holistic approach, so the problems are being discussed in an interdisciplinary manner. There has been increasing awareness among oncology professionals on assessment and management of the problems related with cancer or anticancer therapies. The interdisciplinary team approach, which was emphasized during all education programs, has been the standard of practice at the pediatric oncology clinic. Since hospice care and home care for terminally ill patients is not available yet in the country, some cancer patients or their families chose the hospital as the place of death. If there are available beds, these patients are hospitalized. The most appropriate rooms at the wards, which are usually not in the middle of the clinic, are given to these families.

The concept of EoL care has been largely changing in pediatric oncology clinic with this program. The patients, whose family chose to stay in hospital, spend their last days at these rooms with their beloved ones instead of being alone and hooked at the machines at intensive care units, . All the symptoms have been aggressively controlled at the EoL without forgetting the principle "minimum/no invasive intervention". The health professionals honor the last wishes of patients and the families; they are getting more sensitive about the cultural /religious needs, and rituals.

Contribution to scientific meetings: The members of the PCWG organized two symposiums on palliative care in collaboration with other colleagues in 2013. One was about pain management in cancer, which was organized as a joint meeting with another hospital in Izmir. The second symposium was on Geriatric Patient Care. The group members took part in nine different national scientific meetings as speakers and they made six oral/poster presentations about palliative care in 2013.

Board for Palliative Cancer Care: On October 2013, the Center has started a new project with an aim to integrate palliative care to the cancer care at the hospital. There have been tumor-specific board reviews at the hospital for almost 20 years. Although palliative chemo/radiotherapy or surgery has been discussed at these boards, PC concept was not integrated to standard cancer care. With an aim to advocate for implementing PC strategies to the anticancer treatment starting from the diagnosis to the EoL, the PCWG members started the Board for Palliative Cancer Care. These meetings are open to all cancer professionals who are interested in discussing his/her cancer patients' management with a focus on interdisciplinary PC. All the professionals at the PCWG are natural members of this board.

Other Activities

The first event at the hospital at which health professionals and patients/parents come together to discuss problematic issues about the patient care, and change ideas about the possible solutions was organized by the Center on February 2013. "The Palliative Care Needs of the Pediatric Cancer Patients: Patients and Families Talking for themselves" panel was open to the pediatric oncology patients and their families as well as all health care providers.

The Center has been working on developing volunteer groups. Some volunteers from the community and some NGOs have been organizing social events for the children on special days, like holy days, New Year, etc. Some cancer survivors also participate to these events. The members of the team have been collaborating with some foundations in order to provide social/economic support for families with limited income.

Relations with another university in Izmir (İzmir University of Economics) have been providing increasing social support. The volunteer teachers and university students raised funds, and donated a variety of art material, tables, chairs, electronic tablets, etc. for kids and adolescents. They helped the team for making some wishes of the pediatric patients possible.

Some volunteer students from Dokuz Eylul University School of Physical Therapy and Rehabilitation and from Izmir State Opera performed live music at the Day Chemotherapy Center during cancer week of Turkey.

Relations with Other Structures

The Center has been developing relations with cancer organizations such as Turkish Pediatric Oncology Group, Turkish Oncology Group, Turkish Association for Lung Cancer, Turkish Foundation for Cancer Research and Control through the members' activities.

There is increasing collaboration with the other major hospitals in the city on palliative care education. Group members are taking place as presenters in joint education meetings. The center has been represented at the Palliative Care Commission established by the Izmir Local Health Authority with an aim to develop a regional palliative care program for education and active patient services.

Barriers to Wholistic Service Development

Appointment and Funding of Professionals: A PC Program needs appointment and funding of professionals, and allocation of space [1]. There are no health professionals exclusively appointed for Palliative Care Center yet. This program has been developed with volunteer professionals, all of whom are staff, having other primary appointments and responsibilities within the hospital and/or the university. No funding is available for compensation of their work at the PC Center.

Lack of Physical Space: The center has no physical space allocated by the hospital yet. The group has been using certain meeting rooms at the hospital. A palliative care inpatient clinic is being planned by the hospital administration.

Understaffing: The number of nurses is very limited in the hospital. The physicians at the group are only from faculty. There is shortage of mental health professionals. These limitations have been leading to serious time constraint for the Palliative Care Center's activities. The team has no social worker and spiritual counselor. Like the majority of other hospitals in the country, there are only 2-3 social workers for the 1000 bed hospital. There aren't any professionals in the country who are trained as spiritual counselors.

Frequent Change at the Administrative Leadership: Starting from the initial step, four different medical directors have been appointed at the hospital. Frequent change at the administrative leadership was an important barrier for service development.

Limited Support from Administrators: The medical director(s) of the hospital, the other administrators, the Dean of Medical School, the Rector of the University have been expressing that palliative care is very important, and a palliative care service development is necessary. However, only very limited support has been given for the program's development. The administrators are unable to commit the necessary resources for the establishment of active patient services.

Lack of Palliative Care Organizations: Lack of palliative care organizations; hospice care and home care in the country are major barriers for the continuum of care. However, the MoH Cancer Control Department has been working on developing a national palliative care service program (4).

Lack of Essential Drugs: Although most of the essential medicines for PCis available in the country, neither immediate nor prolonged release oral morphine is available in the market.

Regulatory Barriers: There are regulatory barriers in terms of reimbursement of services provided by the palliative care team. The interdisciplinary patient evaluation by the team has no code for reimbursement from the Social Security Administration. National standards to establish a PC program should be defined.

Conclusion

A small group of enthusiastic volunteer professionals have been changing the culture in a big teaching hospital by acknowledging PC as an important component in management of cancer, although they have been getting very limited administrative support, and no financial support. The major resource is the group of professionals who believe in holistic care and team work. The positive feed-back from patients and families is the major motivation to go on. The feed-back from the team members is also very encouraging; they express their experience with the PCWG not only as a great way of learning, but also a very effective way to prevent burn-out syndrome, which is very prevalent among oncology staff.

The evidence of dozens of program around the world strongly suggests that, by following simple steps, cultural change can occur, and this will benefit thousands of patients and families (1). All the group members believe that the cultural change will benefit thousands of Turkish cancer patients and families.

References

[1] Bruera E. The development of a palliative care culture. *J Palliat Care* 2004; 20(4): 316-319.

[2] Wright M, Wood J, Lynch T, Clark D. Mapping levels of palliative care development: a global view. International Observatory on End of Life Care. *http://www.eolc-observatory.net/global_analysis/pdf/turkey_country_report.pdf*

[3] Elcigil A. The current status of palliative care in Turkey: a nurse's perspective. *J Pediatr Hematol Oncol.* 2011 Apr;33 Suppl 1:S70-2.

[4] N. Ozgul, M. Gultekin, O. Koc, et al. Turkish community-based palliative care model: a unique design. *Annals Oncol* 2012 ; 23 (suppl 3): iii76–iii78.

[5] Mutafoglu K. Current Palliative Care Practice in a University Hospital. *J Pediatr Hematol Oncol.* 2010;32 (suppl 1):S36–S38.).

[6] Alacacioglu A, Yavuzsen T, Dirioz M, et al. Quality of life, anxiety and depression in Turkish breast cancer patients and in their husbands. *Med Oncol.* 2009;26:415–419.

[7] Kamer Mutafoglu (Uysal). The effects of having a child with cancer on the close family members—the Turkish experience. *J Pediatr Hematol Oncol.* 2008;30(suppl 1): S4–S5.

[8] Alacacioglu A, Yavuzsen T, Dirioz M, Oztop I, Yilmaz U. Burnout in nurses and physicians working at an oncology department. *Psychooncology* 2009;18:543–548.

[9] Mutafoglu Kamer, on Behalf of the DEU Palliative Care Strategy Group. A Palliative Care Initiative in Dokuz Eylul University Hospital. *J Pediatr Hematol Oncol* 2011; 33 (suppl 1): :S73–S76.

[10] Emanuel LL, Ferris FD, von Gunten CF, Von Roenn . *EPEC-O: Education in Palliative and End-of-life Care for Oncology.* © The EPEC Project,™ . Chicago, IL, 2005 ISBN: 0-9714180-9-8

In: Palliative Care to the Cancer Patient
Editor: Michael Silbermann
ISBN: 978-1-63117-709-5

Chapter 18

PALLIATIVE CARE: A NEW AND EMERGING PARADIGM

Rab Razzak, M.D.[1] and Thomas J. Smith, M.D., FACP, FASCO, FAAHPM[2,•]
[1]Cedars-Sinai Medical Center, Los Angeles, CA, US
[2]Sidney Kimmel Comprehensive Cancer Center at Johns Hopkins, Baltimore, MD, US

INTRODUCTION

The world population is now over 7.2 billion and continues to grow and age as infectious disease and other premature deaths decline. [1] The Middle East follows that same trend, with people living longer with more frequent and longer-lived chronic diseases. By 2050, the life expectancy will be more than 70 years of age in all of the region. According to the World Bank, the population over 65 years of age in the Middle East and Northern Africa (MENA) is about 4.7% of the world population. The rate of growth of this population is projected to be 5%, with the oldest patients' growth rate exceeding 5% in 11 Arab countries. In countries like Lebanon, the elder population will double by 2050 and others like Qatar and UAE are expecting a five-fold increase in their geriatric population. [2] As shown in Figure 1, by 2050 the number of people over age 65 will be nearly one third of the population.

Society needs to prepare for this aging population as many will have significant chronic diseases, disabilities and dependency. The longer people live, the more chronic cancer, heart disease, circulation problems, renal failure, etc., and most people will have more than one chronic condition. Healthcare infrastructure will need to change and build around this population as they will need care and support. Healthcare professionals will need to increase their knowledge and understanding of different cultures and understand how patients view their disease, especially cancer. These recommendations are as true in the Middle East as they are in the United States and other highly resourced countries. [3]

• E-mail: tsmit136@jhmi.edu.

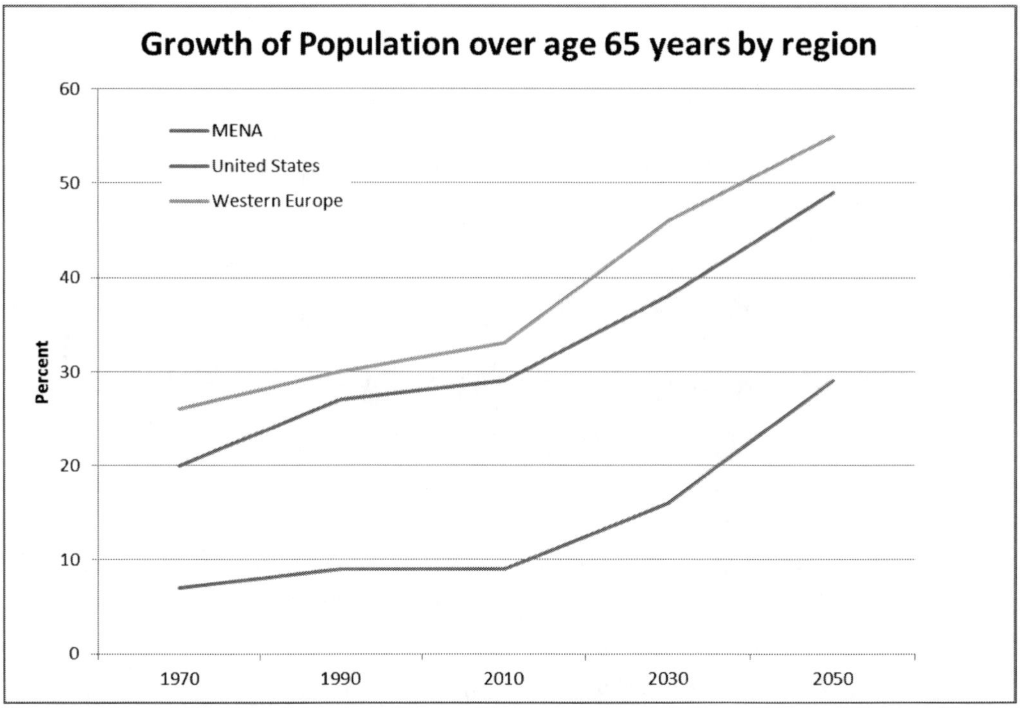

Figure 1. Past and projected growth of population over age 65 years by region.

There will be changes in cancer itself, too. At present, 70% of all cancer patients in the MENA present with grade III or grade IV cancers due to lack of knowledge, fear, stigmatism, low socioeconomic status (SES), and preference for traditional complementary or alternative medicine (CAM) treatments, all of which lead to higher mortality rates. Changing this trend to endorse and actually utilize early cancer screening will lead to greater survivorship and quality of life. Enhancements in cultural sensitivity will provide high-quality care as healthcare professionals will find better ways to explain disease to their patients, which will help ensure patient compliance and understanding with prevention [4, 5] and treatment, [6] and lead to better-nuanced ways of caring for the terminally ill. [7]

In this introduction we will define palliative care, give the clinical and economic justifications, illustrate what practical palliative care looks like, and discuss some barriers.

What Is Palliative Care?

According to the World Health Organization definition, "Palliative care is an approach that improves the quality of life of patients and their families facing the problems associated with life-threatening illness, through the prevention and relief of suffering by means of early identification and impeccable assessment and treatment of pain and other problems: physical, psychological, and spiritual." [8]

We prefer the more detailed definition given in Text Box 1- that emphasizes specialist care (just like nephrology or cardiology, medicine or nursing) delivered by an interdisciplinary team at any time in the illness trajectory.

"Palliative care is specialized medical care for people with serious illnesses. This type of care is focused on providing patients with relief from the symptoms, pain, and stress of a serious illness - whatever the diagnosis.
The goal is to improve quality of life for both the patient and the family.

Palliative care is provided by a team of doctors, nurses, and other specialists who work with a patient's other doctors to provide an extra layer of support.

Palliative care is appropriate at any age and at any stage in a serious illness, and can be provided together with curative treatment."

– Diane Meier, MD, Director, Center to Advance Palliative Care, New York, New York, July 1, 2011 (www.capc.org)

Text Box 1. Definition of Palliative Care.

Primary palliative care [9] is provided by the longitudinal oncologist or other doctor, and care team. *Secondary palliative care* is provided by teams of dedicated palliative care specialists, either in outpatient programs or in an inpatient unit. *Tertiary palliative care* is provided by specialized palliative care providers with advanced expertise in the management of symptoms and pain, including but not limited to implantable drug delivery systems, palliative sedation, and management of advanced delirium. We would now add palliative radiation and chemotherapy, and advanced heart failure management – often the best palliation is treating the illness.

Although palliative care is most thought of as related to cancer care, there are increasing data showing benefit in almost any illness. [9] At our own institutions, for instance, we do palliative care consultations for the dying, but also for those who are on extracorporeal membrane oxygenation (ECMO) for acute cardiac and respiratory failure, left ventricular assist devices (LVAD) awaiting curative heart transplants [10], bone marrow transplantation patients being treated with curative intent, [11] and even patients on Phase I experimental drugs.

We have recently described the identity crisis of palliative care. [12, 13] Palliative care grew from hospice care, which is clearly for those at the end of life. Hospice care is defined as "… a type and philosophy of care that focuses on the palliation of a terminally ill or seriously ill patient's pain and symptoms, and attending to their emotional and spiritual needs." [12] Originating in the 11th century as places to go do die, hospice is inextricably linked to dying. However, palliative care can be given anytime during an illness; however, in practice most patients are referred with days or weeks to live. [14] We must be mindful to continue to promote the good attributes of hospice and palliative care together, while at the same time expanding the number and types of patients seen.

WHY PALLIATIVE CARE?

The Clinical Case

Palliative care is superior to usual care by providing for emotional/spiritual support, information/communication, care at time of death, access to services in community, well-being, dignity, care and setting concordant with patient preference, better pain control and less PTSD symptoms. [15] The data come from multiple randomized trials and all reach the same conclusion: interdisciplinary palliative care added to usual care improves care, improves the quality of care, does no harm, gives equal or better survival (not worse), and does not raise costs. [13] In fact, no studies have shown decreased survival or increased costs – even with all the other benefits. We have listed some of the relevant recent trials in Table 1. Note that it is NOT all cancer patients.

Patients who receive palliative care alongside their usual care, compared to those who receive usual care along, have lower rates of hospitalization, die more frequently at their place of choice, have LESS depression and anxiety, and may even live longer. [16] In the Temel trial with lung cancer patients, those who better understood their prognosis (not curable, going to die of the disease) and goal of treatment (cannot cure, with a goal of improving quantity and quality of life) actually were not as likely to be depressed or anxious, had better quality of life, and lived 2.7 months longer. [17] Telling them the truth did not make them depressed or anxious – the exact opposite happened because patients could now plan their future. This was observed in a large prospective trial of 332 patients and their caregivers, as well: better knowledge, and having a discussion about imminent death, was strongly associated with better quality of life and less aggressive end of life care, but no more anxiety or depression. However, only 37% had any such conversation. [18]

But the benefits do not stop with the patient. Palliative care has consistently been associated with less aggressive end of life care and better quality of life for patients. The caregivers whose patients had better quality of life also exhibited better coping mechanisms and better quality of life. [18] When a patient dies with hospice care, and a planned comfort care approach usually at home, the chance of the remaining spouse dying the next year (5% for women, 14% for men) is decreased by almost 1%. [19]

This approach to palliative care calls for a more comprehensive approach to patient care than the episodic care so familiar to all of us. In the trials done at Kaiser-Permanente, a team with a nurse or nurse practitioner, doctor, social worker and chaplain was assigned to help the patient alongside his or her usual care. [20, 21] Imagine having a team whose job it was to improve your quality of life, answer the phone, and answer your questions, rather than support a practice by piecework billing! We have urged adoption of a framework that emphasizes palliative care from diagnosis with progressive more as the illness progresses, shown in Figure 2.

Much has been written in the recent lay [22, 23] and professional press about how physicians (and nurses) face serious illness and die. A uniform theme has been full and honest information, knowing the risks and benefits of treatments, declining treatments with little chance of benefit, and having a sense of control – along with good symptom management. In essence, palliative care seeks to have that for all patients.

The Financial Case

What health care system does not want to provide better care at lower cost? All the data show that palliative care programs are helpful in reducing readmissions and lowering health care system costs. Palliative care reduces the cost of inpatient stays [24-26] and allows each hospital to calculate the financial savings from adding or expanding their palliative care team. We posted a free calculator for each health care system in the U.S. to estimate the savings from integrated palliative care on the Center to Advance Palliative Care website http://www.capc.org/impact_calculator_basic/.

Table 1. Outcomes from randomized trials of palliative care performed in the last 10 years

First Author, Year Citation		Outcomes							
	Type of patient	Symptoms	Quality of Life	Mood	Satisfaction	Resource Use	Advance Care Planning	Survival	Costs
Zimmermann, C et al. PC Team intervention in OP clinics. Lancet 2014 [51]	Cancer	Improved at 4 months (P = .05)	Improved at 4 months (P = .003)	NR	Improved at 4 months (P < .0001)	NR	NR	NR	NR
Higginson, I et al. Improved med. Post Grad 2011 [52]	Multiple sclerosis	Improved	Improved	NR	NR	Lower with PC	NR	NR	Lower
Temel, J, et al. PC Team intervention NEJM 2010 [16]	Advanced lung cancer	Improved P=.04	Improved P=.03	Less depression P=0.01	Not measured	Less aggressive care P=0.05, $2200 per person savings	More ADs documented in PC group P=0.05	11.6 v 8.9 months P=.02	Lower
Bakitas M, et al: JAMA 2009 [53] Nurse-led intervention	Lung and colorectal cancer	Improved P = .06	Improved P = .02	Improved P = .02	Not measured	No difference	No difference	No difference	Costs
Gade, G, et al. JPM 2008 PC Team Intervention [21]	Any serious illness that could cause death in < 1 year; 1/3 with cancer	No difference	No difference	No difference	IPCS greater satisfaction with care (P=0.04) and communication (P=0.0004)	Costs $6,766 less P <0.001). Net cost savings of $4,855 ((P <0.001). Longer median hospice stays (24 vs 12 days, P=0.04).	IPCS patients had more ADs at discharge than UC patients (91.1% vs. 77.8%; P< 0.001)	No difference	Lower

Table 1. (Continued)

First Author, Year Citation		Outcomes							
	Type of patient	Symptoms	Quality of Life	Mood	Satisfaction	Resource Use	Advance Care Planning	Survival	Costs
Brumley, R, et al. JAGS 2007 PC Team intervention[20]	Any serious illness that could cause death in < 1 year; 1/3 with cancer	Not measured	Not measured	Not measured	Improved, P < .05	Cost $7500 less, P=.03 Hospital days reduced by 4.36 (P<.001) ED visits reduced by 0.35 (P=.02)	Not measured	No difference	No difference

Abbreviations: OR, odds ratio; ED, emergency department; IPCS, Interdisciplinary palliative care service; UC, usual care; AD, advance directive; PC, palliative care; NR, not reported; OP, outpatient.

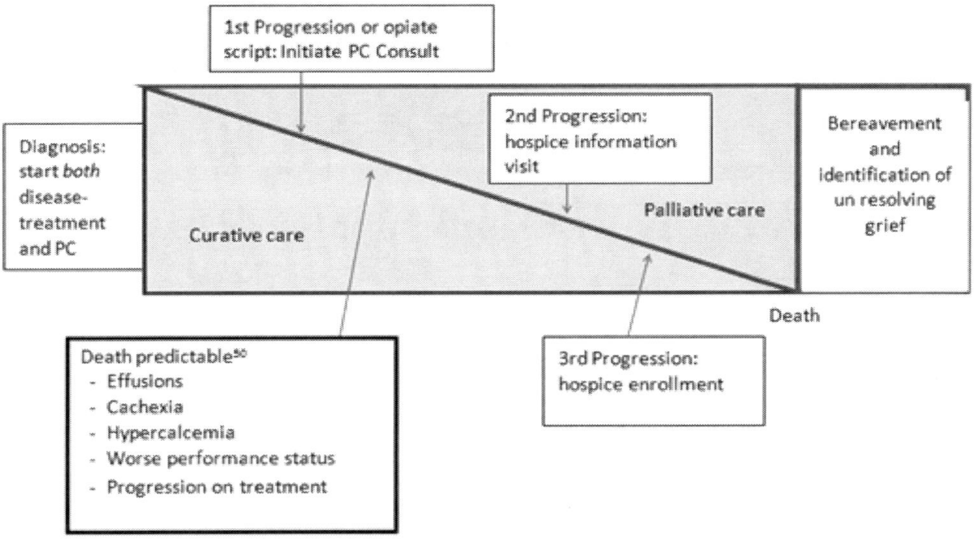

Figure 2. Using the natural history of the illness to guide PC involvement.

Where do the savings arise? The savings are due to reduced inpatient length of stay, and also includes savings from moving a patient from a high-cost venue such as the intensive care unit ($5000 US per day) to a lower-cost setting such as usual or palliative care ($2000 US per day, or $3000 of saving) which we called "cost avoidance." [27] Morrison and colleagues estimated that if the state of New York had palliative care programs in all its hospitals, the government health care program for the poor, Medicaid, would save $84 to $252 million annually.

Reducing preventable readmissions is part of several national strategies to reduce health care costs, with the main target being 30 day readmission rates for patients with congestive heart failure, myocardial infarction, and pneumonia. Palliative care programs appear to reduce readmissions by half, [28] partly by increasing referrals to hospice and home based care, [29] decrease stress to caregivers, [28] and lower overall health care costs. [26] We reassured hospital administrators – who may be judged on hospital mortality rates -- that palliative care programs do not increase hospital mortality rates, because palliative care is better at getting people home and preventing admissions. [30]

The financial link of palliative care to higher use of hospice reduces costs. At one large hospital, only 14% of hospital decedents who were hospice eligible were offered hospice on their penultimate admission, because doctors failed to recognize their eligibility. [31] When hospice was offered and accepted, the patients in hospice were re-admitted half as often, and their end of life hospitalization cost one-tenth as much. [32] Other data show that patients discharged home with hospice have a 5% 30-day readmission rate, those with palliative care an 8% rate, and those with no services in place a 25% rate. [33] In the randomized trial of palliative care for lung cancer patients, hospice use and length of stay were increased in the group that had concurrent palliative care. [16]

The evidence shows that oncology practices can be changed to incorporate more hospice. A study of interdisciplinary palliative care with a "before you need hospice, let's get it in place" referral and meeting the palliative care team increased hospice length of stay from 14 to 48 days. [34, 35] Hoverman and colleagues at U.S. Oncology made evidence-based clinical pathways that reward good advance directive use, and data from colon and lung cancer patients shows equal or better survival, double the use of hospice, length of stay in hospice of over 30 days, and one-third less cost of care for the illness – over $30,000 savings per patient. [36, 37]

WHY PALLIATIVE CARE IN THE MIDDLE EAST?

There are several good reasons. [38] First, palliative care is relatively low tech and low cost and can be utilized anywhere. [39] With less resourced countries that may not have radiation and the most modern chemotherapy available, palliative care should always be possible even within a limited state budget.

Second, opiate consumption is low, but not consistent across the region, as shown in Table 2. For most of these countries, opiates are simply not available to the average patient.

Third, cultural practices such as truth-telling vary considerably across the region as well. There is nowhere in the world currently where patients consistently get as much information as the doctors have, or as doctors would want if they were sick.

Table 2. Opiate consumption by country in the region, mg/person

Country	Morphine consumption (mg/person)
Tunisia	2.36
Cyprus	2.20
Libya	No data
Egypt	0.18
Italy	3.94
Israel	4.08
Jordon	1.88
Greece	O.39
Saudi Arabia	0.58
Iraq	0.047
Iran	No data
Lebanon	1.46
turkey	0.096
Greece	0.36
Albania	0.94
Qatar	0.39
UAE	0.16
Yemen	0.014
Oman	0.55
Syria	0.12

Modified from Opioid Consumption Maps — Morphine, mg/capita, 2010, University of Wisconsin, http://ppsg-production.heroku.com/.

Even in the United States, where truth-telling about cancer has been practiced for about 40 years, only about 37% of cancer patients remember any doctor describing their imminent death. [18] Only 22% of charts of lung cancer patients have any physician note about imminent death, and if such conversations happen they take place just 33 days before death. [40]

For many of us in the health professions, truth telling is confounded by religion, although it is usually culture rather than religion that restricts information. From our practices in many different cultures, doctors and other health care professionals in all religions appear to get more information and be able to plan better than their patients. A better understanding of Islamic beliefs may help and harness better communication with patients. Islam reminds believers to be prepared for death, as it cannot be delayed.

When a patient and family realize death is coming, they are encouraged to pray that death comes with as little suffering as possible. They are encouraged to accept death and have no anger toward Allah for suffering and/or death. However, it is acceptable to be disappointed or frustrated with limitations of medical interventions. [7] Palliative care and hospice and Muslim perspectives on death go hand in hand and should work in conjunction, rather than opposition.

Fourth, in the past 50 years and two generations there has been a dramatic shift in the world and MENA to death in the hospital rather than at home. This is simply unsustainable given the current cost of hospital care in all countries. And, the hospital is not where most people want to die. [41] There are certain groups of patients who will continue to use the hospital for death: the elderly especially those with cognitive impairment, [42], and cancer patients with many symptoms. [41] But this hospital-death trend can be blunted: there has been a downward trend in hospital deaths and increase in home deaths after 2005, coinciding with the launch of the National End of Life Care Program in 2004 in England.

WHAT SHOULD PALLIATIVE CARE LOOK LIKE AND DO?

We have recently written a proposal for "how to do palliative care in the office" since so many of our colleagues stated "We already *do* palliative care." That is the situation – we are all doing palliative care whether we call it that or not, with various levels of training, and many oncologists are not good at real palliative care. [43]

In Table 3 we have listed some of the components of good palliative care that should be standard. Note the use of some standardized assessment instrument such as the Edmonton Symptom Assessment Scale or the Memorial Symptom Assessment Scale-Condensed version. And, beyond symptoms, we must ASK patients what they want to know about their illness, TELL in understandable terms, and ASK again "what is your understanding?" [44] The optimal type of palliative care program has not been identified but inpatient consults, inpatient units, and outpatient programs all are effective. Inpatient units may be more effective because the palliative care team assumes control of the day to day care of the patient, with more families ranking the care as "excellent" than the care received with a consultative team. [45, 46]

Outpatient programs also are effective in reducing symptoms for cancer patients, with highly satisfied referring oncologists. [45]

Table 3. Components of Good Primary Palliative Care in any Setting

1. Remember to always "Ask, Tell, Ask." Always ASK people how much they want to know and what they do know. This works in any culture, and avoids the practitioner guessing how much information the patient or family wants. Then TELL, in understandable words. Then ASK again: "What is your understanding of your situation?" This is much better than "Any questions?"
2. Remember to re-address at transition points. At each transition point (when performance status, treatment, or prognosis changes), ask: "What are you hoping for?" and "What is your understanding of your situation?"
3. Always do a symptom assessment using a valid symptom assessment tool such as the MSAS or ESAS. This is simple to do and will tell you what is bothering the patient.
4. At least some of the time, do a spiritual assessment. Ask "Is religion or spirituality important to you? Would you like the health care team to help with spiritual needs?"
5. Make a "hospice information referral" when the patient still has 3-6 months left to live. In countries with no hospice in the community, this is a major barrier.
6. Use some "palliative care pearls" in your practice. There are increasing specialist palliative care helps for symptom management, such as olanzapine for nausea, ginger for chemotherapy induced nausea, [54] ginseng [55] or dexamethasone for fatigue [56] and better quality of life, and gabapentin for refractory cough. [57]

BARRIERS TO PALLIATIVE CARE IN THE MIDDLE EAST AND NORTH AFRICA

Half of the Middle Eastern countries have established PC programs, whereas the other half is either in the planning or building phase. Political and military instability have been barriers to advancing healthcare, and in particular, palliative care. Lack of funding, education, support and approval from governments, and challenges of services such as having expertise and medications available are common barriers seen with ME countries. Saudi Arabia has the most developed PC programs in the ME.

Palliative care can be improved in this region through private organizations that promote cross-border collaborations such as the Middle East Cancer Consortium (MECC) [12] and educational pursuits through workshops and conferences. [47]

The availability of knowledge should not be an issue. There are excellent resources available free of charge from the National Comprehensive Cancer Centers Network (http: //www.nccn.org/professionals/physician_gls/f_guidelines.asp#palliative), the Multinational Association for Supportive Care in Cancer (MASCC http:// www.mascc.org/guidelines-and-tools), and The European society of Medical Oncology (ESMO). There are excellent resources for a wide variety of palliative care topics at websites such as EPERC (Education Palliative and End of Life Resource Center) http://www.eperc.mcw.edu/EPERC /FastFactsandConcepts.

A significant barrier is the low doctor to patient ratio in most of MENA, [48] with a particular lack of palliative care trained professionals. In Oil-rich countries ratios are still higher than developed nations. In Kuwait, the ratio is 1:667, 1:714 in Saudi Arabia, 1:769 in Oman, and 1:625 in Bahrain. In the US, the ratio is 1:182, which is significantly better than the MENA region. It is hard to do even primary palliative care, if there is no primary care doctor available.

In most countries, the disparities in income are increasing, with well to-do people able to purchase anything on the open market. In Portugal, patients who could afford private hospitalization could receive patient controlled analgesia morphine, whereas those at state-funded hospitals would often receive tramadol and paracetamol. Like with expensive cancer medications, palliative care might become only available to those who can pay out of pocket, which is unnecessary given the relative low cost of palliative interventions.

A significant barrier in the region is the lack of hospice and home care programs. The need for these has been recognized for decades [49] but few are in place. Given that care can be improved at lower cost, the region will need some pilot programs to show these findings in MENA.

SUMMARY POINTS

Palliative care can be justified because it provides better quality of life and care, at a lower cost because it reduces hospitalizations especially near the end of life. For palliative care to be fully effective, it must partner with hospice and home care programs to ensure smooth transitions and in-home deaths for patients and families.

REFERENCES

[1] United Nations N. World population to 2030. http://www.un.org/esa/population/ publications/longrange2/WorldPop2300final.pdf. 2014. 1-5-2014. Ref Type: Online Source.

[2] Hajjar R. R., Atli T., Al-Mandhari Z., Oudrhiri M., Balducci L., Silbermann M. Prevalence of aging population in the Middle East and its implications on cancer incidence and care. *Annals of Oncology,* 2013;24:vii11-vii24.

[3] Ganz P. A., Cohen H. J., Eberlein T. J., Feeley T. W., Ferrell B., Hayman J. A. et al. Delivering high-quality cancer care: Charting a new course for a system in crisis. 2013. Washington, DC, Institute of Medicine. 10-8-2013. Ref Type: Report

[4] Guimond M. E., Salman K. Modesty Matters: Cultural Sensitivity and Cervical Cancer Prevention in Muslim Women in the United States. *Nursing for Women's Health,* 2013;17:210-217.

[5] Shirazi M., Shirazi A., Bloom J. Developing a culturally competent faith-based framework to promote breast cancer screening among Afghan immigrant women. *J. Relig. Health,* 2013;[epub ahead of print].

[6] Tay K. J., Mohamad Zam N. A., Cheng C. W. Prevailing attitudes towards cancer: a multicultural survey in a tertiary outpatient setting. *Ann. Acad. Med. Singapore,* 2013;42:492-498.

[7] Sarhill N., LeGrand S., Islambouli R., Davis M. P., Walsh D. The terminally ill Muslim: Death and dying from the Muslim perspective. *American Journal of Hospice and Palliative Medicine,* 2001;18:251-255.

[8] World Health Organisation. Definition of Palliative Care. http://www.who.int/cancer/palliative/definition/en/. 2012. Ref Type: Online Source.

[9] Hughes M. T., Smith T. J. The growth of palliative care in the United States. *Annu. Rev. Public Health, 2014* 2014;35:1-26.

[10] Swetz K. M., Freeman M. R., AbouEzzeddine OF et al. Palliative Medicine Consultation for Preparedness Planning in Patients Receiving Left Ventricular Assist Devices as Destination Therapy. *Mayo Clinic Proceedings,* 2011;86:493-500.

[11] Chung H. M., Lyckholm L. J., Smith T. J. Palliative care in BMT. *Bone Marrow Transplantation,* 2009;43:265-273.

[12] http://en.wikipedia.org/wiki/Palliative_care . 2014. Ref Type: Online Source.

[13] Parikh R. B., Kirch R. A., Smith T. J., Temel J. S. Early Specialty Palliative Care – Translating Data in Oncology into Practice and Policy. *NEJM* 2013;In press.

[14] Reville B., Miller M. N., Toner R. W., Reifsnyder J. End-of-Life Care for Hospitalized Patients with Lung Cancer: Utilization of a Palliative Care Service. *Journal of Palliative Medicine,* 2010;13:1261-1266.

[15] Casarett D., Pickard A., Bailey F. A. et al. Do palliative consultations improve patient outcomes? *Journal of the American Geriatrics Society,* 2008;56:593-599.

[16] Temel J. S., Greer J. A., Muzikansky A., Gallagher E. R., Admane S., Jackson V. A. et al. Early Palliative Care for Patients with Metastatic Non Small-Cell Lung Cancer. New England Journal of Medicine. *New England Journal of Medicine*, 363[8], 733-742. 8-18-2010. Massachusetts Medical Society. 1-17-2012. Ref Type: Journal (Full).

[17] Temel J. S., Greer J. A., Admane S. et al. Longitudinal Perceptions of Prognosis and Goals of Therapy in Patients With Metastatic Non-Small-Cell Lung Cancer: Results of a Randomized Study of Early Palliative Care. *Journal of Clinical Oncology,* 2011;29:2319-2326.

[18] Wright A. A., Zhang B., Ray A. et al. Associations Between End-of-Life Discussions, Patient Mental Health, Medical Care Near Death, and Caregiver Bereavement Adjustment. *JAMA: The Journal of the American Medical Association,* 2008;300:1665-1673.

[19] Christakis N. A., Iwashyna T. J. The health impact of health care on families: a matched cohort study of hospice use by decedents and mortality outcomes in surviving, widowed spouses. *Social Science and Medicine,* 2003;57:465-475.

[20] Brumley R., Enguidanos S., Jamison P. et al. Increased satisfaction with care and lower costs: results of a randomized trial of in-home palliative care. *Journal of the American Geriatrics Society,* 2007;55:993-1000.

[21] Gade G., Venohr I., Conner D. et al. Impact of an Inpatient Palliative Care Team: A Randomized Control Trial. *Journal of Palliative Medicine,* 2008;11:180-190.

[22] Murray K. How doctors die - It's not like th rest of us, but it should be. http://www.zocalopublicsquare.org/2011/11/30/how-doctors-die/ideas/nexus/. 11-30-2011. Nexus. 1-5-2014. Ref Type: Online Source.

[23] How doctors die - showing others the way. *NY Times,* 2014.

[24] Morrison R. S., Penrod J. D., Cassel J. B. et al. Palliative Care Leadership Centers' Outcomes Group. Cost savings associated with US hospital palliative care consultation programs. *Arch. Intern. Med.,* 2008;16-1783.

[25] Morrison R. S., Dietrich J., Ladwig S. et al. Palliative Care Consultation Teams Cut Hospital Costs For Medicaid Beneficiaries. *Health Affairs,* 2011;30:454-463.

[26] Smith T. J., Cassel J. B., Coyne P. J., Hager M. A. A High-Volume Specialist Palliative Care Unit and Team May Reduce In-Hospital End-of-Life Care Costs. *Journal of Palliative Medicine,* 2003;6:699-705.

[27] Smith T. J., Cassel J. B. Cost and Non-Clinical Outcomes of Palliative Care. *Journal of Pain and Symptom Management,* 2009;38:32-44.

[28] Nelson C., Chand P., Soratais J., Oloimooja J., Rembert G. Inpatient palliative care consults and the probability of hospital readmission. *Perm. J.,* 2011;15:48-51.

[29] Meyer H. Changing The Conversation In California About Care Near The End Of Life. *Health Affairs,* 2011;30:390-393.

[30] Cassel J. B., Hager M. A., Clark R. R. et al. Concentrating Hospital-Wide Deaths in a Palliative Care Unit: The Effect on Place of Death and System-Wide Mortality. *Journal of Palliative Medicine,* 2010;13:371-374.

[31] Freund K., Weckmann M. T., Casarett D. J., Swanson K., Brooks M. K., Broderick A. Hospice eligibility in patients who died in a tertiary care center. *J. Hosp. Med.,* 2012;7:218-223.

[32] Weckmann M. T., Freund K., Bay C., Broderick A. Medical Manuscripts Impact of Hospice Enrollment on Cost and Length of Stay of a Terminal Admission. *American Journal of Hospice and Palliative Medicine,* 2012;1-3.

[33] Equidanos S., Vesper E., Lorenz K. 30-Day Readmissions among Seriously Ill Older Adults. *J. Palliat. Med.,* 2012;15:1356-1361.

[34] Sivec H. D., Pitorak E. F., Armor M. Project Safe Conduct Integrates Palliative Goals into Comprehensive Cancer Care. *Journal of Palliative Medicine,* 2003;6:645-655.

[35] Pitorak E., Armor M., Sivec H. Project Safe Conduct integrates palliative goals into comprehensive cancer care: An interview with Elizabeth Ford Pitorak and Meri Armour. *Innovations in End-of-Life Care,* [serial online] 2002;4.

[36] Hoverman J. R., Cartwright T. H., Patt D. A. et al. Pathways, Outcomes, and Costs in Colon Cancer: Retrospective Evaluations in Two Distinct Databases. *Journal of Oncology Practice,* 2011;7:52s-59s.

[37] Kolodziej M., Hoverman J. R., Garey J. S. et al. Benchmarks for Value in Cancer Care: An Analysis of a Large Commercial Population. *Journal of Oncology Practice,* 2011;7:301-306.

[38] Harford J. B., Aljawa D. M. The need for more and better palliative care for Muslim patients. *Palliat. Support Care,* 2013;11:1-4.

[39] Hannon B., Librach S. L., Zimmerman C. Palliative care program development: an itnernational perspective. *Curr. Opin. Support Palliat. Care,* 2013;7:192-194.

[40] Mack J. W., Cronin A., Taback N. et al. End-of-Life Care Discussions Among Patients With Advanced Cancer. *Annals of Internal Medicine,* 2012;156:204-20W.

[41] Higginson I. J., Sarmento V. P., Calanzani N., Benalia H., Gomes B. Dying at home -- is it better: A narrative appraisal of the state of the science. *Palliative Medicine,* 2013;27:918-924.

[42] Perrels A. J., Fleming J., Zhao J. et al. Place of death and end-of-life transitions experienced by very old people with differing cognitive status: Retrospective analysis of a prospective population-based cohort aged 85 and over. *Palliative Medicine,* 2013.

[43] Having the Difficult Conversation Powerpoint Presentation: UCLA Department of Medicine Grand Rounds.: Division of Adult Palliative Care, Dana-Farber Cancer Institute, 2013.

[44] Smith T. J., Longo D. L. Talking with Patients about Dying. *N. Engl. J. Med.,* 2012;367:1651-1652.

[45] Alesi E., Fletcher D. S., Muir C., Beveridge R., Smith T. J. Palliative care and oncology partnerships in real practice. Oncology Williston Park [In Press]. 1-11-2012. Ref Type: Journal (Full).

[46] Casarett D., Johnson M., Smith D., Richardson D. The Optimal Delivery of Palliative Care: A National Comparison of the Outcomes of Consultation Teams vs Inpatient Units. *Arch. Intern. Med.,* 2011;171:649-655.

[47] Zeinah G. F. A., Al-Kindi S. G., Hassan A. A. Middle East Experience in Palliative Care. *American Journal of Hospice and Palliative Medicine,* 2013;30:94-99.

[48] An assessment of healthcare delivery. http://www.middleeasthealthmag.com/cgi-bin/index.cgi?http://www.middleeasthealthmag.com/may2011/feature5.htm [Emery, Callen]. 7-10-2011. National Institutes of Health. Ref Type: Online Source.

[49] Almuzaini A. S., Salek M. S., Nicholls P. J., Alomar B. A. The attitude of health care professionals toward the availability of hospice services for cancer patients and their carers in Saudi Arabia. *Palliative Medicine,* 1998;12:365-373.

[50] Salpeter S. R., Malter D. S., Luo E. J., Lin A. Y., Stuart B. Systematic review of cancer presentations with a median survival of six months or less. *J. Palliat. Med.,* 2012;15:175-185.

[51] Zimmermann C, Swami N, Krzyzanowska M, Hannon B, Leighl N, Oza A, Moore M, Rydall A, Rodin G, Tannock I, Donner A, Lo C. Early palliative care for patients with advanced cancer: a cluster-randomised controlled trial. Lancet. 2014 Feb 18. pii: S0140-6736(13)62416-2. doi: 10.1016/S0140-6736(13)62416-2. [Epub ahead of print]

[52] Higginson I. J., Costantini M., Silber E., Burman R., Edmonds P. Evaluation of a new model of short-term palliative care for people severely affected with multiple sclerosis: a randomised fast-track trial to test timing of referral and how long the effect is maintained. *Postgraduate Medical Journal,* 2011;87:769-775.

[53] Bakitas M., Lyons K. D. S. O., Hegel M. T. et al. Effects of a Palliative Care Intervention on Clinical Outcomes in Patients With Advanced Cancer: The Project ENABLE II Randomized Controlled Trial. *JAMA,* 2009;302:741.

[54] Ryan J. L., Heckler C. E., Roscoe J. A. et al. Ginger (Zingiber officinale) reduces acute chemotherapy-induced nausea: a URCC CCOP study of 576 patients. *Supportive Care in Cancer,* 2012;20:1479-1489.

[55] Barton D. L., Liu H., Dakhil S. R. et al. Wisconsin Ginseng (Panax quinquefolius) to Improve Cancer-Related Fatigue: A Randomized, Double-Blind Trial, N07C2. *Journal of the National Cancer Institute,* 2013;105:1230-1238.

[56] Bruera E., Yennurajalingam S., Palmer J. L. et al. Methylphenidate and/or a Nursing Telephone Intervention for Fatigue in Patients With Advanced Cancer: A Randomized, Placebo-Controlled, Phase II Trial. *Journal of Clinical Oncology,* 2013.

[57] Ryan N. M., Birring S. S., Gibson P. G. Gabapentin for refractory chronic cough: a randomised, double-blind, placebo-controlled trial. *The Lancet,* 2012;380:1583-1589.

In: Palliative Care to the Cancer Patient
Editor: Michael Silbermann

ISBN: 978-1-63117-709-5

Chapter 19

EFFORTS OF THE AMERICAN SOCIETY OF CLINICAL ONCOLOGY TO FURTHER GLOBAL PALLIATIVE CARE

Vanessa Eaton**, *M.I.M. and Doug Pyle, M.B.A.
ASCO International Affairs, Alexandria, VA, US

INTRODUCTION

The American Society of Clinical Oncology (ASCO) is an international organization of oncology health care providers with a strong interest in supporting the development of palliative care around the world as well as the integration of palliative care into the continuum of cancer treatment received by patients. In addition to its own online training modules and guidelines, ASCO is active in supporting the work of other organizations to develop training materials in palliative care, to deliver education through jointly organized live meetings, and to incorporate palliative care into oncology training programs. ASCO International Palliative Care Workshops organized in collaboration with local and regional organizations have shown positive indicators for improvements in communication and symptom management skills among its participants.

Palliative care, defined by the American Society of Clinical Oncology (ASCO) as simply "the relief of suffering, in all of its dimensions, throughout the course of a patient's illness [1]" is an essential part of cancer care, particularly for patients diagnosed with advanced disease. It is estimated that more than half of new cancer cases occur in low-to-middle income (LMC) countries [2], and this is expected to rise to nearly two-thirds of all new cases by 2020 [3]. Of the patients who are diagnosed in LMCs, 80% are in an advanced stage of disease [4], where curative treatment is often not a possibility, where "moderate to severe pain" is common and palliation can offer significant benefits [5]. Furthermore, the evidence base shows that palliative care can result in improved outcomes for all patients with cancer, not only those with advanced disease; results from a phase three randomized clinical trial showed positive outcomes from providing early palliative care to patients with advanced metastatic

* Address for correspondence: vanessa.eaton@asco.org

non-small lung cancer. Improved quality of life, better control of symptoms, and increased overall satisfaction from patients and their care givers were reported in this study [6]. Yet, despite a growing cancer patient population whose cancers are often diagnosed at advanced stages and for whom palliation could offer significant patient quality of life improvements, access to palliative care in LMCs remains very limited. For example, whereas per capita annual consumption of morphine in the United States is about 75 mg, in Brazil it is about 5 mg and in China less than 1 mg [7].

American Society of Clinical Oncology and Palliative Care

The American Society of Clinical Oncology (ASCO) is a professional oncology association of over 30,000 members around the world. Membership is multidisciplinary, including all major oncology subspecialties, and represents over 125 countries. Nearly 5% of international membership is practicing in the Middle East and Northern Africa (MENA) region.

ASCO has advocated for many years for the integration of palliative care into cancer care. In 1998, ASCO published recommendations for palliative care stressing the responsibility of the oncologist to care for their patients throughout their experience, to control symptoms and to provide psychosocial support [8]. Then in 2009 an ASCO Task Force published a series of recommendations for ASCO to advance the integration of palliative care into the standard of care [9]. The recommendations include the integration of palliative care into the cancer care delivery system to help address the multiple needs of patients and their families; the development of guidelines and quality improvement strategies; advocating for increased access to opioid medications; and the provision of educational resources and training. These recommendations continue to guide ASCO's programs and resources for palliative care today, and as will be described later in this article, many of these recommendations have been put into action.

Integration of Palliative Care into Practice

The goals of palliation are to give comfort from all forms of suffering, and benefits can be derived at all stages of the disease. The integration of palliative care into the standard of cancer care is underlined in all of ASCO's palliative care programs and efforts.

ASCO offers guidelines for supportive care and quality of life. As a response to the emerging evidence of the underutilization of hospice care and the demonstrated benefits of early palliative care, ASCO published a clinical opinion paper in 2012 to further advocate for the integration of palliative care for all patients with cancer [10]. Indeed, ASCO views the integration of palliative care as an important component of overall quality care, and has incorporated palliative care in its cancer care improvement programs. For example, ASCO includes palliative care measures in its Quality Oncology Practice Initiative (QOPI), a program that assesses the quality of a practice based on self-examination, improvement tools, and feedback. Measures for pain control and timely referral to hospice programs are included in the overall assessment process.

EDUCATION AND TRAINING

The integration of palliative care into cancer care requires not only guidelines and quality tools, but also education and training interventions. ASCO has incorporated palliative care training into its international training programs, as well as broader educational offerings.

The value of palliative care integration is built into ASCO training programs, like the Multidisciplinary Cancer Management Course (MCMC) where a patient is followed from presentation, through diagnosis, treatment, and end of life care. Concepts of communication and symptom management are built into the program to emphasize the message that palliative care is a fundamental component to quality cancer care. MCMCs have been held in Egypt, Turkey, and Abu Dhabi.

Additional palliative care training is conducted in-depth through the ASCO International Palliative Care Workshop (IPCW), a course that uses locally relevant content as well as the Education in Palliative and End-of-life Care for Oncology (EPEC-O) developed by Northwestern University and the US National Cancer Institute. The IPCW covers topics such as pain and symptom management and includes role playing to practice patient communications. Communication skills are required for delivering quality palliative care, and feasible for all to immediately put into practice, regardless of the resources that are available.

Since the first palliative care workshop was held in Cairo, Egypt, in 2009, ASCO has presented its International Palliative Care Workshop in five countries in collaboration with local and regional partners. Over half have been presented in the Middle East.

In 2012 and 2013, ASCO and the Middle East Cancer Consortium held two workshops in Ankara, Turkey, and Muscat, Oman. The goals of these workshops were to provide a forum for participants to discuss culturally sensitive issues related to palliative care, to learn skills in symptom management, and to increase communication skills for participants to be able to talk with patients and their families about palliative and end of life care. In an on-site evaluation, 74% of participants indicated that they would make a change in how they work as a result of what was learned with most of these changes being in increased communication with patients and their families, symptom management, or psychosocial support.

In recognition of the central importance of palliative care as part of standard oncology practice, ASCO and the European Society of Medical Oncology (ESMO) added in 2010 significant new sections on palliative care to their joint Recommendations for a Global Curriculum in Medical Oncology, which is intended to be the global benchmark for medical oncology training around the world. The Curriculum has been adopted by 11 countries and continues to be a resource for many more.

More recently, ASCO has partnered with American Academy of Hospice Medicine (AAHPM) to create a Virtual Learning Collaborative (VLC) that aims to support the delivery of high-quality palliative care in medical oncology. The initiative is funded by a grant from the Agency for Health Care Research Quality, and it is scheduled to be implemented in 2016. The VLC is an online learning platform that will include a variety of tools to teach evidence-based approaches to palliative care in oncology. ASCO also offers online training modules and includes palliative care in its Maintenance of Certification exam and Self-Assessment modules available on ASCO University.

In 2014, the first ASCO Palliative Care Symposium will be held in an effort to provide a forum for scientific exchange in the field. The aim is to continue to focus on the integration of palliative care into patient care starting from the time of diagnosis, and to discuss symptom management, healthcare models, toxicity, pharmacogenomics, and quality of life issues.

Advocacy for Access to Pain Medications

In addition to educational efforts to address the stigma associated with opioid use, ASCO supports the efforts of the UICC Global Access to Pain Relief (GAPRI) project to reduce or eliminate barriers to accessing essential pain medications. GAPRI brings together governments and non-profit organizations to create awareness and facilitate action [11].

Professional Development

ASCO not only delivers education in palliative care through workshops, it also offers mentoring opportunities for early-career oncologists practicing in low and middle income countries through its International Development in Education Award in palliative care. In 2011-2013, thirteen awards were given with one recipient from the MENA region.

Conclusion

Palliative care is an important part of delivering quality patient care. Through a variety of educational meetings and materials, as well as mentorship opportunities, ASCO supports the development of palliative care in the Middle East and throughout the world. Additional information can be found at www.asco.org/international or by contacting international@asco.org

References

[1] F. Ferris et al. (2009). Palliative cancer care a decade later: Accomplishments, the need, next steps – From the American Society of Clinical Oncology. 27(18). Journal of Clinical Oncology.

[2] IARC GLOBOCAN Database, 2008.

[3] Economist Intelligence Unit, 2009.

[4] F. Ferris et al. (2009). Palliative cancer care a decade later: Accomplishments, the need, next steps – From the American Society of Clinical Oncology. 27(18). Journal of Clinical Oncology.

[5] T. Smith et. al. (2012). ASCO provisional clinical opinion: The integration of palliative care into standard oncology care. 30(8). Journal of Clinical Oncology. 880-887.

[6] F. Ferris et al. (2009). Palliative cancer care a decade later: Accomplishments, the need, next steps – From the American Society of Clinical Oncology. 27(18). Journal of Clinical Oncology.

[7] Pain & Policy Studies Group, University of Wisconsin/WHO Collaborating Center, 2012.

[8] The American Society of Clinical Oncology. (1998). Cancer care during the last phase of life. Journal of Clinical Oncology 16(5). 1986-1996.

[9] F. Ferris et al. (2009). Palliative cancer care a decade later: Accomplishments, the need, next steps – From the American Society of Clinical Oncology. 27(18). Journal of Clinical Oncology.

[10] T. Smith et. al. (2012). ASCO provisional clinical opinion: The integration of palliative care into standard oncology care. 30(8). Journal of Clinical Oncology. 880-887.

[11] UICC (n.d.). Global Access to Pain Relief Initiative. Taken from http://www.uicc.org /programmes/gapri/activities.

In: Palliative Care to the Cancer Patient
Editor: Michael Silbermann

ISBN: 978-1-63117-709-5

Chapter 20

INVOLVEMENT OF THE ONCOLOGY NURSING SOCIETY (ONS) IN PALLIATIVE CARE AND EDUCATIONAL PROGRAMS IN THE MIDDLE EAST

Carol Long, Ph.D., R.N., FPCN[2], Carlton Brown, Ph.D., R.N., AOCN[3], Kathleen Murphy-Ende, R.N., Ph.D., Psy.D., AOCNP[4], Susan Newton, R.N., M.S., AOCN, AOCNS[5], Catherine Glennon, R.N., MHS, NE-BC, OCN[6] Kate Shaughnessy Hankle, M.B.A., CVA*[*,1] and Barbara Lubejko, R.N., M.S.[1]

[1]Oncology Nursing Society, Pittsburgh, PA, US
[2]Capstone Healthcare, Phoenix, AZ, US
[3]Memorial Sloan Kettering Cancer Center, New York, NY US
[4]Meriter Hospital, Madison, WI, US
[5]Quintiles, Health Management Solutions, OH, US
[6]Cancer Center, University of Kansas, Kansas City KS, US

ABSTRACT

The Oncology Nursing Society (ONS) is a professional organization of more than 35,000 registered nurses and other healthcare providers around the world who are dedicated to excellence in patient care, education, research, and administration in oncology nursing.

Palliative and end-of-life care is an important component to the physical, spiritual, psychological, and social care of the patient with cancer, and a topic on which ONS provides evidence-based literature, research, continuing education, and collaborative opportunities for partnership. The contribution of nurses in providing clinical palliative care and research has been extensive throughout the history of the profession and continues to be a growing role in the Middle East.

[*] Address for correspondence: kshaughnessy@ons.org

ONS has been involved in education and training in the Middle East for many years, equipping nurses and other healthcare professionals to build clinical capacity and leadership development. Sustainable outcomes are facilitated through the identification of practice and policy improvement strategies in participants' institutions and communities. Working in tandem with local and regional partners, such as the Middle East Cancer Consortium (MECC), ONS ensures culturally-relevant and meaningful instruction. In palliative care in particular, numerous cultural factors must be considered and addressed when preparing and delivering information. ONS presenters have learned a great deal from the interdisciplinary and nurse participants through multilateral discussions and case studies. The achievements made and barriers faced by the interdisciplinary care teams in the region are multifaceted, and there are a number of strategies being implemented to ensure quality improvements in patient care.

Experiences gained from those who have taught and learned in the region, as well as initiatives led by ministries of health and other local organizations, serve as excellent reference and guidance for other countries in the world seeking to implement such practices. It is essential that nurses embrace the initiative to take the problems and solutions to their professional peers, leaders, policy makers, and the public. It is the hope of ONS that nurses globally will continue their quest to provide comprehensive and compassionate care to patients and families with cancer through their clinical practice and to pursue focused projects, leadership skills, coordination of care, advanced education, and research.

Introduction

The Oncology Nursing Society (ONS) is a professional organization of more than 35,000 registered nurses and other healthcare providers around the world who are dedicated to excellence in patient care, education, research, and administration in oncology nursing. ONS members are a diverse group of professionals who represent a variety of professional roles, practice settings, and subspecialty practice areas. Since its official incorporation in 1975, ONS has become a leader in cancer care. It has grown to include 231 chapters and 27 special interest groups and provides information and education to nurses around the world. In addition, the Society plays an active role in advocacy activities at the local, state, national, and international levels. Our mission is to promote excellence in oncology nursing and quality cancer care.

Within ONS's four strategic pillars—Knowledge, Technology, Leadership, and Quality—both the Knowledge and Leadership pillars specifically articulate our commitment to disseminate knowledge and educate nurse leaders outside the United States to promote evidence-based cancer care. Palliative care is an integral component to the cancer care continuum and a topic on which ONS provides evidence-based literature, research, continuing education, and collaborative opportunities for partnership. All of our international education and training is conducted with a local or regional partner, who, among many other roles, helps ONS presenters to provide culturally relevant and meaningful training. In palliative care in particular, numerous cultural factors must be considered and addressed when preparing and delivering information. Localized content, usage of discussion groups, and trainers with a high level of emotional intelligence and cultural awareness are needed to effectively conduct education and training outside the United States.

The Middle East is an area of the world where ONS has a long-standing involvement in education and training, equipping nurses and other healthcare professionals to build clinical capacity and leadership development. The healthcare landscape is such that governments, advocacy groups, educators, administrators, and physicians recognize the tremendous value of nurses as members of the interdisciplinary team and have identified the need for nursing education and clinical training, particularly in palliative care. According to the World Health Organization (WHO), the majority of patients with cancer in most of the world have advanced-stage disease at the time of presentation, and their "only realistic treatment option is pain relief and palliative care" (WHO, 2013). These services are directed toward improving the quality of life for those with cancer and their family members by providing physical, psychological, social, and spiritual support. This late-stage diagnosis is common in the Middle East, and nurses play a key role in the provision and coordination of palliative care to those with life-threatening illnesses such as cancer. The Gulf Cooperation Council (GCC) countries (Bahrain, Kuwait, Oman, Qatar, Saudi Arabia, and the United Arab Emirates) "will face an unparalleled and unprecedented rise in demand for health care over the course of the next two decades . . . with the simultaneous need to realign its healthcare systems to be able to treat the disorders of affluence" (Mourshed, Hediger, & Lambert et al., n.d., p. 55). This is one reason for the strong emphasis among each state's government agendas to promote the employment of nationals within the private sector (Khoja, 2013). These factors, among others, are significant contributors to the strong desire and growing need to increase the capacity of national healthcare teams, within which the nurse plays a vital role, through training and education.

ONS Educational Approach

Globally, nurses are on the forefront of patient care. They assess, educate, and provide treatment and continuity of care among the members of the interdisciplinary team. They manage the majority of the family care and communication. Nurses are also on the forefront of patient advocacy and play an integral role in delivering and ensuring quality care from diagnosis through bereavement and survivorship. In palliative care, the nurse addresses the psychosocial, physical, spiritual, and emotional needs of the patient and family.

As a leader in oncology nursing education, ONS has coordinated nurse training and education globally for decades, but began more actively and consistently working in the Middle East in 2007. ONS's partnership with the Middle East Cancer Consortium (MECC) began with a leadership development workshop for nurses from MECC countries. One of the key strategies to effect real change and increase the quality of patient care is to equip nurses in a culturally conscientious manner to be change agents within their institutions and communities. This is accomplished by incorporating leadership training into clinical content. Since the first leadership workshop in Israel in December 2007, MECC and ONS have partnered with local organizations and ministries of health to conduct more than six conferences and educational programs covering topics such as symptom management, pain control, spiritual care, and many other nursing-sensitive aspects of cancer care. In 2012 and 2013, MECC, ONS, the Ministry of Health in the Sultanate of Oman, and the National Association for Cancer Awareness in Oman implemented two intensive palliative care courses for nurses—the first, a basic palliative care course, and the second, an advanced palliative care course.

Developing these educational programs in the Middle East required evaluation of typical program planning procedures with a focus on meeting the unique cultural perspectives of nurses practicing in this region. MECC and ONS staff worked closely with nurses and other healthcare professionals in the Middle East to clearly identify the knowledge and skills needed by those who would be attending the program. Information used to plan these programs included not just the perceived need, but also detail about the educational background, amount of experience and current practice settings of the projected attendees. And since nurses attending the MECC-ONS programs have come from countries and communities that are very different from that of most ONS faculty, it was essential to learn as much as possible about the cultural context within which projected attendees live and practice. Faculty was then chosen based not just on their content expertise but also on their interest and experience in teaching and collaborating with nurses in other countries.

The educational approaches utilized in the MECC-ONS programs have changed over time to provide more opportunities for faculty and attendees to explore the program content and learn together. This has led to a carefully planned balance of didactic presentation and interactive activities. Recent programs have relied much more heavily on large and small group activities, such as integrated learning assessments, role play, analysis of case studies and development of plans for change. The use of Liberating Structures, such as 1-2-4-all, Conversation Café and Celebrity Interview, has also been very helpful in encouraging participation by all group members and creating a safe environment for sharing of opinions and ideas.

One of the key lessons learned by faculty from the MECC-ONS programs is that we all have much to learn from each other. While each country and region may have different access to education and patient care resources, all nurses have the same focus – the highest quality care and the best outcomes for their patients. The most important role that ONS can play in the Middle East is to support quality cancer care through sharing of knowledge and development of skills needed to facilitate change to current practice.

Regional Strategies, Achievements and Barriers

Catherine (Cath) Glennon, RN, MHS, NE-BC, OCN®, from the University of Kansas Cancer Center, served as an ONS presenter in Turkey in 2009. The program she co-led focused on pain control and the development of leadership skills needed to advocate for improvements in pain control administration. Cath noted that the key strength of nurses in the Middle East was resiliency, and the faculty learned so much from them. "When faced with adversity, these nurses creatively found a means to attain the desired patient outcome," she said. "They were extremely bright and positive in their approach to nursing and patient care." Other attributes that Cath noted were their passion for patient care and advocacy for quality and access improvements. Her lecture included a discussion of change management. When asked to address a challenge as a case study, the nurses quickly identified obstacles in pain management: obtaining an order for narcotics and then securing the narcotics, which are in limited supply. "Through the discussion of how to influence such a major change, they were able to identify the stakeholders; manage the conversation and request in a positive framework; apply change methodology; and most importantly, display a passion to care for the patient by meeting their needs, however basic they may appear to others."

ONS presenters Carol Long, PhD, RN, FPCN, Geriatric and Palliative Care Educator and Researcher at Capstone Healthcare Group, and Carlton Brown, PhD, RN, AOCN®, FAAN, from Memorial Sloan-Kettering Cancer Center, noted during their experience teaching in the region that although palliative care nursing is not well developed in most Middle Eastern countries, the MECC and Ministries of Health have employed several strategies to propel the palliative care movement forward. These efforts pave the way for significant achievements to be generatively developed by national practitioners that will improve patient care and interprofessional (as well as patient/family/practitioner) communication. The strategies are augmented by programs and resources provided by ONS and other organizations.

The first strategy, a focus on education, has been pivotal to increasing the understanding of the principles of palliative care nursing. ONS is fortunate to have taken part in many of these educational programs and has learned a tremendous amount from the nurses and other professionals who participated. In addition, thanks to the facilitation of MECC, nurses have come to the United States to learn about hospice and palliative care nursing at Calvary Hospital, designated as an International Center for Training by the National Cancer Institute (Calvary Hospital, n.d.). Many countries in the region are discussing additional educational preparation at the master's level as one way to move nurses into leadership positions so that they can influence the policies and rules that affect how palliative care programs can be developed and sustained.

The second strategy is the enablement of nurses from academia and practice settings to forge new pathways in the care of patients with cancer by creating or enhancing palliative care programs within hospitals or community-based settings. In many situations, the nurse has become a leader and champion of comfort to ensure that patients receive needed palliative care. Nursing research and palliative care programs are rapidly developing in Middle Eastern countries, according to the MECC-ONS Middle Eastern Survey on Palliative Care Needs Assessment feedback.

The third strategy is to encourage nurses to work cohesively within the interdisciplinary team to achieve patient goals of care. With this collaboration among all team members, the patient with cancer has the most to gain from the expertise of all disciplines and the united expertise in promoting quality of life during treatment and through the end of life.

These achievements and advancements in cancer treatment in the region have led to the need for continual symptom management, psychological support, and health education throughout the course of the disease. Nurses and physicians in the Middle East recognize that nurses are in a prime position to provide this level of specialized care; however, the lack of distinction between hope for cure and recognition of terminal illness often results in a delay of providing palliative care services. There is often limited information available about palliative care, a very limited number of formal palliative care units, and a misconception about what palliative care means.

A common barrier encountered by ONS presenters is the reticence among healthcare providers to openly dialogue about the cancer diagnosis and treatment with the family, and especially the patient. Susan (Susie) Newton, RN, MS, AOCN®, AOCNS®, from Dayton Cancer Center, co-presented several palliative care training programs in the Middle East, including two in the Palestinian Authority. Susie noted that a common communication barrier was that the word *cancer* is rarely used in conversation with the family and patient. Patients are not always told that they have cancer, and when cancer is referred to, it is called "that disease." Susie was told that the primary reason for not discussing a cancer diagnosis with patients is that healthcare providers do not want to give bad news, so they leave it up to the family to inform the patient. Additionally, they believe that such a diagnosis will diminish a patient's desire, and therefore fight, to live. Families do not want to take away their loved one's hope because of the stigma associated with cancer. Additionally, concerns often exist about daughters not being able to find husbands if there is cancer in the family or husbands leaving them if their diagnosis becomes public.

Kathleen Murphy-Ende, PhD, PsyD, RN, AOCNP®, from Meriter Hospital, was one of four ONS presenters who led the advanced palliative care course for nurses in the Sultanate of Oman. She, like Susie, observed that patient and family concerns in the Middle East are often multiple and complex, and asserted that communication is an essential component to effective care. The common patient/family issues identified as preventing the acceptance of palliative care included misconceptions about treatment and prognosis; mistrust of healthcare providers; lack of knowledge about the disease and treatment; and cultural, religious, and personal values. Patient and family trust of the nurse is absolutely critical. Communicating effectively and sensitively is a primary way to instill this trust and to manage these complex patient/family concerns. Nurses in Oman reported that families who were able to trust the bedside nurse were able to understand, appreciate, and allow a palliative care approach with the result of a comfortable and peaceful end-of-life experience.

As mentioned previously, one of the most commonly discussed barriers to effective care in the Middle East has been regarding pain management, specifically with limited access to and stigmas around the use of narcotics. For example, during one of Susie's presentations in the Palestinian Authority, one nurse shared a story about a patient with metastatic colorectal cancer from her village who was heard screaming through the night because of uncontrolled pain. During the cancer journey, pain is a common and often undertreated problem requiring pharmacologic and nonpharmacologic intervention. With the high restriction on the use of morphine throughout the region, physicians often are reluctant to prescribe it. Susie also received a question from a pharmacist asking, "What is the dose of morphine reached when patients become addicted?" The concern and misconceptions about addiction have arisen in almost every educational program, and ONS presenters have addressed these concerns in a culturally sensitive way through discussion groups, case studies, and evidence-based research addressing the recommendations on drug administration. Carol asserted that knowing before she gave her presentation on palliative care in Turkey that pain management was an issue, especially due to lack of available drugs, she was able to tailor her curriculum. She spoke to an interdisciplinary audience from multiple countries about pain management theory; knowledge and assessment skills; and importantly, how to advocate for, intervene in, and ensure pain control. She stated that nurses in this region are extremely intelligent with superb patient care skills. Validation of this promotes confidence to enable peer-to-peer communication and interdisciplinary collaboration to ensure evidence-based practice.

An additional barrier, and one that exists globally and is certainly not limited to the Middle East, is one that ONS has labeled *caregiver strain and burden*. While teaching in the Palestinian Authority, Susie was asked, "How long can nurses in the U.S. work in oncology?" The woman then explained that nurses in the Palestinian Authority do not choose where they work; rather, they are assigned a unit based on where there is an opening. The oncology unit is often referred to as the "death unit," and nurses tend to become depressed over time and burn out.

Sometimes barriers can be overcome through use of culturally appropriate terminology. For example, Susie encountered one nurse who had previously worked in maternity and needed to educate Muslim women about family planning. However, *family planning* sounded like birth control, which is against their religion, so the nurse used the term *birth spacing* instead, which was accepted. Do-not-resuscitate orders are against the law in many Middle Eastern countries and are culturally taboo in others. However, practitioners could discuss "allowing a natural death" to address the same topics. Using the phrase *palliative sedation* rather than *terminal sedation* was another suggested change that helped to gain a comfort level among the practitioners in one workshop.

RECOMMENDATIONS

Based on their experience teaching and speaking at length with nurses in the region, ONS presenters made several recommendations to enhance the continuing development of palliative care services in the Middle East and throughout the world.

Nurses around the world and in the Middle East are innovators in the practice of palliative care. Those working in academic and practice institutions, such as hospitals and clinics, see the needs of the patients they serve and are crafting programs and services to meet those needs. They are developing systematic symptom assessment and documentation charts, including flow sheets, as evidence of the nurse's objective assessment and treatment and will enable an evaluation of the effectiveness of care. This will improve the quality of care and ensure accurate communication and a mutual trust with patients, families, and other healthcare providers. Nurses have expressed their conclusion that when the patient, family, other healthcare providers, and administrators trust nurses' assessment and recommendations, positive changes occurred. ONS has developed resources to equip nurses with evidence-based symptom management interventions as part of its Putting Evidence Into Practice initiative (see www.ons.org/Research/PEP).

Patient and family education is often an effective way of providing information that helps those suffering to see beyond their emotional grief and to move toward a palliative approach. Many nurses shared stories of families that spent their time focusing on chasing a cure, and hence missed the opportunity to provide quality time with family or to have a peaceful death. Participants during various meetings identified the need to develop written patient and family educational materials that can be used as an adjunct to the nurse's and physician's explanation of the disease process and the purpose of palliative care. Nurses who are able to address patient and family concerns by answering questions and providing accurate educational materials are likely to be seen as trusted people whom patients and families can seek out again as other concerns arise.

Regarding the development of effective and cohesive interdisciplinary palliative care teams, nurses around the world should be acknowledged as key collaborators. Nurses are the ones at the bedside of a patient dying with cancer. They know how to initiate comfort practices to ensure a good quality of life at the end of life. Thus, it is essential to the development of effective palliative care teams that nurses work with the entire interdisciplinary team to ensure that the physical, psychological, social, and spiritual needs of patients with cancer are attended to.

Ministries of health, in partnership with MECC (2009), can join hands in targeting academic institutions, where nurses receive initial training, and through community or agency/hospital-based educational programs to ensure that continuing education of nurses in palliative care is addressed (Silbermann et al., 2013). Local professional nursing societies or associations should be encouraged to endorse palliative care education of nurses. However, this starts with early awareness and education about cancer and wellness perspectives.

Core competencies in palliative care nursing should be added to nursing curricula in undergraduate and graduate programs in schools of nursing (Bingley & Clark, 2009). Emphasis on pain and symptom management and supportive care for the patient and family is essential. Physical, psychological, social, and spiritual components need to be addressed within the cultural context of each country. Train-the-trainer programs can improve capacity-building and promote sustainability of evidence-based palliative care practice as a means of providing postgraduate continuing education for nurses.

Country-specific palliative care plans should include nurses in the planning and execution of vital palliative care services to high-risk cancer populations in urban as well as rural areas. Dissemination of palliative care education and services needs to occur across age groups, across cancer diagnoses, and for nurses working in all settings where they are likely to encounter individuals with a cancer diagnosis.

There should be continued discussion on change methodology and management, leadership skills, and establishment of an adequate infrastructure to support concepts learned. A critical strategy to ensure sustainability in the training and education is to reinforce participants' tremendous contribution to nursing and health care. ONS teaches that every nurse is a leader, and within their cultural context, nurses can use evidence-based practice to effect change. They are experts, and sharing their wisdom is key. Education should not be a one-way dialogue but rather a dynamic conversation.

An essential outcome of ONS trainings in the region have been the action plans that are developed based on the material discussed during the training programs. These ideas that participants have drafted would be wonderful concepts for other countries to adapt.

They include:

- Recommendation to have a physician and a nurse focused only on palliative care in the hospital (Pakistan and Iraq)
- Designation of specific rooms in a medical ward to oncology and palliative care (Sultanate of Oman)
- Incorporation of palliative care into the BSN curricula (Sultanate of Oman)
- Creation of a palliative home care team (Egypt)
- Implementation of a pain resource nurse (PRN) program in the hospital for every nursing unit (Saudi Arabia)
- Development of a palliative care specialty program into a master's degree nursing program (Saudi Arabia)
- Implementation of a telephone triage program for oncology patients by specially trained oncology nurses (Sultanate of Oman).

ONS and the Association of Oncology Social Work (AOSW) wrote a joint position on palliative and end-of-life care, which may serve as ONS's recommendations to countries wishing to develop palliative care services and increase the capacity of their healthcare teams to promote higher quality patient care. The position addresses "patient and family care," "integrated care systems," and "public advocacy" and can be found on the ONS website at www.ons.org/Publications/Positions/EndOfLife. Highlights from this position include the following (ONS, 2010. Reprinted with permission).

- Palliative care, as appropriate, should begin at the time of diagnosis and continue through bereavement (WHO, 2007).
- Palliative care addresses the physical, psychological, social, and spiritual aspects of the patient and family experience and attends to values, preferences, goals, and needs of the patient and family (Berzoff & Silverman, 2004; NCPQPC, 2009).
- Physical, psychological, social, and spiritual elements are comprehensively assessed, and symptoms are measured, managed, and documented using available standardized scales.
- A comprehensive care plan is implemented and adjusted according to the patient's and family's goals of care through all phases of the illness experience, including loss, grief, and bereavement.
- Effective communication between the patient, family, and care team is facilitated and prioritized (Institute of Medicine, 2008). Family conferences that include the patient (when possible), family members, caregivers, and relevant members of the interdisciplinary care team are encouraged to enhance communication and empower families.
- Care is provided by an interdisciplinary team that includes at least physicians, nurses, social workers, and spiritual care professionals and ideally also includes pharmacists, nursing aides, bioethicists, volunteers, and allied personnel who are skilled, credentialed, or certified in the essentials of palliative care.
- Healthcare professionals recognize the complexity of the patient and family experience that builds on a preexisting family history, requires ongoing role adaptation, demands adjustment to altered goals of care, and includes difficult decision making. Healthcare providers advocate and support for patients' and families' participation in care and decision making, in accordance with the patient's goals of care and the needs of families and caregivers (National Association of Social Workers, 2004; NCPQPC, 2009).
- Care is provided using evidence-based practice that reflects quality research in palliative care.

CONCLUSION

The contribution of nurses in providing clinical palliative care and research has been extensive throughout the history of the profession and continues to be a growing role in the Middle East. ONS educational programs have sought to develop leadership skills and clinical capacity in nurses across the region by having course participants identify practice and policy improvement strategies in their institutions and communities. It is essential that nurses embrace the initiative to take the problems and solutions discussed during these programs to their professional peers, leaders, policy makers, and the public. It is the hope of ONS that nurses globally will continue their quest to provide comprehensive and compassionate care to patients and families with cancer through their clinical practice and to pursue focused projects, leadership skills, coordination of care, advanced education, and research.

It has been, and continues to be, an honor for ONS to be a part of the multilateral education and development of nurse leaders around the world.

"We assume most men and women choose to become nurses because they want to help people live well. Our hope is that they will see the unlimited possibilities of nursing to change the world" (Dreher, Shapiro, & Asselin, 2006, p 254).

REFERENCES

Berzoff, J., & Silverman, P.R. (Eds.). (2004). *Living with dying: A handbook for end-of-life healthcare practitioners.* New York, NY: Columbia University Press.

Bingley, A., & Clark, D. (2009). A comparative review of palliative care development in six countries represented by the Middle East Cancer Consortium (MECC). Journal of Pain and Symptom Management, 37, 287–296. doi:10.1016/j.jpainsymman.2008.02.014

Calvary Hospital. (n.d.). Awards and accolades. Retrieved from http://www.calvaryhospital.org/site/pp.asp?c=ktJUJ9MPIsE&b=3266477

Dreher, M., Shapiro, D., & Asselin, M. (2006). Healthy places, healthy people: A handbook for culturally competent community nursing practice. Indianapolis, IN: Sigma Theta Tau International. Pg 254.

Institute of Medicine. (2008). Cancer care for the whole patient: Meeting psychosocial health needs. Washington, DC: National Academies Press.

Khoja, S. (2013, April 29). Can GCC workforce nationalization succeed? Retrieved from http://www.zawya.com/story/Can_GCC_workforce_nationalization_succeed-ZAWYA20130429085608

Middle East Cancer Consortium. (2009, September). Welcome to the Middle East Cancer Consortium (MECC) Web site. Retrieved from http://www.mecc.cancer.gov

Mourshed, M., Hediger, V., & Lambert, T. (n.d.). Gulf Cooperation Council health care: Challenges and opportunities. In Global competitiveness reports. Retrieved from http://www.weforum.org/pdf/Global_Competitiveness_Reports/Reports/chapters/2_1.pdf

National Association of Social Workers. (2004). NASW standards for palliative and end of life care. Washington, DC: Author.

National Consensus Project for Quality Palliative Care. (2009). Clinical practice guidelines for quality palliative care (2nd ed.). Retrieved from http://www.nationalconsensusproject.org

Oncology Nursing Society and Association of Oncology Social Work Joint Position on Palliative and End-of-Life Care (2010). Retrieved from www.ons.org/Publications/Positions/EndOfLife.

Silbermann, M. (2012). Impressions and experiences of a palliative care course to nurses in the Sultanate of Oman. *Journal of Palliative Care and Medicine*, 2(3). doi:10.4172/2165-7386.1000e116

Silbermann, M., & Al-Zadjali, M. (2013). Nurses paving the way to improving palliative care services in the Middle East. *Journal of Palliative Care and Medicine*, 3(2). doi:10.4172/2165-7386.1000e125

Silbermann, M., Epner, D. E., Charalambous, H., Baider, L., Puchalski, C. M., Balducci, L., Smith, T. J. (2013). Promoting new approaches for cancer care in the Middle East. *Annals of Oncology*, 24(Suppl. 7), vii5–vii10. doi:10.1093/annonc/mdt267

World Health Organization. (2007). Cancer control: Knowledge into action. *WHO guide for effective programmes: Palliative care.* Geneva, Switzerland: WHO Press.

World Health Organization. (2010). *WHO definition of palliative care.* Retrieved from http://www.who.int/cancer/palliative/definition/en

World Health Organization. (2013). *Palliative care is an essential part of cancer control.* Retrieved from http://www.who.int/cancer/palliative/en

INDEX

#

A

B

C

D

E

F

I

J

K

L

M

N

O

P

Q

R

S

T